See Saw

Part II of the Albert Plevier Trilogy
By Jayne Kelly

Jayne Kelly

For Al, Elaine, their family, my family, and the fans that have patiently waited for this next installment.

Jayne Kelly

Table of Contents:
Introduction

Introduction:

*C*ontrasts are what make life interesting and beautiful.

Beach sand meets ocean waves washing against one another people drawing people to the shore line. Each wave pulls back and then crashes forward in a wonderful moment in time soon replaced by the next or most beachgoers, but not all.

Today, on this New Jersey beach, a toddler is smiling as his mother chases him around the area they have established as their spot on the sand. The little boy's father sits on the blanket at the center of this miniature mayhem holding a baby. The man marvels at how the sun sparkling over the Atlantic Ocean in late August is so different from its winter slate blue color the last time he saw it.

The toddler darts away from the blanket toward the water's edge as his mother grabs his giggling, squirming body and they both return to the blanket. She looks at the man, shrugging her shoulders and smiling in surrender. "Al, there will be no rest for me today."

He responds with an even larger smile. "I think I'm going to have to agree with you, Hon."

Al's thoughts wander as the baby in his arms grabs his hands, wanting to join his big brother and Mommy. *I will remember this day. It's a gift. I had forgotten how bright, clear and crisp the colors are. Thank you, God for allowing me to have my sight back. How beautiful Elaine is today with her tan skin against the soft blue form-fitting swimsuit. How many men are as lucky as I am to have a wife so beautiful and a body so perfect after two pregnancies?* His back stiffens as he straightens in his seated position on the beach blanket. *I won't let her know I'm sad. I don't want to ruin this perfect day or the five months I have left to see them.* He thought back to the previous month. *She cried when she saw the look on my face when I first saw baby Larry. She needs this time. I can't tell her how scared I am. I can't tell her how afraid I am to go to sleep at night, knowing there will be a morning I wake up again in permanent darkness.*

Baby Larry looks up at his Dad, smiles broadly and makes a happy sound drawing Al's attention to him. "You like this day, huh little man? No eating sand, now. Your mama won't like that." Al pulls the baby up a little higher on his lap.

Elaine dashes after Albert, catches him and walks to the blanket, trying to hold him as he twists his body in positions only a determined toddler can form. "Albert is wearing me out."

Al looks at his wife closely as Albert throws his head in a tantrum, arching his back and letting loose with a scream that draws the attention of sunbathers on nearby blankets. "Wow, where is that coming from? Maybe it's naptime for someone."

Albert's head snaps up at the word nap and as fear flashes over his face. "No, no. No nap!"

Al and Elaine laugh together and then the smile fades from her face. "Al, do you think we should get you out of the sun? Dr. Grove said you shouldn't be in the sun even if you are under an umbrella. It can't be good for your burns."

The stubborn streak in his personality came out in a blast. "I'm fine. Trust me. I have my Jobe Shirt on, I'm under the umbrella, and it's a quick dash to the car from here." Al obeyed his doctor when it came to the pressure garment therapy the Jobe shirt offered to aid his healing burns.

Elaine gave in to both her husband and the temperamental three-year-old in her arms. "It's not quite two years since the accident. We've had a lot of miracles, the first being your survival. I just don't want to tempt fate any further."

Albert continued to squirm until finally loosening his mother's grip. He threw himself unceremoniously on the sand next to the beach blanket, rolling as far away from his parents as his mother allowed.

Al looked over at his namesake and shook his head amiably. "I get it Albert. Naps stink. There is too much to look at." He realized what he had said and quickly moved past the comment. "But think how much fun you will have and how great everything will be when you wake up well rested."

Elaine looked at the thick dark sunglasses Al wore that wrapped around the sides of his eyes. Underneath them were a completely white, blind left eye and the clear, temporary, sight of the right. She watched the contented smile on his face as he looked from one child to the other and then directly into her eyes. She knew in her heart he fully appreciated the moment and was not bitter about the darkness he would gradually be plunged back into. The man she loved accepted life on its terms regardless of the good, the bad, the happy, the sad, the light or the dark.

Jayne Kelly

Chapter I: Clarity

Al sat on the toilet staring at the wallpaper. Each day the edges of the flower petals were becoming clearer and more defined as his recent corneal transplant healed. The mornings were his favorite time to check the progress of his vision. The rising sun streaming through the eastern facing bathroom window on mornings with clear skies allowed the maximum natural light needed to aid the artificial lens cap that no longer allowed his pupils to dilate.

After rising from the toilet Al turned toward the sink to wash his hands. Over the sink was the full wall mirror. Every morning, as he gauged the progress of his sight, the view of his scarred body became more distinct. The thrill of the vision he enjoyed was tempered as he shuddered at what he knew Elaine had been looking at for two years. Seeing the initial blurred images of his body, anger rose inside him and he felt the courage of himself and his family. The scars were the physical confirmation that they all had moved past something horrible.

Movement and noise in the master bedroom told him Elaine was up with their two boys. Albert Junior was a non-stop tornado of energy at three and a half years old, constantly testing the boundaries of his world. He was, in his parent's opinion, a sponge soaking up all the information the world offered to him. His six-month old baby brother, Larry, watched Albert with eyes shaped like saucers, drinking in the activity as he patiently waited for the time when he could physically keep up. Al knew in his heart that he would get to see Larry's first steps before the eye transplant began its inevitable descent to failure and returned him to complete darkness.

There was a soft knock on the bathroom door. "Al? I'm taking the boys outside. Albert is driving me crazy."

Al fought the urge to grab his robe or a towel to cover up the scars. "That's polite of you to knock. Come on in. I'm getting ready to take a shower."

Elaine pushed the unlocked door fully open. "Come outside when you're done." Larry, perched on her hip, leaned back over her shoulder to watch Albert jump on the bed.

"I will." Al turned to the mirror and ran a hand over his scarred chest, arms and sides. "These scars are awful." He dropped his hand to the counter. "The discoloration, the raised lumpy, bumpiness, the bleeding spots where I've rubbed or scratched, the surgery scars from my chest rebuilding and even my oily hair create a real horror show for you. My skin looks angry." Al felt Elaine's hand in his as she moved next to him. "I guess I'm lucky my face healed normally. It looks like it did before the accident." His hair was oily to the touch and he ran his free hand over it. "How do you like being married to a brunette now?"

Elaine squeezed his hand. "You're just as handsome as you were when we married. Don't worry about the chest scars." She looked steadily into the mirror with him. "To be honest, I'm used to them. For the rest of the world, you always have your Jobe shirt on. No one except the doctors and I will ever see them." She looked at him playfully. "At least no one else better see them."

Larry giggled and squirmed in Elaine's arms as Albert squeezed into the bathroom. "Daddy! Daddy!" When he was blocked from joining everyone in front of the sink Albert threw a full throttle tantrum.

Al laughed. "Mommy's coming right out. I'll be out in a couple minutes. Daddy needs a shower."

Albert kept pushing and tried to step around Elaine. She scooped him up with her free arm, put him back down on his feet and patted his bottom as he ran giggling into the master bedroom to jump on the bed. Larry began to fuss waving his arms.

She turned to the bouncing toddler and walked out of the bathroom. "Come on, Albert. I'm taking you and Larry outside to the swing. It's a nice warm day. Since you ate all your breakfast I'll bring cookies."

"Cookies!" At the sound of the offer Albert rolled off the bed and onto his feet. He ran for the door flanking his mother and almost bringing her to the floor.

Elaine regained her balance and saw Larry entranced by his big brother. "I'm beginning to see what I'll be up against when you're walking. It will be all I can do to stand aside and not get run over by the both of you."

In the bathroom Al stepped into the shower, anxious to finish quickly so he could put his Jobe shirt back on. Even several minutes without it returned him to uncomfortable itching. As soon as he was done he toweled himself off, sprinkled talcum powder all over his body especially under his arms to replace deodorant, and worked his body into the Jobe shirt.

When he first received the elastic pressure garment therapy shirt from Dr. Grove, he needed Elaine's assistance to put it on. After more than a year of wearing the prescription pressure garment, he was now able to climb into the undersized, elastic, form fitting garment unaided. As he slipped his arms into the sleeves he took one last look at his scarred torso before pulling the Velcro strips that held the shirt into place to hug his body tightly. Once the pressure was in place against his scars, the relief from the itching, healing skin was immediate. He breathed deeply, feeling the fabric and allowing the comfort it brought him. The T-shirt he pulled over the Jobe shirt left the Jobe shirt sleeves showing, but since they were home he didn't care. In public, he always wore long sleeves to cover the evidence of his still recovering body.

He reached for his glasses, stared for a moment into the mirror at the completely white left eye and then placed them over the miracle of his returned sight in the clear, normal, right eye. The left lens of the glasses was dark to hide his disfigured left eye and the right lens was clear to protect and aid his new vision. If the outside world wondered about the strange glasses, the tilt and turn of his head was evidence to his ability to see out of his right eye only. Even with the ability to see, he continued to move with thoughtfulness and purpose as he found himself maneuvering around scattered toys and family paraphenalia. Walking through doorways, he would still reach out and touch the doorframe as if he might need to know it was there. This morning was no exception.

Halfway across the living room, he looked up from watching the steps he took and kicking toys out of his way, to absorb the sight of Albert on his swing through the porch windows. Then he stubbed his left foot on the coffee table.

"Ouch!" Al regained his balance and composure and spied his cane where it hung on the staircase hand rail.

Standing tall, he walked straight for the cane, grabbed it exuberantly, opened the front door and hesitated a half second before jumping off the top step. Keeping the cane tucked under his arm, he reached the side of the road, paused and leaned he head back. Glimpses of cirrus clouds came into view for him against the beautiful blue. From his vantage point, the bright green leaves of the trees layered the colors. In awe, he did not move until the sound of a car rattled him back to the present moment and he once again felt the cane under his arm. After the car disappeared, he held the cane in front of him and in one movement whipped it into the wooded area on his right, watching it fly like the rotor on a helicopter. Instantly he regretted the spontaneity knowing that he would either have to buy another or find he one he had just thrown somewhere among the branches, vines and poison ivy.

I'll deal with that another day.

He walked back up the road, strolled into the driveway and was drawn to the laughter of Albert.

I could find him without sight, but not today. Today I can see him.

Al walked up to Elaine who was pushing Albert as high as she could on the swing. "You want me to take over? You know I can push him higher."

Elaine stepped aside for Al. "Absolutely." Larry, still perched on her hip, began to fuss the minute she stepped away from Albert. "We're not going back in the house, Little One. Just over here to give Daddy room."

Al smiled brightly as Albert squealed with delight. He watched the back of his son's head fly into the air and then come back toward him. He pushed back just in time before the swing nailed him across the middle of his body. "Elaine, for the life of me I can't believe the attorney actually thought I would consider not having the corneal transplant based on his advice. Was he kidding?"

Elaine's brow furrowed. "He was just doing his job. He thought it might have a negative impact on our legal case if a jury thought there was any kind of hope you could see." She paused and measured her next words. "It didn't seem to matter if it would only be a temporary fix."

Al swallowed hard. "I know. He's good at what he does, but he was too involved in trying to be a part of my decision making." Al realized what he said and tried to back pedal. "I'm sorry, sweetheart. I mean our decision making."

Elaine looked at Albert's smiling face and tried to freeze it in time. "This is one of those amazing days. Do you think we can keep the world out for twenty-four hours?"

Just then a car pulled into the driveway and Elaine watched her parents park their car. "Mom and Dad wanted to come by and spend some time with the kids." She looked apologetically at Al. "It's Saturday. They work so hard during the week. This is their down time."

Al laughed good naturedly as Albert looked over his shoulder at his grandpa getting out of the car and firmly slamming the door shut. "Pop, Pop!"

13

The swing began to twist with Albert as he attempted to get down in mid-air. "Whoa, little man." Al stopped the swing short and Albert hopped off to run to his Grandpa.

Mr. Hinds scooped up his grandson and tossed him in the air. "Hey!" He looked at his daughter and Al. "How's everybody doing today? Al, you look like the cat that swallowed the canary."

"Hey Dad." Al gave a deep belly laugh, walked over to the picnic table and sat down. "What a day, huh?"

Mr. Hinds gave Albert another toss, as his wife walked up next to him with bags in her hands. "I'm going to put all this in the kitchen. Elaine, you want to come with me?"

Elaine handed Larry off to Al. "Little man, you stay out here with the boys. It's too nice of a day to be inside. I'll be right back." Larry looked into Al's face and smiled.

Al's stomach tightened as he looked into Larry's face and returned the smile before boosting him onto his left shoulder. "I got him, Mama."

"Al, are you supposed to be out in the sun? It can't be good for your burns?" Mr. Hinds focused on Al's shirt front.

"I'm covered up, Dad. The Jobe shirt's sleeves are effective on their own even with only a T-shirt. I put it on the minute I'm dried off from the shower. I sleep in it too." He rubbed his right hand stiffly over his chest. "Dr. Grove says I'm healing nicely."

Mr. Hinds swung Albert around again and then faced Al. "That shirt is a simple miracle. Who would have thought." Both men smiled.

"An engineer Dad. You have a problem, you solve it. The simplest solution always makes the most sense. Trick the body into thinking it already did its job healing the wounded skin by putting pressure on it. The body stops sending the fluid to heal the skin and the scarring is reduced. It's simple genius." Al rubbed his chest again as Larry shoved a fist in his mouth.

Mr. Hinds put Albert on the ground and watched the little boy run circles around them. He watched Al following

Albert with his good eye. "Son, I am so happy for you. I know your sight is temporary, but it's a gift you fought for and won."

Al smiled broadly. "It feels like I've been fighting everybody, even the people that are on my side." Al rubbed his finger over Larry's cheek and in return the baby rubbed his running nose all over his dad's shirt. "Thanks pal." He smiled gently at the baby. "Elaine and I were just talking about the lawyer."

Mr. Hinds looked cautiously at Al. "Everything good?"

"Oh, yeah, yeah. We're good. We were talking about how over involved he is in our personal decision making."

"How so?" Mr. Hinds had a look of concentration and worry.

Al measured his words, aware that the lawyer was referred to him by his father-in-law. "Dad, I understand that he is good at what he does, but to tell me that I should reconsider having the transplant because it might hurt the monetary reward in my lawsuit is stepping over his boundaries." Al's tone changed as his frustration began to build. "He's the lawyer. It's his job to work with the facts."

Mr. Hinds took a moment to gather his thoughts. "Son, he cares about you and your family. He's a good man who has taken a personal interest in seeing that you are able to move on with your life and the life of your family."

Al breathed in and out deeply. "I realize that. But, I need a lawyer not a friend. I want to fight this to the bitter end. He's already talking about if we have to settle this at some point. I mean, Dad, really? We're just getting started." Al stopped for a moment to compose himself. "I understand that he is a very caring, conservative man who knows something terrible happened to my family and me. We're good people and he likes us." Al stopped again briefly. "Sometimes I want to scream at him 'don't like me, fight for me!' I'm running into the same thing with Dr. Westmont and Dr. Leesville." Al laughed good naturedly. "Why does everybody like me?"

Mr. Hinds joined his laughter as Albert stopped running circles and ran to join the two men. "It's a curse."

Al continued in the same vein. "He and I both hope this will end quickly." He held up his right hand in surrender. "Not because of the fight. I'm always willing to fight." He dropped his hand. "It's just that it would be better to settle quickly because I'm going to have to pay back any Worker's Compensation that I'm being paid now out of the award money. I'd rather it be less, than to have it add up to ten years of payments." He shook his head slowly as Larry stared at him and the change in his face. "He has already brought up settling out of court as a possibility because if we win with a jury, the companies who lost will file appeals that could drag on for years. He wants us to move on with our lives."

Mr. Hinds face took on a granite façade. "I want you to consider all possibilities. Settling out of court is one of them. You are young and you've been through hell. There's a quality of life issue here."

Al was thoughtful for a moment and his father-in-law gave him space while he let Albert dragged him over to the picnic table where he proceeded to climb on the older man's back as soon as he sat down. The two wrestled until Al broke the silence.

"I'm all about quality of life, Dad. Part of my quality of life is not to change who I am. I'm a fighter." His wounded pride came through even as he tried to sound tough.

Mr. Hinds pulled Albert around to his front and set him on his feet again. "That will never change. You will always meet life on its terms and fight when you have to. The point is that you have to decide what it is you want to win."

"I can see, Dad. I can see! If there is a chance for that, even temporarily, I'm going for it. I don't care what a lawyer tells me." Al's voice began to rise, not aggressively but passionately. "I will get to see Larry take his first steps. This is September. It's been two months since the surgery and I figure I will have my sight at least until Christmas. Even if it starts to fade, I will see Larry's first Christmas to a degree."

Mr. Hinds saw Larry watching Albert as he ran in circles, bored and working off his extra energy. "I do believe you're right, Al. That little power house in your arms will be up and walking before his first birthday. He's anxious to keep up with his big brother. He watches him like a hawk."

Al stood with his chest out, as much as he could, holding Larry as he expressed his pride. "These two are real boys. They wear me out during the day so much that I'm back on a regular sleep schedule. It was hard to sleep normally without sight." He thought back to the movie he and Elaine had gone to several months before the corneal transplant when he had fallen asleep. "Elaine and I would be out somewhere and I'll fall asleep out of boredom. Watching TV with her in the evening was the worst. Without the visual stimuli, I was out almost instantly and then I was well rested and couldn't sleep at night. It was a constant struggle." He paused to change the subject and looked first at Larry and then Albert. "Kids are blessings in so many ways. I can't wait to coach them in baseball."

Mr. Hinds gave Al a quizzical look. "Al, what are you planning?"

"Dad, the way I figure it, I'm going to keep doing corneal transplants for as long as I can. Once this one goes bad, as predicted, I'll ask to be put back on the list again. I'll leave the left eye as my spare tire in case something goes wrong with the right eye. I won't have any transplants done to it for now. As long as Dr. Leesville says it's okay, I'm going to keep trying." Al turned his head to watch Albert, who by this time had grown bored with the conversation the two men were having and began hanging over his swing on his belly. "Dad, I don't want to miss anything if I don't have to."

"I understand." The older man paused. "I know you, Al. What's your backup plan? You always have one."

Al walked over to the swing as Larry began to fuss, squirming relentlessly and trying to get his father to put him down onto the grass. "I'll let you down after we push Albert."

Mr. Hinds stood. "Al, you play with Albert. I'll follow Larry on the ground and make sure he doesn't eat anything."

Al put Larry on the ground and immediately the eight-month old reached up to the bench at the picnic table, pulling himself up. "Dad, you better stay with him. Elaine will kill me if he puts something gross in his mouth." The white fence at the edge of the river caught Al's attention. The contrast between the white fence and the grass that met it held his gaze.

"Daddy!" Albert hung over the swing on his stomach and began to push off with his feet, impatient for his Dad's attention.

Al tore his gaze away from the grass, turned Albert over placing him bottom down on the swing and gave him a soft push. "Dad, the colors are amazing and crisp. I can't believe I never noticed them before. Look at the white fence against the green grass. It's amazing."

Mr. Hinds looked over at the scenery. "I guess we all take things for granted until we don't have them." For a moment, he saw what Al saw. "I'm going to try and appreciate these things with you."

Both men continued to look at the fencing until Al broke the trance. "You know, Dad, I will continue with my plan for teaching the boys baseball. I'm not losing that dream. I don't have to." He pushed Albert a little stronger each time until the little boy swung high in the air.

"I figured you still had a plan. I can still see you on the kitchen floor with Albert rolling the ball back and forth a year after the accident." Larry babbled non-stop carrying on an imaginary conversation with his grandfather. "I can't wait to see what you're going to do next." He realized what he had said.

"It's just a matter of planning and strategizing. I'm not saying I won't get hit in the head with a baseball now and again, but it will work." Al gave Albert an extra hard push and the little boy squealed loud with joy. "I'm not missing a minute with my kids. They're not taking that away from me." Al's face became stoic. "Before the surgery last month, I started to

take Albert behind the garage and toss the baseball. I kept a hand on the wall as a guide. The wall also helped keep the balls from getting away. I made sure I had at least four in my pockets." He was thoughtful for a moment. "Now I'm thrilled to be able to make eye contact with Albert when I toss to him. He's even starting to make contact, sort of, with the plastic bat." Al spoke with pride. "I'm glad we had this time together in the warm weather. When I'm working with him next spring I'll go back behind the garage and that will be okay. We're learning together, he and I."

Mr. Hinds started to laugh. "Just don't make it like the basement near electrocution incident. No close misses." Both men shrugged and laughed nervously. "You get hurt playing baseball, and my daughter is never going to let you forget it."

"Elaine's given up trying to stop me from doing anything." He paused for a moment, realizing he was talking to his wife's father. "We have an unspoken agreement. Together we decided we weren't going to let the accident and its aftermath change the life path we chose and, well, I'm still the same man I was before. She's accepted it. She already has two little boys, there is no need for her to add a third one she didn't give birth to." He struggled to take the edge out of his voice. "I was trying to teach Albert to ride a bike while I can see, but he isn't ready yet. I know he's only three, but I thought since he's so active, it might have worked." Al held in the real reason for the effort which was the joy he knew he would feel seeing Albert ride for the first time.

Albert looked over his shoulder. "My bike!"

Al slowed down his pushes. "I know Pal. Daddy doesn't want your bike. I just want to teach you to ride without training wheels."

Mr. Hinds watched Al tilt his head to the left. "Do you see better if you tilt your head?"

"The earth tilts at a five-degree angle. I'm just trying to compensate." Al deadpanned.

Mr. Hinds had an expression on his face as if he had just heard a great nugget of truth he never knew before. "Is that true? Wow, that's something."

Al turned his head away from his father to keep from laughing. "Do you know how I keep an eye on the corneal transplant's progression?" He continued to push Albert as he talked. The little boy squealed as he flew higher and higher on the swing.

The older man looked straight at Al, anxious for a new fun fact from Al.

"I look at the wallpaper in front of the john every morning. I don't tilt my head then. Too dangerous." He stared straight ahead waiting for a response from the older man.

Mr. Hinds finally let out a belly laugh. "Here comes your better half."

"Al, Dad and I can watch the boys." She caught the swing in the middle of its arch and handed a snack to Albert, who immediately let go of the ropes and grabbed at the cookie. "Do you want to go for a bike ride? The weather is great."

Al gave her a quick hug. "Albert I'll be back in a little while."

Albert hardly gave his dad a thought as he finished eating the first cookie and looked anxiously at Elaine for a second.

"Nice to know where I rate next to cookies." He walked quickly toward the garage smiling.

Al let the bright sunlight saturate him. When reached the garage door he yanked it open wider than necessary and grabbed at the ten-speed bike his father-in-law had lent him. He stood alone in the garage for a moment absorbing the fact that he could go for a bike ride on his own. Looking around the former small horse stable he breathed in the smell of the river behind the house and listened to birds, crickets and leaves in the breeze. This was the suburban life he dreamed of as a kid growing up in the heart of Patterson and he never tired of it. It was quiet at night and easy in the day. The large, old trees created a canopy of darkness that created a sharp contrast to the hot, bright, continuous cement of a city. He threw one leg over the bar, shook himself out of his trance, jumped onto the seat and peddled out of the garage.

Elaine called as he picked up speed. "Be careful."

He waved over his shoulder in the direction of her voice as he peddled faster and shifted up in the gears. The bike took a sharp right turn out of the driveway, keeping him on the shoulder of the road, but not slowing if a car had been approaching. The flatness of this section of Lake Road allowed him to gather the momentum he needed to get up the hill ahead of him. The birds were active this time of the day as evening approached, but he didn't notice. He was too busy taking in the scenery that flew by. With his glasses on he did not feel the wind burn his eyes. The color of the trees kept him in the moment and did not let his mind wander as it used to when he rode his bike before the accident. His hair did not fly freely due to the oily consistency even after showering.

Smiling, he crested the top of the hill that was ahead of him only a moment before. Leaning forward he held his chin close to the cross bar, letting his hands slip into the curves of the ten, speed handlebars. He felt like the lead man in the Tour de France, cool and sleek on his black racer. In front of him he saw a car traveling in the same direction as him. In no time at all he overtook the car and began to fly past it.

The passenger window was down and as he reached the front tire a woman's voice began to yell, calling his name. "Al! Al! What are you doing? You can't see!"

Al recognized the voice as Donna from Audubon Parkway. He never stopped or yelled back to her. He was joyful, free and flying. There was no one else in front of him and all stop signs were for the cross traffic. The black top under his tires fully supported his freedom as he leaned into the curve at the bottom of the hill and continued on the circular ride home. The warm air was cool on his face and his body was strong as his legs pumped ferociously with the speed he had created.

Three weeks later he would hold the same pace and speed right before he crashed into a rail fence. It would be his last bike ride alone for five years.

Chapter II: Torture

 *T*he ringing phone startled Al. He was deep in thought remembering a dream he had during his first hospital stay after the accident.   Jumping up from the red couch and making an end zone dash for the receiver that hung next to the breakfast bar, he tripped over the stool Elaine had moved earlier and nearly fell.

He grabbed at the phone cursing under his breath. "Hello?"

"Hi Al. It's Fred Potter. How ya doing?" Fred's positive attitude and gregarious nature usually lifted Al's spirits, but today he found it irritating.

"I'm doing alright. What's up by you?" Momentarily Al forgot about the stool he never saw lurking in the shadows that had begun to invade his deteriorating vision but, took a defensive stance against the man's innocent and caring question.

"Do you still have some free time?"   Fred was very good at prefacing his questions.

Al paused a moment knowing what was coming next. "To tell you the truth Elaine is keeping me pretty busy with babysitting. Two little guys make for twice the trouble even when one is pint sized."

Fred laughed good naturedly. "I understand, but the invitation to join our Bible study on Tueday nights is still open. I can pick you up."

Al paused before answering, clenching his jaw and misplacing his frustration. "I appreciate it, Fred. I'll give it some thought." Al didn't want to hurt the man whom he considered a friend. "Right now, I want to enjoy my sight while I have it. By Christmas I may be back in the dark again."

Fred took a breath on the other end of the phone. "We have a Braille Bible one of the group members found for you."

Surprised and touched, Al felt his welled, up anger deflate. "Well, if you guys are going to all that trouble you must really want me as a member."

"I just want you to know you have a place you can come to when you need to make sense of all that's happened to you. A place to clear the air when life becomes overwhelming." Fred hoped his friend knew he wasn't trying to preach to him.

"I appreciate it, Fred, but I don't ask why this happened. It just did. It's done. I have to keep moving." Deadpanning, he hoped his friend would not be hurt.

"That's what makes you who you are. I just want you to know you have a support system here." There were several seconds of uncomfortable silence between the men. "We've known each other for a long time. You're a strong man." Fred was silent briefly again. "Let your faith help you."

Al tightened his grip on the phone. "Fred, when my sight is completely gone again, I promise I will come to one of your meetings. You have my word." Hearing himself say the words of the impending darkness added another weight to his shoulders.

"I believe you and I want you to believe that we will help you." Fred's resolute tone resounded.

"Alright." Al's typical drawn out 'go to' phrase left an unintentional void of sarcasm he realized he needed to quickly fill. "Fred, I don't know if you're going to believe me, but I had what I thought was a dream in the hospital that I now believe was a vision." Fred was silent. "I actually didn't remember it until this afternoon." Al began to stumble over his words. "I don't know, maybe it was a dream. It seemed real, like I could touch the man in it."

Fred's voice became excited. "Who was the man?"

Al hesitated now, afraid his friend would think he was just placating him or worse, making fun of his beliefs. "It was Christ."

"Al, what happened in the vision?" Fred asked levelly.

The words came out slowly and deliberately. "We were in a graveyard. The Lord stood on my left and to my right there was a sky with different shades of gray that seemed to go on forever. There were no trees or vegetation of any kind to the right. There was nothing else either except for a cross in the sky. I had peripheral vision and to the left I could see a brilliant shade of green I knew to be grass." Al paused to give Fred a chance to comment and when he did not, he continued. "We were on a gravel path that was edged with red bricks. The huge cross was laid against the dismal gray sky with a man hanging on it. It hung horizontally with the man's head toward the path and his feet seemed to extend forever into the sky that had no horizon. The man on the cross had been beaten. He did not have long hair but he did have a beard. I felt overwhelmed by the presence of the man on the cross and the man walking next to me. I cast my eyes down. There were headstones placed intermittently in the dirt. It was not a graveyard like the kind we know. There was no landscaping or writing on the headstones. Just barrenness and gray, lifeless dirt. Not even what you would call soil, just dirt." Al shuddered involuntarily at the memory. "I could not bear the emptiness I felt coming from the gray sky and found the courage to look to my left and saw a great wall with three gates on it. The gates were rounded at the top. They were closed but I somehow knew they weren't locked. It was then that I looked up at the man who was intently watching me." He felt his throat constrict. "He spoke to me in a low gravelly voice that vibrated. He said, *'It's not your time. Go back and do your job.'* He had white hair that was short like an afro and a beard. He was not an old man, but ageless with tan, weathered skin. He was strange looking if I had to use an adjective."

Fred's voice became a whisper. "What happened next?"

"I just stared at him for a moment because his eyes changed color with the ferocity of fire and with brilliance. The light to his left beyond the city was very bright. I knew this was a city because of the activity I could hear taking place behind the high walls that were flat at the top. The gates did not open and there was no one around but myself, the man next to me and the dead person on the cross. The walls and the gates had a shimmering effect with more colors than a rainbow. There was no sun and there was a definitive line between the dismal gray sky and the bright blue sky above the city. The clouds above the walled city were drifting and were not the type of clouds we see here." He stopped speaking, no longer able to find his voice.

Fred's voice was level again. "Did you ever tell Elaine about this?"

"She told me the first time she came to see me in the hospital, the day after the accident I somehow spoke to her through my banged, up face and lips. I told her that the Lord came to me and said everything would be okay, but I don't remember talking to her. The man in the vision told me: *'go back and do your job'* he never told me everything would be okay." Standing up he began to shift his weight from foot to foot.

"You made a choice to live. The misery and pain you went through to be with your family and to continue to love them and life is testimony of the incredible strength of your soul and spirit. You obviously did not want to leave your family alone." Fred gave his words time to be absorbed before continuing. "You and your family do not have to face any of this alone. Your extended family, friends and our group are here to support you. You know you can count on me whenever you need a car ride somewhere or a shoulder to lean on."

Touched by Fred's sincere gesture, Al took a moment to respond. Any residual frustration, fear or anger over his diminishing sight dissipated completely. "You've been there from the day of the accident, Fred. I never doubted your support for my family."

"You are the main support for your family. It reminds me of a thought I used while counseling one of my friends: 'A good parent triumphs in their vocation no matter what the circumstances. A bad parent fails in the best and most convenient circumstances'. The vision you had is proof you came back to be the father to your son that your own father never had the chance to be. No matter what happens, you will not fail at that." Fred wondered if he was preaching or building up his friend. "For a man who lost his father at five and then his grandfather at nine and overcame being a latchkey kid in the fifties, the fact that your determination to be a good father to your own boys is outstanding. Your fight to live is remarkable."

"Fred?" Al needed Fred to understand the truth.

Fred became aprrehensive and afraid he went too far with Al. "Yes?"

"I'd give my right arm, literally, to be able to see again permanently. I can live with one arm. But if the lesson I had is that I will never take my family or my love for them for granted, then well, I will find a way to live without my sight." Empowered, he couldn't stop himself or slow down. "I've been on both sides of the materialistic fence. Elaine and I have had nice things. I grew up poor, I grew up alone, and I'll never be alone or allow my family to live without me." He looked over his shoulder into the great room and the huge stone fireplace. On the mantel sat the copy of the picture of Babe Ruth surrounded by children in front of the fireplace when it was a lodge. His gaze fell downward to the open, empty fireplace. Fear gripped him for a second and then sadness. He knew he could and would never allow a fireplace in his home to be utilized again.

Fred misunderstood the momentary pause. "I believe you're beginning to make peace with the whole mess."

Al shrugged his shoulders as he tore his gaze away from the fireplace. "Yeah. I thought I already had but maybe what I was doing was just accepting it. Honestly, it may be a while longer before I can say I am at peace. I have learned not to take anything for granted. That's a gift in and of itself." He rubbed at his chest where the scars lay beneath his Jobe shirt.

"Some people never get that. They spend their whole lives wanting the unreachable or unattainable and never seeing what is right in front of them." Fred realized what he said and quickly circled the conversation back to Al's vision. "If you don't mind I'm going to send you some material on tape to listen to for our class sessions. It's Revelations 21 and 22. I think it may surprise you." Fred thought he would get Al's standard 'Thanks, but no thanks'.

"Sure Fred. That would be great." Al felt any resistance he had to Fred's 'helpful suggestions' dissipating slightly.

"I had a similar experience to what you shared with me. I'll tell you about it another time." Fred wanted to keep the focus on Al's spirits.

Al wasn't sure if Fred was telling the truth or creating a lead in for further conversation. "That would be great. It would be nice to know I'm not crazy." Both men laughed lightly before Al brought the conversation back to topic. "I suppose in a sick way, I lost my sight to be able to see clearly. It's amazing what you see when you can't see. I would have preferred an easier route to my epiphany, but I'm where I'm at and that is the way it is." He gave a stretch with his free hand and looked across the kitchen at the clock. "I haven't been listening to the radio since I got my sight back. It was my way of keeping track of the time."

"What are you doing now?"

"Looking at the clock."

Fred laughed and let the moment unravel. "Got it."

Al spotted the newspaper on the counter. "Fred, I forgot how much I used to enjoy doing the crossword puzzles. I was sitting on my mom's porch the other day doing one. It was a bright, sunny day and some neighbors who were walking by knew me and couldn't believe it. I had to go through the explanation of the transplant and that the doctor had put a plastic lens in place. Since the eye does not adjust, the brighter the day the better I see. It's tunnel vision but I ride my bike pretty well."

"You're riding a bike?" Fred asked incredulously.

"Of, course. I started cutting the grass again too. Elaine had a fit, but it felt good. I think I'm the only man on the planet who's glad to cut his grass." He sat back down on the breakfast bar stool. "I think this was the last cut of the season. Maybe not. Next year I'm going to work out a system with ropes as guides. Why should we have to pay someone or ask my father-in-law to cut it? He was a great help that first summer after the accident."

"You think you can come up with some way to do it alone?" Fred was impressed with his friend's ability to overcome anything.

"Sure. It can't be that hard. Now that I have my sight back I see things I forgot about in the yard and I can plan my strategy-dimensions, grading, pitch and obstacles. I'll make a concentrated effort to memorize all of it before I lose my sight completely." This time the thought of the impending darkness did not hurt as much. "There are days when I think it would be easier to just wake up six months from now in complete darkness but have clear sight up to that point. The loss of sight after my accident was like ripping off a band aid. No choices. I had to deal with it immediately. It took several weeks after the surgery to have clear vision, and now it is beginning to go the other way. Each day a little bit is lost. The loss is very faint now, but it's there. Every day I'm trying to hang on." There was a pause before Al continued. "It's like when Dr. Leesville removed the staples in my eye after the transplant. It's this pinging sound and a feeling I can't describe. Not exactly pain, but it hurts. I was willing to go through it because I knew I was starting to gradually see. It was slow and frustrating, but there was a positive reward. Now I'm heading down a very gradual descent, a little each day. It's not painful, but it still hurts."

Fred felt his friend's frustration building. "You're talking about it. That's as important as the focus you have with moving forward and planning for the eventual loss. With the Bible study group, you gain and enhance your faith." Fred circled back around to his objective.

"Fred, there's a chance I could have a new corneal transplanted every five years. I would be okay with that. It would be like seeing snapshots of my family as I watch them grow. Since I can only have three to each eye I'm keeping my left eye as a spare tire." The sight of a smiling Larry pulling himself up on the coffee table this morning and hanging on was forefront in Al's mind as he continued. "I'll see Larry take his first steps. That child has no desire to crawl. He goes from sitting up to pulling himself up on all the furniture."

"That boy wants to keep up with his big brother, no doubt." Fred smiled.

"I'm grateful for the gifts, but if I had to list what I miss when I don't have sight the first thing would be eye contact. You can know what a person is thinking a lot of the time through their eye contact or lack of it." Al leaned back and looked up at the vaulted ceiling of the great room behind him. "The eyes can tell you the truth and the eyes can lie."

"That could be frustrating, but I'm sure you're able to pick up more in the tone of voice than I could." Fred was more curious about this rather than just stating a fact.

"I suppose. Sometimes I'm concentrating so much on reminding myself not to slump over that I'm hardly paying attention to what someone is saying. People without sight tend to slump from fear without realizing they're doing it. Can't really blame them." Al spotted a stain on the ceiling that could only mean a small roof leak. He knew Elaine probably hadn't noticed it.

Fred decided to change the subject. "A friend of mine has a '71 Corvette he just picked up. You want to take it out for a joy ride with me?"

Al started to laugh. "Are we *borrowing* it?"

Fred gave a long belly laugh. "I don't steal. It's a real beauty and I'd like for you to see it. The weather is perfect for us to take it down a back road and let you drive."

Suddenly Al felt a surge of enthusiasm and treachery. "When do you want to do this?"

"What are you doing now?" Fred was feeling his own excitement and also knew that his good friend was out of town.

Al jumped off the stool. "Can you pick me up in twenty minutes?"

Elaine came into the room carrying a sleepy Albert. "Hey, what's up?"

Al heard Fred's voice and looked at Elaine at the same time. "Give me forty-five minutes. I have to go get the car." He hung up without saying goodbye or giving Al a chance to change his mind.

Elaine watched Al hang up the phone. "Who was that?"

"Fred. He's taking me for a car ride in a Corvette. Do you mind?" He purposely left out the part of his driving.

Elaine laughed good naturedly. "Go enjoy yourself. Maybe he'll let you drive. I know how much you miss that."

Trying desperately not to smile, he felt like a kid who just got away with skipping school and hanging out for the day. "Yeah, I hope so. That would be great."

An hour later he was at the wheel of the Corvette staring down the empty, two lane straight road driving thirty miles an hour. Fred was in the passenger seat, calm and smiling as he watched his friend keep his hands at two and ten on the steering wheel. The power of the engine ran through him. He didn't think about the future, about loss or how careful he found himself driving. There was still time for things like this.

"Hey Fred, you better not tell your buddy about this. He might not feel so charitable toward people with handicaps!" Al yelled over the sound of the car.

"Keep your eye on the road! We can talk later." Fred laughed and leaned back in the car.

Al caught the literal meaning to what Fred yelled at him.

There were no obstacles in front of him, what was behind him couldn't stop him and whatever lay in his peripheral vision could not be seen. At this moment, that was enough.

Chapter III: Dreams

$\mathcal{L}$arry snuggled in Al's lap in the passenger seat and Albert happily played behind them in the back seat of the station wagon without the constraints of seatbelts. The year 1976 was winding down as an early ice storm rolled into the area. All morning, as he and Elaine prepared the boys for the trip to Dr. Grove's office, Al would steal moments to stare out the window at the beauty the storm had created. Although the streets were clear, they had been unable to find someone to come and watch the boys for the day. The appointment with Dr. Grove to check on the progress of the Jobe shirt could not be postponed any longer.

Larry drifted off to sleep and Al was able to enjoy the passing scenery. "Elaine, it's so beautiful. Everything is shimmering."

"It's gorgeous." She smiled and then took a moment to catch a glimpse of Albert pretending his army guys were talking to each other. "Al thanks for painting the great room. The stain from the leak was bugging me after you pointed it out."

He continued to stare out the window as they spoke. "No problem." He gave her a second to complete the compliment and when she didn't he finished it for her. "You're welcome for fixing the leak too."

She gave him a smirk that he could still see even in the muted light inside the station wagon. "Sorry. Thank you for catching the leak. I never look up."

31

"I'm glad I caught it before the weather turned cold. That might have been a problem with snow." Secretly he was also glad he caught it before his vision faded. He hated paying contractors and he knew without sight he would not have been able to repair the leak. "Glad you like the paint job, Sweetheart."

"Are you using the same system to paint that you're going to use to cut the lawn next year?" She was glad the storm had kept most people home today. Driving always had been a chore for her and during bad weather it became unnerving.

Al smiled and turned away from the window for a moment. "You were watching me?"

"The strings were hanging down. I almost yanked down the first one I walked into. Albert was jumping up trying to grab at them." She saw Albert look up quickly at the sound of his name. "Albert, did you get any of Daddy's strings?"

"Daddy you dipped paint all over." Albert gave the back of Al's head a stern look.

Elaine tried to laugh at Albert's comment, knowing the fact that his sight was fading was a heavy strain on Al. The cuteness of Albert's absent letter 'r' from words still made her smile.

Al tried to sound serious. "Sorry buddy. Dad does his best."

"Al, the ceiling looks good. I'm amazed how much you were able to finish in the house this year." The scenic ice wonderland was beginning to break up as the sun rose higher. Water gathered on the roadway and Elaine's thoughts went to the condition of the road for the drive home.

Adjusting himself in the seat so he could look at her through the fading vision of his right eye, Al felt Larry stir. "When we get home, I'll put the finishing touches on the paint in Larry's new room. We'll be home hours before the sun sets so I'll have plenty of natural light to help me." Al knew Elaine would be concerned about driving home.

Elaine gave him a conspiratorial glance. "I think Albert has noticed the difference in having his brother share his room.

It would have been a challenge as they grew and fought over the space." She smiled. "Fortunately, I have a husband who is an extraordinary carpenter. I never would have thought to divide the floor plan the way you did to make it work. Making the porch part of the great room so that we did not lose that common area when we made Larry's bedroom was genius."

Al shifted Larry again on his lap as he began to fuss. "I can live with you thinking I'm a genius." He turned to stare at the passing scenery again. "You know how much I missed construction when I took the job at A&K. I used to feel like my office was a prison. I would much rather have been out in the fresh air. It was always for the money and security." He shook his head at the realities of his former life. "I was always pushing and pushing to make myself enjoy it."

"You were taking care of us. I think eventually, like in any industry, there would have been lay-offs and you may have gone back to work in construction full time. Probably would have started your own company." Elaine and Al looked thoughtfully at each other before she turned back to the road and took the exit to the doctor's office.

The appointment with Dr. Grove was uneventful, routine and necessary. He checked the progress of Al's scar tissue and was happy with the Jobe shirt's ability to slow and in some places, halt the scar tissue from building further. Al expressed his continued thanks for the relief the shirt offered and promised the doctor he would continue to utilize it as directed-wearing it constantly except when he showered. Although it was difficult to get used to wearing it at night he did. Sleeping through the night no longer required medication to ease the pain, discomfort and itching from the healing burn tissue.

When they arrived home later that afternoon, Al changed his mind about painting and decided to hang the Christmas lights early. He was pulling lights out of the boxes in the basement when Elaine came down.

"I thought you were going to paint?"

Al lifted a twisted mound of light strings. "This seems like a better idea. My sight is fading and I don't want to leave this to the last minute when we have so many other things to do around the holidays. You didn't have Christmas lights for two years. I want you to have them now."

A yell from Albert carried through to the basement and Elaine reacted immediately. "I better go see what's going on. Be careful. If you need me, yell like your son. I'll come running."

He nodded his head in agreement before dropping the light strings into the box he was going to carry outside. Al turned and went up the stairs to grab the ladder he kept in the garage. The sun was just dropping below the top of the tree line and he began to rush. After the ladder was set against the house he climbed up with the enthusiasm he had from his early days in construction. He reached the top to contemplate where he would begin the strings and found the original hooks and markers he had set up when they bought the house. Pangs of regret struck him as he wondered what might have been had the accident not happened, but they lasted for only a moment as he stood three rungs from the top of the ladder at the edge of the roof. Shaking off the regrets, he realized with gratitude that because he had set these markers up four years ago and found them today, he would be able to hang the lights every year with or without sight. He climbed down, gathered a string of lights and finished the job with the ease of a professional. Before calling to Elaine to come see the lights he snuck inside the house, flipped the switch to turn on the lights and jogged to the end of the driveway to stared at the lights as the sun dropped below the horizon. Their beauty captivated him. The strings shimmered, each color complimenting the other in a way he decided an engineer must have planned and created. The red, green, blue, and yellow accentuated the house line perfectly. Pride filled him as he realized he alone had set these lines up four years ago never knowing he would be doing it for himself at a moment when he needed it.

The kitchen door swung open and Elaine came out to join him. Looking over her shoulder as she walked, she slipped her arm through his when they met. "Wow, they look great."

A look of satisfaction spread across his face. "This Christmas will be special."

"They're all special as long as we're together." She leaned her head on his shoulder.

"I guess it's really just about finding the joy that is life. The simple joy of being able to be together and appreciating it." He kissed the side of her forehead. "Where are the boys? We should bring them out to look at this."

Elaine reluctantly left his side. "I'll get them and Mom." Elaine talked over her shoulder as she walked away. "Rose was having so much fun playing with the boys I didn't want to tell her I was coming out to take a peak."

Secretly glad for the solitude, Al continued to stand and stare at the sparkling multicolored lights becoming more prominent as twilight darkened the sky.

Elaine came back several minutes later carrying Larry with Al's mother trailing behind pulling Albert as he fought to stay with his toy pile. Elaine looked at Al apologetically. "Sorry Al. He was in the middle of building a skyscraper."

In the growing darkness, Al saw his son as only a shadow. "Hey Albert, turn around. Look at the pretty Christmas lights."

Albert pulled his hand out of his grandmother's, twisted his head to see the lights and immediately stopped fussing. "Kismas lights! Is Santa here?"

The three adults laughed lightly. "Not yet, buddy. A few more weeks and Santa will bring you lots of presents, so you better be good." Al took hold of Elaine's free hand.

Rose Plevier stared at the lights. "They look beautiful son. I am so glad to be living here with you this Christmas."

Elaine looked over at her mother-in-law. "We are too, Mom. There was no way we would ever let you live alone after being robbed." She stared at the lights along the roof line of the second floor. "The room upstairs is perfect for you but I wish it was bigger. I know it was an adjustment to live in one small bedroom." Elaine knew Rose felt like she was intruding since she moved and she went to great lengths to make her feel comfortable.

"Mom, the boys love you being here. Christmas will be extra special." Al thought ahead to the holidays. "I can't wait to see the boy's faces Christmas morning."

Tears filled Rose Plevier's eyes and she looked away from the group until she could find her voice. "It will be a very special holiday."

Al thought about the gifts he and Elaine had hidden upstairs in his mother's closet far away from where the boys might accidentally find them. Watching the lights twinkle in the approaching night he thought about everyone who had and was still helping them.

"We have a lot of people to give to this year. I think they will appreciate the handmade gifts I created before and after I got my sight back this year. I still have that shot gun and barrel rifle I carved out of wood last spring for Mr. Bayplaza. He was so impressed that I could carve the little pistol I gave him that I figured I'd make him something bigger. He'll really enjoy getting them for Christmas and I don't think he'll expect a Christmas gift from a client. I have to see him next week before the New Year starts." He paused allowing the beauty of the lights back into his awareness. "We need to go over the case strategy."

A worried look passed between Elaine and Rose. "Son, where are you with all that?"

Al realized that what he had said might have cast a pall over the holiday preparations. "Don't worry about it, Mom. This lawyer is sharp. He cares too much personally about us, but he is an excellent attorney. Tough as nails. I think if he didn't care so much he'd share my attitude of going for the throat." He felt himself going down the spiral he had discussed with Mr. Hinds and he decided to stop. "We are just going over the next stage, and I have to update him on the private detective the defending company hired to follow me. Elaine has been keeping a log book that the attorney's secretary photocopies when we go in." When his mother's worried look did not change, he continued. "It's all good. He has said from the beginning that if a settlement is offered we should consider it seriously since we are young and have a family." Al now felt a complete change of subject was in order. "I'm seeing Dr. Leesville next week. He needs to check the progression of the cornea. Not sure if I'm riding in with Dave or if Elaine is taking me. I'd like to give her a break from driving." Al saw the look on his mother's face and knew he went from a bad subject to a worse subject and he became desperate to bring back the enthusiasm of a few minutes ago. Albert took care of that for him.

"Daddy you make good lights." Albert pointed at the house and began to jump up and down giggling.

"Yeah, buddy. Daddy makes the lights shine. Pretty lights for all the pretty ladies in our life." He saw Elaine and Rose relax a little again.

Elaine spoke up also eager for a subject change. "I'll take you, Al. I hate to see you stuck there all day waiting for Dave to get out of work. Especially after last time." She shifted a squirming Larry again while one chubby hand held her shoulder and the other pointed to the lights.

Rose looked over at Al. "What happened last time?"

Al began to shift nervously, from one foot to the other. "Nothing really, Mom. More aggravating than anything. Dave dropped me off and I was getting ready to cross the street. A woman saw my cane and grabbed my arm, practically dragging me across the intersection. She never asked, just said hurry before the light changes. There was a cop there who always let me know when to cross, and besides I can hear the traffic and my sight was better than now." He could see that this was not helping assuage his mother's worry. He was losing the magic of the evening. "I'll tell you what would really be helpful is a schematic of the men's room in Braille outside the door. Do you know how many times I poked someone with my cane? They are never happy campers, I can tell you that."

Both women rolled their eyes as Larry began to laugh at his brother's antics and squirmed to get out of Elaine's arms. "This one will be walking in no time at all. All he wants to do is chase his brother."

Al looked at his family and knew prayers are always answered and dreams do come true. He turned back to the lights that shimmered for him in the early evening darkness not worrying about tomorrow. It would have to take care of itself.

"Elaine, Mr. Bayplaza asked me at the beginning of the month when he could take the Sylvania's and us out to dinner. Completely his treat. The holiday is coming up so quickly. Should we have him and his wife over to see the lights and the tree, maybe for cocktails?" In truth, Al had completely forgotten about the invitation until this moment with the realization that he had an impending appointment with his attorney.

Larry gave up trying to escape from Elaine and, losing interest in the Christmas lights, satisfied himself by watching Albert. "Let's wait until after the New Year. It will be something nice to look forward to in January. To be honest, we're not in a position to entertain."

Al agreed. "I know. As long as he wants to take us out, I believe Bob Sylvania would agree that it would be rude not to accept." Al thought again about how he had forgotten. "I think it was supposed to be a holiday gift. When I talk to him tomorrow I'll use the holidays and having my sight as an excuse. I've been trying to squeeze in as much as possible, so that isn't a lie."

The family enjoyed the beauty of the lights until the chill of the evening drove them inside. After the boys were in bed Elaine found Al outside without his jacket staring at the lights. She joined him and they stood together, holding one another as they saw Rose turn out the interior lights upstairs.

Early the next morning as the sun began to rise, Al woke before Elaine and the boys. Unable to go back to sleep he decided to take a walk around the neighborhood. Unsure of how much longer he would have the marginal sight, he wanted to remember and mark a few places along the driveway and road with objects that he would easily find without sight. The dim morning light was not helpful and he found himself utilizing his cane for navigation so that he didn't have to count his steps. Moving quickly, he was anxious to be back before Elaine woke. Thinking he was leaving his driveway he turned hard into the low holly tree branch at the driveway entrance. Angry and scratched, he swung the cane so hard into the tree he broke the tip.

Well, that's another cane I'll have to replace. Elaine is not going to be happy with me.

Turning around he walked back toward the house. The sun was brightening up the sky that had a cloud cover. He thought about last night and the crystalline appearance of the Christmas lights. The closer he got to the back door the stronger the memory was.

That's what will carry me when I can't see my family.

Chapter IV: Light and Movement

ℐhe blinds in Larry's room were fully raised and December's morning sunshine streamed into the room. Al worked at changing the diaper of the eleven-month-old with the precision of a pit crew. He knew he had a small window of time before the pint size bundle of energy would be twisting to get back to play time. Without bright sunshine, Al's world had returned to shadows. In the middle of the night he was returned to changing diapers by feel only and he knew that shortly this would be the norm during the day hours. Even with the streaming daylight he placed Larry's cloth diaper cover over his thigh and the little boy giggled with joy as his father's shirt was covered in pee.

"Thanks pal. Now Daddy needs to be change too." Al spotted what he knew was the small pot of fresh soapy water and hand towels Elaine had discretely placed at the corner of the changing table, where they had always kept it before his transplant surgery. He pinned the diaper solidly, feeling each pin slide firmly into its holder before he released his hold on it. Slipping the warm jumper onto his son, Al lifted Larry off the table and placed him on the floor while he washed his hands. "Don't go anywhere." Larry pulled himself up, hanging onto the changing table and watching his father intently. "Almost done." He picked up the happy baby and the two of them walked into the great room to greet an impatient Elaine.

"Thank you for changing him, Al." She watched him place Larry next to his brother on the carpet. "We really have to get going. Dr. Leesville won't appreciate it if we're late." She walked over to kiss Albert goodbye. The little boy hardly noticed her as he pulled his toys away from his little brother. "You boys be good for Grandma."

Al inclined his chin to his mom. "Thanks, Mom. We should be back by two at the latest."

Rose walked over with her morning coffee and sat down on the sofa watching the boys as they played near the Christmas tree. "Take your time. Albert has been refusing to move from under the tree all morning. I think he's hoping Santa will come before Christmas morning."

Al and Elaine made a hasty exit. An hour later they were inside the examination room with Dr. Leesville discussing the progression of the corneal transplant after his full examination of the eye.

"Albert the deterioration of the transplanted cornea is happening along the timeline we expected." Dr. Leesville was always perfunctory in his explanations to Al. He knew the emotional toll the immediate loss, then the miraculous return and now the gradual loss of his sight was having on his patient but his job was to explain the facts without any false hope. Experience had taught him that, as cold as he might appear, knowledge and facts were what allowed his patients to cope. "As you are aware the optic nerve was damaged by the chemical but not completely severed from the retina. This will allow for another transplant. However, there are a limit to the number of corneal transplants that can be performed on each eye. My analogy of planting a tree in the desert is as accurate as I can be in layman's terms." The expression he viewed on Elaine's face was not fear. Al's expression was unreadable as he looked directly at Dr. Leesville. "Let's talk about the failure process again and the ability for more transplants." He looked at his hands folded over the medical file on his desk. "The little piece of the old cornea that we had to leave in order to attach a donor cornea is not allowing the nutrients from the blood to turn the fluid completely clear. The cloudy fluid passing to the donor cornea does not have the nutrients necessary to keep the donated cornea healthy and eventually it will fail. The slow failure may be harder for you to accept as your world grows darker." There was still no reaction from the couple in front of him. "The ability we have to perform another transplant is due primarily to our success in removing the floating chemical debris and some of the scar tissue. The plastic implant we replaced your lens with will not be changed if another transplant happens. Again, your optic nerve is performing even though the nerve endings were split and altered the sight you had for a short time." Dr. Leesville watched Al follow him as he stood up from behind his desk and walked around the brightly lit office. "The shadow vision you have now may last a while longer according to what I saw in the exam. I believe you will have this limited vision into the beginning of January." Dr. Leesville was careful not to make a reference to the holidays.

Al absorbed what Dr. Leesville said. "That's what I expected. I've continued to use the wallpaper in the bathroom as a gauge. It isn't blurry, but it has a shadow now. Nighttime was never as clear as daytime because the eye can't adjust. My tunnel vision has never changed, of course. I knew that was never possible because of the damage and the surgery." Al spoke as antiseptically as the doctor in order to hold his sanity together. "I'm holding off using my cane consistently for as long as possible."

Dr. Leesville looked defensively down at the medical chart he held as he spoke. "Have you been able to enjoy doing things you thought you would never do again?"

Al shook his head thoughtfully. "Sure. I rode a bike until I crashed it into a fence." The doctor smiled, knowing the humor Al used to survive. "I look forward to ice skating on the neighborhood pond if my sight holds on until the end of January. The ice storm was pretty wonderful to see and got me thinking about skating. I could probably do that without sight, but it was wonderful to imagine watching a winter wonderland."

"I'm really happy for you. The rest of us were busy complaining about the inconvenience of the early snow and ice. You might want to go on a motivational speaking tour." He finished writing in the chart.

Al snorted good naturedly. "How much does it pay?"

The doctor smiled and closed the chart. "Pretty well, from what I hear. I think you'd have a large audience."

Elaine had remained silent during the exam up to this point. "We're so grateful Al can see both boys. I have to agree with you in all sincerity that Al could inspire others with everything he has endured."

Al couldn't tell if the doctor was serious, placating him or just being as sarcastic as he was. He didn't want to burst Elaine's bubble about his ability to speak in public so he just agreed. "I'll give it serious consideration and let you both know my decision."

Doctor Leesville looked soberly first at Al and then Elaine. "I'm sure I don't have to say this, but please enjoy this Christmas together. You will still have sight. In the daylight, it will be a Christmas to remember and not shadows."

"I intend to enjoy Christmas and all the moments surrounding it, Dr. Leesville. I've been prepared for the inevitable return to living without sight." Al wondered if either Elaine or the doctor believed the lie.

Two weeks later Dr. Leesville's prediction became reality. The entire family, including Rose, Mr. and Mrs. Hinds, Ronnie, Al, Elaine and the boys sat around the Christmas tree late Christmas morning enjoying the aftermath of the chaos. Even Larry, who did not yet understand who Santa was, understood the excitement and the toys underneath the colorful paper. Christmas music blared all over the house through the speaker system Al had installed as a project to keep him busy after the accident and before the cornea surgery.

Al sipped his tea and stared at the tree. "Once we lit the tree and put the presents under it, everything looked so sharp and bright. I'll never forget that sight." Al reached for Elaine's hand.

At that moment Albert walked over, took a toy from Larry and carried it back to his 'nest'. Instead of crying, Larry pushed himself into a standing position.

Elaine had a short intake of breath. "Oh, I think he might walk."

"Shhh." Al squeezed her hand.

Tottering for a brief moment Larry took one step without smiling. He looked only at where Albert sat, not at anyone else in the room. The second step came and then the next ones until finally he reached Albert. Larry squatted down, took his toy back and then walked back to his own toy nest where he plopped himself down and began to babble. The adults sat speechless and smiling with their mugs halfway to their mouths.

Fighting to talk over the lump in his throat, Al broke the silence. "It's all over now Elaine. Us against them. I think they're going to win."

Everyone started to laugh including Albert who looked over at the big people on the couch and wanted to be a part of the joke.

"I think that will be the last time Albert dares to take something from his brother." Mr. Hinds looked proudly over at the two boys.

Al looked at his father-in-law. "Ha! I think the wrestling matches will get more intense as they grow."

Ronnie broke out in laughter. "How are the temper tantrums going with Albert? I had to chase him around the house for ten minutes the other day trying to get his clothes on."

"Ronnie, if you think I'm chasing a little pint of stubbornness around the house with or without sight you're wrong. I scoop him up and give him a pat on the bottom." Al gave a gross look. "The joke used to be on me when he had a full diaper that exploded.

"An exploding diaper?" Ronnie rolled her eyes. "Never did that one."

Al laughed. "I forgot about that until this minute. Albert was out of diapers soon after we found out Elaine was pregnant with Larry. He didn't fuss at all. I think he was as ready as we are. One in diapers at a time is enough."

Elaine got up from the couch. "Would anyone like eggnog or more coffee? If you want something light I could get sweet-breads out."

Rose stood next to Elaine. "I'll help, Honey. It's your Christmas too."

As Rose and Elaine worked in the kitchen Al walked around the torn paper, empty boxes and toys strewn about the carpet and stood in front of the window that looked over the back yard. A light snow had been falling and was now clinging to the evergreen trees. Icicles were hanging from the gutters and the entire yard looked like the winter wonderland he remembered from childhood. The indoor lights he had strung around the great room sparkled in competition with the Christmas tree lights. He kept switching his gaze back and forth between the two scenes memorizing the smallest detail.

Elaine crept up quietly behind him and wrapped her arms around his waist. She felt the edge of the Jobe shirt under his oxford, always there as a reminder. "Merry Christmas."

"Merry Christmas Sweetheart." He pulled her arms tighter. "Time is running out. You guys are disappearing into the shadows."

"We'll have this again. You have to believe." She leaned her head against his back.

He breathed out deeply. "Hope is born out of the miracles and progress of modern medicine. As an engineer, I can live with that." They were quiet together watching the snow fall and listening to the activity around them. Everyone in the group, including the children left them alone for those few moments. "No compromising, Elaine. I want to continue to live my life without compromise."

"Why would this next round be any different than the last twenty-six years of your life?" She slipped around to stand next to him and looked into his right eye. Steadfast without emotion, strong in her conviction, she continued. "You'll always be able to find me. I'll be the one closest to you in any room or space

Al felt the fear and the sadness of his return to life without sight leave him as he stood next to his wife, looking down and memorizing her features. On that Christmas Day of 1976 they were crisp.

By early February 1977, even in bright sunlight, he was looking down into a shadow where her features used to be. Every evening, he joined the true minority of those living without sight. His cane was his constant companion as he readjusted to the darkness even inside the house. He looked for diversions to fight the panic he felt rise inside him from time to time. Their life had become a daily routine of talking about the disappearing beauty in front of him.

"Elaine, I spoke to Mr. Bayplaza today. He still would like to take us all out to eat." A night out of the house gave his spirits a lift. "Maybe we should do this before my sight is completely gone."

Sitting next to Al on the couch that evening, Elaine knew their quiet time after the boys went to bed had become melancholic of late. "I agree. We need to get out."

"I never told you, but I pictured the attorney differently." Al thought back to the first time he saw the man who held his family's future within the scope of his talent in August when his sight was perfect.

"How so?" Elaine looked around the room at the scattered, unkempt, happy environment her children were growing up in.

"I anticipated a short, fat, serious little man. Instead, he's of average height and weight." He left off the personality comparison.

She leaned back and looked at the pattern of the paint swirls from Al's work. "Call him tomorrow. My parents can watch the boys. It will be great to see Bob and his wife."

"I would like to see Bob before I can't. We really owe him for connecting us with the right attorney." Al saw Elaine's head tilted back and knew she was looking at the ceiling. "Did I miss a spot?"

"No. As a matter of fact, it's perfect." She closed her eyes and opened them again. "Our life is perfect. We have a beautiful family that is growing." She let the last sentence hang in the air."

Al looked at the shadow of her and knew there was happiness in her face and the sparkle in her eyes. "Really? Are you sure?" Joy ran through him.

"Believe me, I'm sure. I'm beginning to be a professional at knowing when I'm expecting. You and I have this system down perfectly." They both laughed.

He leaned over, lifted her chin and kissed her. "This is wonderful news. We're still moving forward, Sweetheart."

Elaine felt herself getting teary. "I feel the same way."

Al felt giddy inside. "When do you want to tell the family?"

"We're supposed to go to mom and dads for dinner soon. Let's wait until then, just to be sure enough time has passed." She yawned widely. "The first trimester always leaves me tired, especially at the end of the day."

"I'll put away the toys. You should have a fresh house to wake up to." He gave her a sly look to lighten the mood.

Al got up from the couch and felt in front of him for the box of matchbox cars, Hess trucks and various miniature eighteen wheelers that were only Alberts. It was this container that set Albert apart from the younger brother and allowed his individuality to remain intact.

"Elaine, do I have his entire collection?" It was a sweet and a little sarcastic question. Both of them knew Albert kept a mental inventory of his 'treasures'.

"That's all of it." Elaine looked admirably at the large collection.

Al picked up the light, former orange crate and walked backward out of the living room with one hand feeling to his right. He used his back and butt as a guide ensuring that he would not crash into anything.

A sadness came over Elaine as she watched him maneuvering across the room. She saw her husband being returned to the world without sight and how he was forced to cope. It was in this instant that she realized she had been so jubilant over the return of his sight she had forgotten about the parameters they would be forced to work within. He would always reach beyond the parameters and he would succeed but it would take work, ingenuity and four times the amount of time a person with sight would take to complete a project. Life was simpler and kinder when her husband could see.

Quelling her own fears, she circled back to the diversion of dinner with the attorney. "Al, I'm looking forward to the evening out." She hoped socializing and the new addition to their family would help them move past their fears and transition back to living with blindness. "We'll have to tell the lawyer about the new baby or he is going to wonder why I'm able to eat more than everyone else. You know how hungry I get while I'm expecting."

That weekend, in the early evening light, the three couples sat around a private table in a darkened, quiet Italian restaurant. Al knew he was in trouble from the minute they walked inside.

"Al, you've got to try the steak. Mike, the chef, creates a char that is unduplicated, even in the restaurants I've been to in the city." Mr. Bayplaza normally would never mix business with pleasure, but he enjoyed both couples and felt a fatherly need to protect all of them.

Al tried to relax. "That sounds great. I'll let you order for me tonight. We're on your turf." He turned his head from side to side trying to distinguish what were now just dark shadows.

The waitress arrived, immediately noticed Al's dark glasses in the dimly lit room. She turned to Elaine first, asking if she and Al would care for drinks and then counter clockwise around the table finally reaching Al after Mr. Bayplaza had ordered a steak dinner for him.

The waitress looked at Al. "Sir, would you care for an appetizer?" The young girl spoke loudly and drew the attention of diners at the next table.

"No, I'm fine with the steak." Al was used to this reaction, but wondered how his attorney and the others felt.

Increasing her volume and pitch, the young waitress continued. "Soup or salad comes with your steak dinner. Which would you prefer?"

Al leaned closer to her with the side of his head. "I'm sorry, what?" He felt Elaine kick him under the table.

Unaware he was mocking her, the waitress thought she needed to speak louder still. "Would you prefer soup or salad with your dinner? There is bread in the middle of the table if you would care for some." She suddenly looked as if she had forgotten something important. "There's butter too!"

Al no longer felt angry at being treated like a child. He felt guilty for the discomfort the young woman displayed. "I'm good. Trying to lay off the extra calories from the bread."

She shook her head in agreement. "I understand. Me too."

Mr. Bayplaza waited until the young girl left. "Al, you have the patience of a saint."

"Actually, Elaine's the saint in the family." He reached for her hand under the table.

The second his hand touched hers, her irritation deflated. "The waitress is young. Al, do you want me to run interference for you the rest of the evening?"

Bob jumped in. "I can do it, if you want Boss." He was still very protective of his friend's daughter and son-in-law.

"We got it, Bob. But thanks anyway. It's good to know you have our backs." Al settled in, no longer disturbed by behavior he knew he had to readjust to.

By the time the steak arrived, the small amount of evening light streaming through the windows had completely dissipated and he could not see the food or barely discern the location of the dinner plate. He waited until he heard Elaine begin to use her dinnerware, felt for his knife and fork and prepared to eat his steak. As difficult as the night was, Al could not bring himself to disappoint or embarrass his attorney. That man still believed Al had a reasonable amount of sight that would allow him to enjoy a steak. In reality, steak was the one food he never ordered without sight and tonight, for all intents and purposes he did not have sight.

"How's the steak, Al?" Mr. Bayplaza talked between bites.

Al swallowed hard on a piece of steak that was half fat. "Wonderful. You were right, Art. This chef knows his way around a steak." Given the circumstances, there was no avenue for him to graciously dispose of the unpalatable portion.

Elaine noticed the difficulty Al was having and leaned close to him, hoping the others at the table would believe they were only having a private moment. "Al, can I help?"

Curtly but with a smile still trying to make the table believe he was doing fine, he answered. "No. How much of a mess am I making?"

"None. You're fine. The steak came with a potato at two o'clock." She kept a false smile on her face while they spoke. "How about a piece of bread to help push the food onto your fork?"

"No. Just do me a favor and give me a kick under the table if I get messy." He ceremoniously stuck a forked piece of steak into his mouth.

Art, always controlling any situation he was in, spoke up, thinking he was trying to interrupt the couple's private conversation and keep the social evening alive. "Folks, they have the most amazing desserts here. They take Tiramisu, surround it with a cream that is a must."

Al stopped with another fork half way to his mouth. "I can't wait. Let's do it."

They managed to get through the night without food ending up on Al or spilled across the table. Relaxed, they came into the house that night accepting their new reality as Al walked through his own house using his cane.

In the subsequent days he adjusted to descending completely into darkness aided consistently by the cane. The descent was so gradual that when it encompassed him completely he was greeted with a familiarity that colored his days with sadness. Toys were swatted out of his way with his cane in frustration. Occasionally one the boys would chase him grab the cane in play and bring him out of the fog of sadness and into the light of fun.

A giggling Albert snuck up on him one late afternoon two weeks later and grabbed his dad's cane. "Okay you two. Dad needs his cane to move around. You don't want me to accidentally whack your bottom with it, do you?" Both boys laughed harder, even though Larry didn't know what he was laughing at. "Larry you're a little sprinter. I don't even know where you come from half the time." At the sound of his name, the toddler just kept giggling. "Mom and Dad are going over to grandma's house, so if you want to come you have to cooperate with me." Albert immediately dropped his grip on the cane and started to gather toys to bring with him.

Elaine came into the room slipping the strap of a diaper bag over her shoulder. "Al, I'm getting used to the diaper bag being an extension of my body."

"I can understand that." He lifted the cane in her direction. "We both have our appendages."

"I guess we do." She turned to the boys. "Let's go troops. Grandma and grandpa are waiting."

Rose came down the stairs. "Do you two need my help getting out the door?" Sharing a home with Rose made it necessary for her to be the only family member aware of Elaine's pregnancy. She was now trying to help Elaine more than her usual extensive assistance.

"No, we're good, Mom. What are you up to this evening?" Al reached down to where he heard Larry babbling

and picked him up.

"Fenna is coming over to pick me up and then I believe we're having dinner at her house." Rose helped Albert put a few of his toys in the carry bag his parents had given him for outings. "Albert, I don't think you can fit one more truck in there. You'll have to choose."

"Nooooo." Albert, who was starting to be weaned off his afternoon naps, began to cry.

"We're all leaving, Albert. Dad has some sawing work to do for grandpa. No crying among the rank and file." Al turned and started to walk toward the door.

A panicked Albert grabbed at his bag letting extra toys fall out and onto the carpet. "Daddeeee. I coming."

Al smirked and turned toward where he thought his mother stood. "We're telling Elaine's parents tonight about the baby."

Rose smiled broadly and hoped her voice conveyed her excitement to her son. "That's wonderful. I've been so excited for you that I wanted to tell everyone. This family deserves more of this kind of joy."

Al held a wiggling Larry and heard Albert drag the overfilled bag across the kitchen. "Tomorrow we'll call Fenna and you girls can talk until your hearts are content."

Rose watched Elaine. "Honey, if you need me to do anything extra tomorrow, speak up. I want to help."

"Thanks, Mom. We'll see you later." Elaine had a hard time keeping up with her men as they piled into the station wagon for the drive to her parent's house. She was excited to tell everyone about the new baby and the anticipation that someone else was cooking dinner for her tonight filled her with happiness.

"Elaine what is your Mom cooking tonight?" After the recent dinner debacle with the attorney, Al felt being prepared was the best means of attack.

"Soup and gourmet grilled cheese sandwiches. Mom is always thinking of you. Sandwiches are the next best thing to finger foods. How does that sound?" She started the car and pulled away.

"Perfect. No more unnecessary challenges or avoidable potential disasters. I thought that steak at Bayplaza's dinner was going to end up in my lap." Al's stomach growled in answer to their discussion.

Mr. Hinds was standing in the driveway when they pulled up a half hour later. He was staring at the roof and Elaine started to giggle. "Al, Dad is staring at that branch like it's going to do something." She couldn't stifle her laughter. "He really needs you."

"I love your Dad, but anybody waiting for a blind guy to help them out is in serious trouble." The two of them tried desperately to stop laughing before her father took notice.

Mr. Hinds walked to the passenger side door and opened it for Al. "Hey, boss. Glad you're here. That branch has been rubbing against the roof since the storm last week. I think it's about to break off the tree. It must be hanging by a thread. You're going to need to cut it down piece by piece." He continued without giving Al a chance to comment. "I have the ladder already set up."

"Pop Pop!" Albert jumped over the hump between the driver and passenger seat and out the door almost knocking into Al.

"Hey Little Man. You go inside with Mommy. Dad and I will be in shortly. We got some work that needs to be done." Mr. Hinds patted Albert on the back and shooed him in toward Elaine who was holding Larry's hand. Larry stopped struggling to get out of her grip once he saw Albert was coming with them.

Elaine pulled her open coat around her. "Al we'll be inside. Don't take forever or we'll eat without you." Elaine got both boys in the front door without further fussing. "Brrrr. It's still really cold. I can't wait for March to be over. I'm ready for an early spring."

He heard the door shut and turned to Mr. Hinds. "Nice, real nice. Alright Dad, let's get this over with. I'm starving." Al let Mr. Hinds guide him to the ladder. "Dad, where is the branch and how big is it?"

"It's on the peak." Mr. Hinds looked worried. "Listen, kid, if you don't want to do this, don't. I'll call the tree guys tomorrow. I thought I could do it, but I got halfway up the ladder and knew I'd have problems up there." He touched his right leg absentmindedly.

"Dad I don't want you to spend money if you don't have to. Please, let me do this. You do so much for us." Al felt in front of himself for the ladder. "Where's the ladder positioned against the house from either end of the roofline?" Al zipped up his coat and then with both hands on each side of the extension ladder he prepared to climb.

Mr. Hinds assessed where he placed the ladder. "About halfway across. You will have to go to your right to find the branch." Mr. Hinds looked at the tree branch as he spoke.

"Alright. Give me the handsaw." Al carried the hand saw Mr. Hinds gave him and slowly climbed one rung at a time counting as he went up. He felt in front of him after the tenth rung and found the rain gutter. "Hold the ladder tight, Dad."

Mr. Hinds called from below. "Your hands are next to the roof line."

Al tried not to smile. "Thanks." He continued up slowly and crawled over the top of the ladder. He stopped for a moment on his hands and knees to get his bearings. His stomach growled in aggravation. "Dad, tell me where the branch is."

Mr. Hinds stepped back to get a better look. "You need to climb to the peak and then move to your right. The branch starts about ten feet from where you are." He called up to his son-in-law as he tried to calm his own nerves. "Al, be careful."

"I'm okay. I've been on this roof a hundred times since you bought the place. I spent the afternoon mapping out the roof in my head." Al began to carefully crawl upward. "Thanks Dad."

Mr. Hinds laughed lightly. "If anyone saw the two of us right now I think they would call in the marines."

Al used the saw he carried to help him crawl. When he reached the peak, he shuffled sideways to his right holding onto the peak as he moved. He counted his steps as he went. When he hit the number twelve the tip of the branch poked him in the side of the face.

"That's it." Excitedly, Mr. Hinds saw the possibility of this projects conclusion.

This comment on the obvious from Mr. Hinds almost caused Al to lose his balance. "Thanks." Still on his knees, he carefully grabbed hold of the branch, sawed a small section and whipped it in the direction of the edge of the roof. "Dad did that piece go off the roof?" Al stayed still for a moment and suddenly wished he had remembered to eat something before they left home.

"Yup. You're off to a good start. Take your time. I got the spotlights on for me so I can tell what you're up to there." Mr. Hinds again touched his leg. He stepped back again to get a better view of what Al was doing.

Al moved over one step and felt further down the length of the branch. This time he cut a longer piece, tossing it wide to go over the roof. "Dad let me know if one of the branches doesn't make it over the side."

"Okay. I got a bead on you. Just keep going slowly. No need to rush." He leaned on the picnic table behind him.

Al felt in front of himself, and realized the branch extended on the other side of the peak. Carefully, he climbed over the peak to the other side and inched his way forward until he felt in front of him a length of the branch he wanted to cut. The tree branch was the size of a sapling the closer it was to the roof edge. He knew this was going to take longer than he anticipated and started to rework the map of the roof in his head to move the job along quicker.

Staying in the same spot, he started to saw the next portion of the branch and pushed at it until he felt it fall freely over the roof edge. He felt behind him for the branch with the hand that held the saw, found it, felt for the next section and sawed the remainder.

Satisfied at the job completion, he raised his hand that held the saw to wave at his father-in-law.

Mr. Hinds could only see the saw waving behind the roof peak and yelled out. "You alright up there, Son?"

Al heard Mr. Hinds and yelled back to him. "Dad, I'll be down in a minute."

Without warning he stepped backward into nothingness without time to yell out. At first, he thought he could recover, grabbing at anything. The ground smacked into his upper back first after he had fallen fifteen feet to the ground. He straightened out in pain from head to toe with his calves elevated slightly on a tree root.

Unknown to Al, Albert and Larry had been staring out the window as they played with Albert's small green army men on the sill. "Mommy, Daddy's flying."

Elaine looked up as she heard her father yell outside for help. She and Helen ran outside to find Mr. Hinds leaning over Al on the ground.

Mr. Hinds stared down at the still body of Al. "Call an ambulance! Al! Can you hear me?" The older man tried to stay in control to get the help Al needed, but he was shaking.

Al found his voice around the pain. "Oh man."

Standing over Al, Elaine assessed the situation. "Stay still. Mom's calling an ambulance. Can you feel anything?"

Al tried to lift his head. "Hurts."

"Stay still! Your head is bleeding. Dad, don't let him move." She started to pull off the glasses that had miraculously stayed on his face, broken, but at an angle.

Al spoke to her through a clearing mind. "Elaine cover my eyes." She knew her husband's request was more than mere vanity and she would do nothing to test or challenge his pride.

The ambulance siren started in the distance after what seemed like an hour. "Can you feel pain?" She could see that his right shoulder and side had taken the brunt of the fall.

"Yes." He grimaced. "I'm not hungry anymore."

She looked at him closely. "Al, stay still. You could have broken bones." She was terrified that he might have done serious, permanent damage to his back.

The ámbulance crew did not realize Al could not see even though it was night and he kept his glasses on. When he arrived at the emergency room he was taken immediately in to be seen by the doctor on call. The doctor looked at the immobilized man on the stretcher and couldn't figure out why he was wearing glasses. He pulled them off Al and swore loudly as he saw the white, blind eyes.

"How the hell did you get hurt tonight?" He put the broken glasses on the movable tray next to the stretcher.

"Hey doc, please don't lose those glasses. I know they're broken but so is my spare. I need them for tomorrow." Al touched his cut head. "I was cutting a branch off my father-in-law's roof."

He stared at Al incredulously. "What the hell is wrong with you? Don't you know you're blind?" The doctor stood back shaking his head with anger.

Al didn't know whether to be sarcastic or respond to the doctor with apologetic phrases to ensure that he would fix him up. Already in pain, he chose sarcasm. "The thought occurred to me, but I figured what the hell. How much more could be done to my body. Guess I was wrong."

The doctor didn't laugh. "I see a ring on your finger. Don't you care what kind of pain you put your family through? Do you have a death wish?" The doctor was building into a crescendo loud enough that the other people in the triage area were turning to see what the commotion was about.

Suddenly Al was transported to last year and Dr. Grove was leaning over him yelling at him for ruining all the plastic surgery he had performed on his shoulder. He felt like a child again, being told what he could and could not do. The current doctor did not understand that the limits others put on Al only moved him forward to push through the boundaries.

"No, I don't have a death wish. I just have a wish to live on my terms." Al's sense of humor was gone. Defensive anger began to rise to the surface.

"That's fine as long as you don't take anyone down with

you. I hope you haven't done residual or permanent damage to your back or limbs. How would you like to be blind and in a wheelchair? The doctor turned to get the instruments he needed to stitch Al's head. "Nurse, after I'm finished stitching him take him for a full body x-ray. Keep talking to him. Do not let him drift off. He doesn't have the visual stimulus to keep him conscious while we are taking care of him.

Al laughed derisively. "I'm here and I would be happy to keep you both entertained." He knew he shouldn't smart mouth this guy. "To answer your other comment, I fell off the roof alone. My wife refuses to stop me from living my life. She has two little boys and she is pregnant with our third child. The last thing she needs is another little boy."

The doctor was silent as he tore open Al's shirt exposing the Jobe shirt. Al assumed the doctor was probably exchanging a look with the nurse. He didn't care. All he could think about was whether or not he had broken his shoulder and how many additional doctor's visits would now be necessary as he felt his Jobe shirt being opened.

"What's your name, sir?' The doctor's hands moved to his head.

"Al, Al Plevier." He felt his defenses fall away as the competent doctor did his job.

The doctor pushe and prodded the cut gently. "How old are you, Mr. Plevier?"

Here it comes. He's going to tell me to grow up or act my age. I hate this guy already. "I'm twenty-six."

"I can see that you're wearing a Jobe shirt. Whatever hell you've been through you've earned the right to live any way you want. You obviously do not have fear or else you at least believe in facing any fears you have." He began to stitch Al's forehead. "What you may be forgetting is that as much as you may want to prove to yourself that nothing can stop you, there are other people involved. Whatever happens to you they have to live with also." The doctor continued to lecture while he worked, partially to keep the blind patient in front of him from losing consciousness. "You're not a kid anymore. You have kids of your own." He slipped another stitch into the head wound.

Al flinched. "Ouch!"

The doctor stopped and held the needle mid-air. "Really? Seriously?"

Al leaned back into the stretcher. "Do whatever you want." Once again, a doctor had his body and he believed God had his soul.

Chapter V: Endings and Continuations

Fortunately, the latest misadventure of the roof fall didn't do any permanent damage and miraculously there were no broken bones. The shoulder muscles were torn and the right side of his body was very bruised. Al recovered slower that he would have preferred and after a follow up visit to Dr. Grove that included being screamed at, he was relegated to a sling and his recovery was monitored until April.

The morning after Al fell off the roof most of the family, gathered around his hospital bed chastising him for the latest debacle. Elaine and Al exchanged looks as they ranted at him and decided this was a good time to tell everyone about the new baby. Momentarily caught off guard, they literally cheered at his bedside and then utilized the blessed event as fuel for their cause.

Mr. Hinds went on the defense. "I'll take responsibility for coaxing you up there. It was a stupid idea. You should have told me to forget it."

Al moaned in his bed and Elaine jumped in. "We have names picked out already. Christopher if this is a boy and Pamela if this is a girl. It would be nice to have a little girl among all the men in my house."

Fenna shook her head. "Al, you have to start being realistic. You can do anything you did before you lost your sight, but a roof? Are you kidding? You're about to add another child to your family. Start thinking."

Al moaned again in the bed. "I'm always thinking."

In order to regain the mobility in his injured right shoulder and arm, he practiced throwing darts when he was alone in the basement. He would tell Elaine he had work to do sorting laundry, always pretending he was using his left arm. He tied one end of a string to the dart board and the other to a dart with a bell attached and walked until he reached the end of the string. Before he threw the dart, he would pull on the string making the bell ring to get a distance approximation. He then untied the string and threw the dart. The first couple of times he did this the dart went everywhere except to its intended target. Several weeks passed after he started this in mid March and both his arm and his game were improving. Left handed in everything he did, he found that this practice had enabled him to throw equally well with both hands. It was the only activity he performed ampidexitriously. After the initial accident, the recovery of his mobility had been confined to his right side. That fact allowed him to function as a left-handed person uninterrupted.

Today he thought his ruse was still intact as the laundry swished in the washer on the right side of the basement and he prepared to throw his next dart. "Yes!" Al heard the dart hit the board and walked over to feel how he did.

"You're getting better." Elaine stood leaning on the basement doorframe.

Al jumped. "Whoa, where did you come from?"

"I've been watching you the last couple of times you snuck down here." Elaine watched him try to regain his composure.

"Do the boys know where I am? I don't want them following me down here." All pulled the last dart out of the board.

Elaine took a step toward him. "Not yet."

"I started doing this to keep my shoulder and arm active and get them back into shape, but I realize I miss darts." He stopped in front of her. "It's been such a crazy couple of years, I'd forgotten how good it felt to relax with a beer, music and darts after work."

"Whatever makes you happy in your down time is fine with me." Elaine leaned in for a kiss.

"The dart practice is helping with my aim for teaching Albert baseball. I'm working through scenarios in my mind." Al went for a second kiss.

The kitchen screen door opened and banged shut. "Elaine?" called Rose.

"We better see what's up." Walking out of the basement he placed all the darts on a high shelf over the washer. "I don't think Albert and I will have any trouble practicing throws. It's when he starts to connect with the ball that I'm worried about."

Elaine turned to him at the top of the stairs. "I can understand that. It makes sense that you want to practice lining up distances. Ingenious."

"I'm full of ingenious ideas. Look how well the car refurbishing business is going." The sarcastic tone of his voice led Elaine away from the topic.

Rose stood outside the kitchen door. "I figured you two were off somewhere together." She gave Elaine a strange look. "The basement is not the most pleasant of places. Were you helping with laundry, Son, or getting stuff together for electrical work today?"

Al felt like a person caught with his pants down. He had been trying to put off the work he had scheduled around the house as long as he could. Now that Elaine was aware that he was almost completely healed from the fall off the roof he could no longer hide.

"We were going over a few things. I'm going to start switching out the light fixtures tomorrow." He followed Elaine into the house.

"Thank you darling." There was a generous amount of sarcasm in Elaine's tone.

He answered her with an equal amount of sarcasm. "You're very welcome. I need to get all of the projects out of the way before the new baby arrives." Al walked straight for the phone.

His mother watched him. "I have lunch ready. Can it wait?"

"No. This is the middle of my work day with the car refurbishing business. I have to stay on top of Sammy and Luke. Something is not right. Two months into owning this business and the nonsense has started." He pressed the buttons on the new phone Elaine has the telephone company install last week. It was an adjustment at first to remember and feel the buttons for each digit, but he now preferred this to a rotary phone. "I'm not sure what these guys are up to but I'm getting stone walled by a couple of the dealerships."

Elaine and Rose shared a look. "Luke is Carol's husband, right?"

Al snorted derisively as he listened to the ringing tone of the number he dialed. "Yeah, family. I mean, they're second cousins but they're still family. You would think I wouldn't have to worry about getting screwed by family, especially family I hired to help after he got laid off. He's slow and lazy, but I think Sammy is doing jobs on the side. I'm getting screwed by both of them in different ways."

A male voice answered on the other end. "Chrysler dodge. Can I help you?"

Al recognized the voice immediately. "Hey Tony, it's Al Plevier."

A slight hesitation in the man's voice told Al all he needed to know. "Hi Al. What's up?"

Al paused before continuing. "I wanted to check in to see if you had work that needed to be done before the new car line was rolled out."

Now the man didn't hesitate at all. "No, we're good. I'll call you if I need anything." Tony hung up before Al could respond.

He held the phone in his hand. "That clinches it. Sammy is definitely doing car refurbishing work on the side. A gallon of the chemicals I'm buying generates $600 to $800 worth of work. He's only been bringing in $200 the last couple of weeks. I've been splitting the profits with him 50/50, but the chemicals are costing me $100. He's been telling me he's making mistakes and spilling it." He clenched his fists. "I'm not going to use him anymore. Let him chase me for work. He may have built up a couple dealership relationships on his own and thinks he can carry the cost of running a business, but wait until he's paying for the chemical himself. He'll have to raise the prices he's probably charging them and he won't be able to get the price discount I'm getting for the chemicals." Al let himself have the outburst. "I still have Luke. As slow as he is, it will still carry me over until I find a replacement."

The business had been opened for about two months. Al organized and started it up while the corneal transplant was in the final stages of failing. He wanted to bring in money for the family with a business that required phone calls to generate clients. In the beginning, he went on the sales calls with Sammy and Luke to bridge the relationship with the dealerships and establish credibility. Bringing a family member into the business was the final element of his plan that he believed insured its success as he utilized slow working Luke as a safety net. Extended family members were aware of the problems he and Elaine were working through, but they knew that Al was a dependable businessman. He thought this would be enough to ensure loyalty.

"Let Sammy start his own little business if he thinks he's so slick. He'll never be able to keep it running. He doesn't have the stamina or the ethics to maintain it long term." The bitterness in Al's voice was biting.

Elaine put a plate in front of him. "It was a good idea and still is. This would have happened regardless of our situation." She did not voice the fact that this man was taking advantage of a man without sight. "It's the cost of doing business. Sometimes it works, sometimes it doesn't."

He nodded. "You're right. I probably wouldn't even bother with this type of business if I wasn't trying to be creative in pursuing avenues of income." Al reached in front to see what he was being fed. "Thank you for the sandwich."

Rose knew the plunge back into darkness was still a fresh wound and any more experimental surgeries were far out on the horizon. "Some people are no good. It doesn't matter what opportunities you give them or how long you've known each other. Family can be the worst, so keep an eye on Luke." It angered her to know Sammy would kick her family when they were struggling.

Suddenly Al felt guilty. "Mom, don't worry about me." A memory of playing stick ball with Sammy as a child flashed through his mind. "We're not kids anymore. If this is what the guy has to do to survive, it will catch up with him eventually. He dropped out of High School so his options are limited."

She shook her head in agreement. "It's really too bad."

"Mom, let it go. At this point I'm cutting him loose so I can look for someone else while I keep the business going with Luke." He ate the sandwich like a determined man.

Elaine stopped eating her own sandwich. "Luke has never been a hard worker. Can you count on him alone until you find a replacement for Sammy?"

He swallowed hard after barely chewing half the sandwich. "I have no choice."

Al worked diligently with Luke over the next two months. He had an account with the local Chevy dealership that paid well and kept the company going. Local ads in the newspapers had not produced an employee yet that would be both trustworthy and dependable. Fortunately, Luke was still laid off from his factory job. It was not unusual for Al to get last minute calls from the dealership for repairs on new car interiors. He noticed lately that Luke would take longer to either get to the dealership or spend a lengthy period of time doing the repair. It was not costing the refurbishing business money, but was irritating to the dealership and to Al. It seemed to be more of a headache than it was worth, but with a new baby coming, he wanted to continue the income source for as long as possible.

On a hot June morning, when Al was concerned that Elaine may be taking on too much as her pregnancy progressed, an emergency call had come from the Chevy dealership.

"I want to see how long this job takes Luke. He's on his way over to Wayne Chevy to fix a tear in the front seat of a new delivery before their buyer picks up the car at 2." Al felt the light fixture in front of him that Elaine had wanted him to install several months ago.

Al wouldn't agree to pay an outside contractor for anything in the house that he could do. Their third pregnancy was going well with an expected due date of early September, an Al wanted the status quo to continue. Elaine was showing and glowing. In reality, the projects Elaine had lined up in the house could have been completed after the birth of the newest Plevier, but he agreed to the preparations during her nesting period.

Elaine's voice brought him back to the present moment. "Al, are you ready to mark the wires?" She stood in the center of their bedroom looking at the exposed wires of the pretty yet simple new light fixture they had just purchased.

"Yes." He held a wire. "What do I have in my fingers?"

"The black."

He marked it and felt the next. "Now?"

"The white."

He marked that one. "I assume the green is left."

"Perfect." She stepped out of his way as he reached for the wall mount where the fixture was going to be hung and wires were disconnected and exposed.

He began to feel those wires and prepared to mark them. "The power is off, right?"

She gave him an incredulous click of her tongue. "Are you kidding? You're holding disconnected wires." She cut him off before he could respond. "I can live without power for a couple hours. I'll let you know if you need to stop working and put the power on."

Al wanted to finish this work and get back to monitoring his employee. "What time is it?"

"It's almost ten o'clock. You'll have this done long before dusk."

Al shook his head. "I haven't heard from Luke." The lines on Al's forehead were deeply creased. "The job I sent him on this morning should only take a half hour at most." Al felt the wires. "What is this?"

"White."

He marked it and moved to the next. Electrical work always took him four times as long as it did for a sighted person, but if Elaine didn't mind having the power off, projects went well. "I'll have this done by three. Luke needs to be done at the dealership long before that. I'll close work down and we can relax into our evening." He gave Elaine a weak smile.

She could see the concern on his face for the job Luke was sent to and tried to divert his attention. "I don't care how long the electric takes. It's not like you're working on the toilet." The fact that he had left the water off for the entire day while he had worked on installing a new kitchen fixture still annoyed her two months later.

He concentrated on the wires. "Still not over that one? I can't say I blame you. What color do I have now?"

"Green. It's worth the expense to pay a plumber. There are too many Plevier's these days under this roof who require water without interruption." Elaine watched how carefully he worked.

Al emotionally blackmailed her by debating who was the most inconvenienced. "Hey, I was peeing behind the tree out back."

"So was Albert." And with that last comment, she walked out of the room to answer Albert's call to her and left him alone.

Into the empty space Al spoke loudly, having heard her open the door. "Hey, attitude is eighty percent of the battle living without sight. I may have ingenuity and think any job out thoroughly, but I have to make a concentrated effort not to quit once I start." He knew she was down the hall so he talked louder. "I plan ahead. I anticipate inevitable problems, but I don't let it immobilize me. Patience is not a virtue, it's a requirement." Now he spoke under his breath. "Should be for my family too."

"Heard that." Elaine was walking by the door with Albert in tow.

Elaine, never a passive aggressive personality, would get even with Al over moments like the plumbing fiasco by standing and watching him paint without her help. He never needed her help, but he would not have refused the offer either. She had to admit his system for painting was pure genius, marking the room with tape and utilizing strings to tell him where he stopped and started. Sometimes more paint would get on Al than on the walls, but never did he spill any on the carpet or furniture. He was always very careful to cover everything. If he hadn't covered all surfaces he knew he would never hear the end of it. This project also took him four times longer than a sighted person.

An hour into the electrical work, he heard the phone ring. "Al, its for you. It's the Chevy dealer."

He dropped the wires and walked over to the nightstand and picked up the extension. "Hello?"

"Al, it's Gary at Chevy Main. Where the hell is your guy? It's almost noon."

"He was supposed to be there at 9. I'll call him and get right back to you." Both Al and Gary hung up without pleasantries.

Al dialed Luke's number and the phone rang five times before a sleepy voice answered. "Hello?"

"Luke? What are you doing? The Chevy dealer said you haven't been there yet." Al was furious.

"Uh, I fell asleep. When do I have to be there?"

Al went numb. "Are you shitting me? The client is picking up the car at two. The chemical will take twenty minutes to fully set after you do the patch. You were supposed to be there at nine this morning." Al's anger reached a fever pitch and he yelled. "It takes you over two hours to finish a patch. How the hell do you expect to finish this before two?"

Luke moved around before he responded trying to shake off sleep. "Man, I don't think this is gonna happen today."

Al was speechless. "We're done." He hung up the phone, picked it back up after he knew the call was disconnected and called the Chevy dealer back.

Gary picked up on one ring. "Chevy."

"Gary, it's Al. My guy isn't going to make it there." Al's dialogue was cut off.

"You're wasting my time. I have one of our techs doing the job. I'm not outsourcing anymore work to your company. It costs more under our roof, but at least I know the job is done on time." Gary hung up.

Al sat at the counter for a moment trying to think through the phone call. "Elaine?"

"Yes. I'm still in the kitchen." She had heard Al's side of the conversation. "What do you want to do?"

"Dissolve the business." Al pushed the chair back. "Let the accountant know. Enough is enough."

She put down her cup and walked to the counter. "It was a great idea but that doesn't mean it was going to work. People are always the variable whether on the client side or the employee side. Let it go. We broke even and you still have the income from the woodworking business."

Al breathed out heavily. "I guess. It's hard to let go of an opportunity that I thought would, over a period of years, get us out of the red and make the lawsuit settlement a financial bonus and less of a necessity."

She shrugged her shoulders, watching her reflection in the glass of the cabinet door. "It is what it is. At least you tried. You're always in forward motion. That momentum will carry us financially. Remember, we broke even on this venture. We didn't lose money." She watched him sit wordlessly in front of her. "I need to pick up something at Sears. Want to go for a drive?"

He breathed out heavily. "Can Mom watch the boys after I finish the electric?" Al was grateful to get out of the house and away from the latest debacle

"I'm sure. You finish the electric and I'll let her know we'll be going out later this afternoon. That gives me time to do a few things and set her up with something to do with the boys while we're gone."

Late in the afternoon Al and Elaine found themselves walking in preoccupied steps as they approached the front of Sears department store. They both had been quiet on the car ride distracted by the newest economic loss. Al kept a hand on Elaines shoulder and followed her without question in complete trust as they continued their habit of re-learning their old pattern of walking together with one blind partner. It was a busy spring afternoon in the store as the public had come out spurred on by the warming weather.

Al heard lots of conversation around them in the seconds before his face caught the edge of the doorframe. After the impact, their pace didn't stall or miss a step and Elaine never noticed.

"Whoah! Mommy did you see the shot that guy just took?" A little boy stared at Al's ripped face as his mother pulled at him to keep walking.

Elaine heard the little boy and then felt Al tug slightly on her shoulder. She turned to find him bleeding and readjusting his bent glasses.

"Oh my God! Al what happened?" Elaine looked in horror at the bloodied face of her husband, a cut dripping over his right eye socket.

"I couldn't wait any longer for you to turn around. I think we scared a little kid." Al now touched his head and felt the wet texture of fresh blood. "Get me to the men's room so we can finish shopping."

They both laughed together as other customers started toward them and then backed away. The release they both felt jolted them back to the moment. Al cleaned himself up and after getting approval on his appearance from Elaine, they finished their shopping to the surprise of several employees working the retail area.

Al came home that evening anxious to expand the wood working business he kept going in the garage. It was creating nominal money, but he had not been putting his full attention into it.

"Now that we've decided to shut down the car refurbishing business I'll spend more time in the wood shop starting tonight. Do you mind?" He was trying to be considerate of the fact that she was closing out the second trimester of her pregnancy.

"It's fine. Working on a new wood project will generate some money for us and get you out of the house." She laughed and rubbed a hand over her stomach.

He smirked and held out his hands in front of himself. "Didn't I just finish a project inside the house?"

She opened the fridge and stared. "That was the last one I had on my mind to finish before the baby comes. You can spend all your free time in the garage." She heard Albert running upstairs in Rose's bedroom and felt the family settling in for the evening.

"The natives are restless upstairs. Let's have leftovers." Al's mind started to work out the picnic table he had started to create for a neighbor and was determined to finish by tomorrow.

The one point Elaine would not compromise on was having all wood cutting that needed to be done take place behind a locked garage door. Precision measuring and cutting had to be completed on the ground. Al was then able to crawl and feel around the material he worked on. This method left the children vulnerable to being hurt if they tried to involve themselves with anything and they always did.

He used a wooden ruler that unfolded and if he did not keep it close, Albert would find it and incorporate it into his toy collection along with the clicker that was used as another measuring device. When he first started trying to do carpentry after the accident, Al ordered a framing square that was marked in Braille. These three items, a skill saw, and his years of

71

experience in construction prior to being hurt enabled him to complete just about any job they needed done in the house or his woodworking business. Fred funneled work to Al through the company he was currently on a part time crew with. He told Al that at first the owner agreed out of curiosity as to the quality of work a blind person could produce, but once he had the finished products, the reduced cost from his normal inventory convinced him to put Al on the payroll. Each job that may vary from the previous order gave him a chance to learn a new way of doing the craft.

The day after the refurbishing business' obvious collapse Al bounded out of bed, helped Elaine start the family's day, made several phone calls to officially close that business and headed for the garage. As he worked on finishing the picnic table, his mind worked out how to generate more income from the wood business. The list of individuals still in construction would be his target for phone calls that evening and afternoon. The business' he dealt with were smaller and needed beams and headers cut to order and cheaper than they could buy locally. If he could provide the custom orders under cost to them, he would have a steady income through the summer and fall. When winter slowed that part of the business he could stock pile the inventory to have in place when the custom order cuts came in. Then it would just be a simple cut to fill each order.

He took a lunch break early that afternoon. As he closed and locked the padlock on the garage he heard soft movement behind him. "Hello?"

"Hi Daddy." Albert held a ball in one hand and a cookie in the other.

"Hey Pal. What are you doing out here? Is Mommy with you?"

"Nope." Albert stated this proudly with a chin held high and cheeks stuffed.

Al stood still for a moment. "Where's Mommy?"

Albert shrugged his little shoulders. "Inside."

Al had a knot in his stomach. "Albert, did you come out without telling Mommy?"

Albert looked at his father with wide eyes and then turned to run back in the kitchen. Al heard the kitchen door squeak open and bang shut.

Al followed the path he heard Albert take back to the kitchen door without his cane, stubbing his shoe on small objects. "Elaine?" No one answered and he continued walking into and through the house. "Mom?" Al heard footsteps on the stairs coming down.

"What is it?" Rose stood in the kitchen looking at Al's nervous face.

Al turned his head to Rose. "Where is Elaine and Albert?"

She looked at him quizzically. "Elaine is lying down with the boys."

Al shook his head. "Not both of them. Albert snuck outside looking for me."

Rose's face took on the expression of a knowing mother. "I'll find him." Rose crept into each bedroom until she found Albert pretending to sleep in his bed.

Al came up bedhind her. "Where is he, Mom?"

"Shhhh. You'll wake Elaine. "

"Too late." Elaine stood in the doorway of the master bedroom looking refreshed.

Al turned to her. "We have a problem. Albert's sneaking out of the house."

Albert buried his head in his pillows trying not to giggle as the three adults stared into his room.

Elaine stretched. "There's three of us and one of him. We need a new system."

"The garage door was locked tight while I was working. He must have been standing outside waiting for me." Al shifting from one foot to the other.

Elaine tilted her head in thought. "I think a lock high on the front and back doors will work."

"It will slow him and his brother down, until they figure that out." Al knew that this foreshadowed what the future held for them.

Jayne Kelly

"Do you have a better suggestion?" Elaine was not sarcastic, she was a little scared.

"It is what it is. We have a couple of little boys." He paused in the silence that engulfed. "Welcome to our reality."

Chapter VI: Possibilities

Al missed playing sports, particularly baseball. As a child and then as an adult, whether it was softball or baseball, he was always the first one on the field for games or practices. It was a love he wanted to pass on to his boys.

The weather had become warm earlier than usual that year and he grabbed the opportunity to continue teaching the basic skills of baseball to Albert. After he lost his sight and when he began to feel physically capable, he initially taught Albert by rolling a ball across the floor. Gradually this gave Al the chance to continue to improve his skills at teaching baseball as a blind person. Albert was the first of their boys to learn, and Al was confident that he would be able to help teach his siblings as they grew up.

Today they were using the back of the garage as a guide. It helped Albert learn coordination and gave Al the practice of judging distance and direction using the sound of Albert's voice as he had done with the tiny bell he tied to the darts he threw at the board he hid from the Albert in the basement.

"Daddy you threw that one too high." Albert banged the bat on the back of the garage.

Al had turned his head slightly to get a better indication of Albert's location from his voice. "Sorry Pal. Stay next to the garage. Don't move."

75

Albert's attention was beginning to wane. "I want to go play trucks, Daddy."

Al knew he probably had only a few more throws before Albert would insist on going inside. "Just two more please. We have to keep practicing if you want to do t-ball." The two had been outside for twenty minutes.

Albert knew how to count and his eyes lit up when he saw an end in sight. "Okay Daddy."

Al stepped back one foot. He had been moving backward in small increments each time he felt he had a good idea of height. Staying down on one knee he gave the ball a soft toss toward Albert.

Al heard the ball connect with the bat and felt the ball fly by his right ear. "Very good! Now let's step away from the wall a little bit. Daddy wants to try something different."

Albert felt like he was being tricked to stay out longer and he didn't like it. "Daddy you said we were almost done. That was a good hit."

Al breathed out deeply as he tried to maintain his level of patience. "I said a couple more." He tentatively stepped sideways several feet. "Line up with me, Albert."

Albert gave him a confused look. "Huh?"

"Step sideways and stay right in front of me." Al listened for movement of the little boy's feet. He pointed in front of himself. "Are you there?"

Albert saw a chance to trick his dad. "Yeah." His voice came from Al's right.

Al stood up tall with hands at his side. "Albert, if you want to be done quicker then you have to do what I ask you."

Albert shuffled to a place lined up with his dad. "K, Daddy."

Al pointed in front of him. "Are you there."

This time a small voice was lined up directly in front of Al. "Yes."

"Good. Let's see how we do like this." Al pitched the ball underhand slowly.

The ball reached Albert and again he made contact with the ball. It flew over Al's left and hit the garage wall. "Excellent! You did great, Albert. One more time, please? For me?"

Albert was at the end of his patience. "Just one more, Daddy. This time you promise."

Al laughed lightly. "Yes, this is it." He pointed again at the direction of Albert's voice. "Are you there?"

Albert was getting used to the new approach already. "Here, Daddy. Here."

Al smiled broadly and lightly pitched over hand. "Here it comes."

Albert smacked the ball and it flew close by the right side of Al's head. Grateful the ball didn't smack him in the face, he decided practice was done. "That's enough. You can go inside and play with your trucks."

Albert dropped the bat and ran for the kitchen door leaving his dad on one knee feeling for baseballs. He had trained Albert to bring back the ones he had hit, but he didn't have the heart to interrupt his play time any further.

Elaine walked around the corner of the garage. "Hi. Dinner will be ready soon." She saw Al feeling around for the balls. "Can I help?'

Al lifted his head in her direction. "That would be great."

They gathered up the scattered baseballs and Albert's tossed bat. "How was practice?"

Al stood and leaned against the garage straightening his back. "He's doing great. The enthusiasm he has in the beginning shows he likes it. He stayed with it for almost a half hour. That's not bad for a pint, sized kid." Al lifted his chin proudly.

She grabbed the last ball and stood in front of him. "I'm glad he has you for a Dad. You'll figure out whatever it takes."

Al followed the sound of her voice as she walked. "Speaking of whatever it takes, I tried pitching away from the garage wall and it worked."

Elaine smirked a little. "You're telling me that he didn't try to trick you or anything and sneak away?"

Al laughed. "He's my kid, of course he tried to trick me. Where's the fun in always playing by the rules? I kept him on track, today. He'll realize that if he doesn't do what I ask, practice will take longer."

"Good thing you have patience and love the game." Elaine picked up the last scattered ball.

"I love being with our kids in any activity, but it is also my obligation as their dad. I don't want someone else teaching my son the things that I should." He stood waiting for her to move next to him. "I talked to him a little when we were playing ball about continuing to try and ride his bike without the training wheels."

Elaine dropped the baseballs she had into the bag Al now held and they started to head toward the house. "Give him a little more time. His buddy at preschool just started riding without training wheels. That might be the incentive he needs."

They were quiet for the few moments walking back to the house. Al dropped the bag next to the back steps and followed her inside. "I'll give him a couple weeks and if he doesn't talk about his buddy I'll bring it up. He and I do just fine. I run alongside the bike holding the seat."

Elaine was enamored with Al's tenacity. It reminded her of why she fell in love with him in High School. As they came into the kitchen she saw the flowers Mrs. Hinds had brought over from her garden.

"Al, I can't find the flowers I had laid out to plant. They were next to the flower beds on the west side of the house." Elaine watched him pour himself a glass of water as she waited for a response.

"If you left them next to the beds they're probably mulch." He gulped the water.

"What are you talking about? You mowed yesterday." Elaine felt her aggravation grow.

"No, I almost finished yesterday. I had to finish the

backyard today." He finished the water without pause or apology.

"Al, I am not the boys. I don't leave toys around. I was transplanting them from mom's house. Couldn't you have stopped after you felt something other than grass in the mower?" Elaine was angry, forgetting the pleasant chat about baseball and did not care if this led to an argument. The only time she did not find his ability to do or try anything without sight was when her possessions went missing.

Al was both defensive and annoyed. "If you want to mow the lawn, go ahead. When I mow the lawn, I am too busy keeping track of moving the rope along the anchor line so that my cut comes out even." Al reached for the pretzels he left on the counter earlier and dug in for the fight.

"Oh, come on! You couldn't stop for one minute to see what you ran over? Did you think it was a heavy pile of grass?" She really liked the daisies she anticipated in the summer.

"My job takes twice as long as a normal grass cutting. That lawn mower blade is twenty inches wide, I do ten-inch widths of cuts to make sure they overlap and I don't miss anything. The prep time tying the anchor rope to two solid objects and then lining up my line takes a half hour." He shoved a couple pretzels in his mouth.

"Great. Thanks Mr. Engineer. Now I have to spend twenty minutes driving round trip to my mother's house, a half hour complaining to her about what you did, another half hour listening to her complain about something Dad did, and then twenty minutes eating cake I shouldn't. All because you couldn't stop for five seconds." She crossed her arms knowing he couldn't see, but it made her feel better and then reached for her purse hanging on a kitchen cabinet door handle.

"You're getting the bad end of the deal." He answered her sarcastically and held another fistful of pretzels halfway to his mouth. "The next time you or the kids, and that includes the one in the oven, leave anything in my path I'm running over it five times." He drank another glass of water for effect and heard the door slam loudly behind Elaine.

Quietly Rose came up behind Al. "Really son. You're being so inconsiderate. Elaine is pregnant. Would it have killed you to stop for a moment?" Now she stood in front of Al with her arms crossed. "I see you have no answer for me. I'll continue to take care of the boys for the afternoon. When your wife comes back, take her out even if it's only to McDonalds. She's pregnant so she'll eat anytime or anywhere." Rose did not give Al a chance to respond. She turned on her heel toward the boys.

I've got to move her into my sister's house. Al thought miserably to himself.

He showered off all the dirt and grass from playing outside with Albert while he waited for Elaine's return. The day was very warm for early June and he dressed in a T-shirt over his Jobe shirt and shorts. When she came through the back door, he was standing there waiting and for this one instant was glad he could not see the angry look that was probably still on her face.

"Honey, Mom said she would keep an eye on the kids. Would you like to go for a drive?" Al sounded like he was pleading.

"I just came back from a drive." She dropped her purse angrily on the counter and walked past him.

That went well. "Maybe we could go buy some new plants." He followed the sound of her footsteps and then heard her drop on the couch.

"The plants you mowed over were free." Elaine picked up the magazine she had left on the coffee table this morning.

Al walked over to the couch without his cane deservedly stubbing his toe on several toys. "Elaine, I'm sorry. Really sorry. If you don't want to buy new plants lets go over to your mom's and pull up some new ones."

At this she started to laugh. "Alright, you're off the hook. The sight of you on your knees helping me transplant flowers in the same spot you were flat on your back months ago is too much even for my anger right now." She tossed the magazine on the table again. "I didn't like those particular plants that much. What I wanted was for you to say you were sorry for being inconsiderate of my feelings."

What is she talking about? I thought this was about some plants. What do her feelings have to do with this? "You're right. All I was thinking about was setting a precedent about when I mow the lawn."

"Set it with the kids. I'm sure they'll leave items all over the lawn as the years go by. These were plants not little plastic green army guys."

He was about to give up and walk away when his mother's advice resounded in his mind. "Let's get out of here. Let's go for a drive and get something to eat."

Elaine looked at him and knew all she wanted was to go out to eat and she didn't care what it was. "Food? I'm hungry."

Relief spread across Al's shoulders. "Of course. How about fast food? We can go to the golden arches. It's the closest." Al got up off the couch and decided he better remember to thank his mother. This fight could have gone on through dinner.

He walked to Albert's bedroom where Rose had retreated with the boys when she heard Elaine's car pull up. "Mom, Elaine and I are going to McDonalds."

At the name of his favorite restaurant, Albert jumped up. "Yeah!"

"Sorry, Pal. You stay with Grandmom. We'll bring you back something, I promise." Al turned not knowing where Rose was in the room. "Mom, thanks. You were absolutely right."

Rose laughed softly. "Go have fun and bring me back a cheeseburger and small fries."

Once Al and Elaine were in the car the fight was not even a thought in either of their minds. Elaine was concerned with satisfying her appetite and Al was working through the assembly of Albert's present for his upcoming July birthday. He had kept the project in the garage and covered with a blanket, working on child size work bench at night for two weeks after the boys were asleep.

Elaine pulled into the McDonalds parking lot with tires squealing. "Whoa!" Al smiled and laughed lightly. "Someone is not just hungry, she's starving."

"I really have a craving for two whole beef patties, special sauce, lettuce, cheese, pickles, onions, on a sesame seed bun." Elaine finished the jingle with the tune from the McDonald's commercial.

"Make it two and large fries. Don't forget the coke." Suddenly he found himself with a craving of his own.

After they got their food and were seated, Elaine left the table to order the fried apple pie she had forgotten. The moment she left a small voice spoke over Al's right shoulder.

"Hey Mister."

Al thought he could pretend he didn't hear it and maybe the kid's parent would hush him. No such luck, although the parent tried.

"Joseph leave the man alone. He's eating." The embarrassed mother knew her little boy saw that Al was blind.

Little Joseph turned back around for a second, but bored with his food he turned back to Al. "Hey Mister?"

Al decided by ignoring the little voice he might hurt Joseph's feelings. "Yes?"

Now excited that Al had responded, little Joseph hung over the booth partition. "What happened to your hand?"

Curious, the mother tried to peer over the booth herself. She was so polite when she saw him come in with his cane, that she hadn't stared at him like her son. Al's scarred and battered hands stuck out prominently from the white Jobe shirt sleeves that were obviously medical in nature. Once the woman understood the nature and extent of his injuries she involuntarily shuddered.

"Well, that happened to me when I touched something that was hot. So, don't play with matches. Don't touch fire. Be careful." This seemed like more of a teaching moment than telling the little boy he had been doused with bad chemicals.

Elaine returned and saw the little boy hanging over the booth talking to Al. "Hello there. What's your name?"

"Joseph." The boy never took his eyes off Al as he spoke to Elaine. "Hey Mister?"

Al couldn't contain his amusement any longer and figured the next question would be about his eyes. "Yes?"

"Can I ask you another question?" Joseph didn't wait for a reply. "What happened to the other hand?"

Al was a little surprised the boy was focusing on his burns and not his eyes. "I burned that one too."

Joseph paused a moment. "Can I ask you another question?

Joseph's mother spoke up, even more embarrassed now that Elaine was there. "Honey, I think you've bothered the man enough."

Not wanting to stifle any child's curiosity, Al interrupted. "It's okay. Really. Let him ask. Go ahead, Joseph. You can have one last question."

Joseph scrunched up his face in honest bewilderment. "Why'd you touch it twice?"

It took Elaine every ounce of self-control she could muster not to laugh out loud. She knew from her own four-year old how honest, simple and brilliant children could be. This little boy appeared to be about Albert's age.

Al was speechless. "I bet you're smarter than I am, Joseph. You would never even touch it once. Right?"

Joseph's mother rose from the table. "Come on, Joseph. We have to go."

Little Joseph never said good-by. The minute they were out the door Elaine laughed. "How do you like being humbled by a little kid?"

"It happens every day at our house." Al shoved more fries in his mouth.

Elaine watched him with guilt. "Al, I'm sorry I didn't tell you how I set your food up."

He shook his shoulders. "Don't worry about it. I know that when you're expecting and you're hungry nothing else matters."

Stopping what she was doing, she realized he just

evened the score between them. "It's a little late, but your fries are at two o'clock, what's left of the Big Mac is at six and the soda is at eleven. I didn't see you drink it yet."

He slowly reached for the drink and took a long gulp. "No, I was actually afraid to keep feeling around for it. If it spilled onto your side of the table, I think this day might have gone the rest of the way down."

"Can't argue with that logic." She looked shyly at him knowing he couldn't see how calm she was since satisfying her hunger. "How are Albert's tool bench and his big boy bike assembly going?"

Al raised his eyebrows appreciatively. "It's going. There's a lot more parts to both than I thought. It took me a week to sort them and to set up the separate spaces I needed in the garage for each toy. Can you believe that?"

"Yes. I watched you this Christmas trying to put together toys with partial sight. It's more than I would have the patience for."

Al thought back to the last clear picture he had from the winter. The snow was falling and the icicles were amazing. "There's no other way to attack it than slowly. Don't ever buy them something a week before their birthdays or Christmas and expect me to have it ready. It will never happen." He took another long sip of soda countering the delicious salty taste of the fries. "I have a three, step process to toy assembly too. Wanna hear it?"

She shook her head to no one. "Sure."

"First I sort the parts making sure I have plenty of room between them so nothing accidentally intermingles. Second, I find out where things go. That takes the longest time. I take plenty of breaks so I don't get frustrated. I feel things out carefully, sometimes several times. The last thing I have to remember is that when I get stuck I need to step back and think about what I need to do to overcome the problem." He leaned back against the booth proudly.

"Sounds like an engineer."

"God bless the training I received. I don't know how

people without sight work through issues without the problem-solving skills I learned in college. Some of it was ingrained already from my background, but my inner confidence came from earning my degree. Everything requires a system. After I got my sight back I actually forgot to keep up with the plan I had made for my clothes. It was just easier to hurry up and do laundry. As my sight began fading I had to slow down one day and redo all the pin positions like the face of the clock on my clothes. I went through my drawers to make sure everything was organized before I lost my sight completely." He gave Elaine a suspicious look. "You'd tell me if I mixed up my socks or shirts, right? Even if you were mad at me you wouldn't let me go out in public looking stupid, would you?"

She paused a second to let him suffer. "Of course, I wouldn't."

"I'm just asking because Ronnie knocked the paper clip off the OJ and I put it in my tea instead of milk. She let Albert play with my shampoo in the tub, and I searched for ten minutes this afternoon before I found my stuff in the shower. Not that I'm complaining. Free babysitting is free babysitting. It's just that being blind is a pain in the ass sometimes. Without my systems in place I lose time." This was as blunt as he thought he could be to let her know his system was being tampered with, and it was slowing him down.

"I got it. I'll speak to her." Elaine felt the baby kick. "Al, do you want to come over to my side? The baby is kicking up a storm."

Immediately he started to slide out his side and join her. "Probably looking for more fries." He placed his hand on her stomach and felt a little foot stick out. "That is amazing. I love this part of parenting. They're trapped in there making us happy and joyful without wearing us out."

"Speak for yourself. I'm exhausted." She moved his hand around to where a little elbow poked. "I love this part too. This little one may be as active as his brothers."

"You said 'his'. Do you have a feeling about this one?" Al knew Elaine was still secretly hoping for a little girl.

She looked sheepishly. "I guess it was habit. So many men in my life."

"Thank you for taking care of us so well." He kissed her lightly on the side of her head. People at the table next to them looked on with envy, replacing the looks of pity they had given them when they first came in. "A special thank you for helping me sort my money this morning before the whole grass cutting incident."

She laughed as the people continued to look and now smiled, misunderstanding her happiness. "No problem. I took a couple of bills, I have to confess."

"I can live with that. Consider it your cut. Everybody should get paid, I always say." He felt her elbow him appreciatively.

"What am I going to do for money when the government finally figures out a system to mark bills for the blind?" She kept moving his hand around her stomach as the baby moved.

He huffed sarcastically. "I don't believe you have to worry about that. It would be a simple system of hole punching or Braille markings, whichever is cheaper to produce, but the wheels of progress either run slowly or not at all." He lifted his chin proudly, something he always did when he had sight. "The world could learn something from the way I mark my yard and house."

Elaine stopped moving his hand around her stomach and looked at him, puzzled. "What are you talking about?"

Al smiled broadly. "You don't even notice what I do. It's brilliant. When you believe I'm going for a walk, I'm labeling." He tried to put his right arm around her as high as his healed injuries allowed. "Walks are boring. I need to be doing stuff." He turned his head to her face.

She raised her eyebrows. "Al, there will be no shortage of things for you to do with another baby on the way. I don't know when you're going to have time to build your models or kits after September. If I'm sitting down for five minutes at night with you, I'm zoned out with the TV."

"That's when I start doing logic problems, Chisanbop or brain teasers, in my head. Listening to TV bores the heck out of me." He moved his hand away from her stomach as the baby started to settle in again. "I think I should sell the wood productions I make that you like. I know you want to keep them, but we could keep the ones with little mistakes and make some money off the rest. The telemarketing job said they would pick me up again whenever I want so that's two sources of income, as little as it may be." The annoyance and anger over the failed car refurbishing business rose back to the surface.

Elaine relaxed into the stiff booth. "That's good but I want to go to nursing school. I've learned a lot in the last two years with all the doctors and insurance questions we've had to handle. I could start next winter after this baby is born. Now that Mom's retired and living with us, she will help with the sitting when you have doctor appointments or are busy with your work." She waited for a response and when she did not get one, she continued. "What do you think? It should take two years for me to complete if I stick with the schedule of classes."

"I think it's a great idea. Sorry, I was just lost in thought figuring out the logistics. This could definitely work and if it's something you like, then go for it. I bet I could get some tutoring work through the nursing school you choose. I should already be doing that for High School kids." The goal setting that they always had in their relationship was reignited.

She started clearing the table. "We might continue living financially month to month for a while until the case is over, but we can do it. The dog houses and wishing wells you have been making seem to get the most attention and requests from people."

They started to walk out of the restaurant. "Don't forget about the headers and beam orders from the construction companies. I can stay busy all summer making things in the garage. I'll build up a nice stock before the baby is born and then have it ready for Christmas orders."

She looked down her expanded stomach. "I wonder if I had the dates right on this little one. He seems so big."

Al smirked. "You said he again."

"Hmmm. I guess I did." She lifted her chin and gave her head a tilt thoughtfully. "I'm so anxious."

As Elaine's due date grew closer, Al worked steadily in the garage to build the stock of items to sell. He had everything from bird houses, dog houses, and wishing wells to carved wooden guns. The real challenge was keeping Albert and a fast, moving Larry from banging on the garage door when he was working in there. He had tried only working at night, but that interfered with time he and Elaine had carved out for each other. Inevitably during the day, Albert would sneak out of the house to see where his dad was. Al felt terrible when he heard Albert banging on the door to come in.

On September second, early in the morning, he covered up his latest finished creation and locked the door. He was halfway to the house when his mother yelled out from the kitchen door.

"Son! Elaine is having contractions. I called the ambulance." She slammed the door and went back inside to be by Elaine's side.

Al ran for the kitchen door unimpeded by obstacles. Once inside he called out to his mom and Elaine. "Hey! Where are you?"

Rose Plevier yelled from the back of the house. "We're in your bedroom. The boys are playing in Albert's room. Hurry up!"

He had never heard his mom sound this nervous and he quickly made his way across the house kicking toys out of his way. "Mom, can you drive her to the hospital? I'll stay here and keep an eye on the boys until mom or dad can give me a ride."

A weary and uncomfortable Elaine answered. "Al, it's too late. I don't want to take the chance of having the baby on the side of the road in a car. If I don't make it to the hospital at least I'll be in an ambulance."

Al felt a chill come over him. "Hhhhow close are the contractions?"

"About two minutes apart. They came on fast and furious." She stopped talking to breathe through the latest one.

A siren was heard, tires were on the driveway and Al spoke over his shoulder as he went the door. "That sounds like a cop not an ambulance."

He was right. At the back door stood a uniformed officer with a bag in his hand. "Can I come in sir?"

Al waved his hand for the cop to enter. "Yes. Get in here. I don't know how to deliver a baby." Al led the cop who, after realizing Al was blind, was somewhat astounded by his adeptness at moving through the house to the master bedroom.

The first thing the officer did was pull out a flashlight and request to see how far along Elaine was in the delivery process.

Elaine almost jumped off the bed. "No way! The ambulance can't be far behind you. Trust me, this baby will be born in the ambulance." She stopped talking again to breathe through the contraction.

"Ma'am I just want to see if we're going to have to deliver the baby here in your house for both of your safety." The sound of the ambulance could be heard.

"See, the ambulance is coming. Let them decided when they get here." Elaine continued to breathe while Al made a call to his mother and father-in-law.

Fortunately, both Mr. and Mrs. Hinds were still home, not having left for work yet. Mrs. Hinds said she would be right over and would give him a ride to the hospital. At that moment, Albert and Larry broke out of their rooms when they spied a uniformed officer through their door. Immediately both boys, in the excitement of the moment jumped joyfully on the bed around Elaine.

Rose tried to grab Larry, the smaller of the two. "Boys, your Mommy is going to the hospital to get the new baby and she's tired from all the excitement. Albert, get down now."

Al started to become very nervous. "Albert! Off the bed."

Albert jumped down, surprised and a little taken back

by his dad's uncharacteristic yelling. He stared at the officer and then watched in absolute amazement as two men with white uniforms pulled a bed into his Mommy and Daddy's room.

The officer looked into Elaine's eyes. "Ma'am, let's get you in the ambulance." He then turned to the two attendants. "I couldn't give her an exam but she said the contractions are two minutes apart and closing in."

Elaine climbed onto the stretcher and turned to all present. "This baby is coming now. Get me into the ambulance."

Elaine lifted her hand to wave to Al and the boys and was immediately loaded into the ambulance and driven away. Every ten minutes the ambulance pulled over to the side of the road, but made it to the hospital immediately before the baby was born. Al arrived shortly after the birth with Elaine's mom and dad as his escort. The nurses were kind enough to take him immediately upstairs to the maternity room where Elaine laid recovering with their newest family member bundled up and wide awake in his clear bassinet.

"Al, we have another son." Elaine smiled and looked down the little pink bundle who still had not been cleaned by the nurses.

Al was led to her bedside before the nurse left the room. He leaned in to kiss her. "Another boy. I can't believe it. We're starting our own baseball team."

"I can't argue with that logic. We sure seem to be heading in that direction even if it's not our intention." She breathed deeply and leaned back against the pillow. "He's nice and cozy all bundled up in his bassinet on the left side of my bed, Al."

Al's face became serious. "Are you okay, sweetheart?"

"Yes, everything went perfectly well and quickly." She laughed lightly. "I thought Larry was faster than Albert. This little one was anxious to meet everyone. I don't mind telling you I was a little scared." She closed her eyes and tried to relax through the discomfort her body was feeling.

"We better be prepared for the next time." Al started to feel his way around the bed to the bassinet.

"Next time?   Give me a little breather here."   She chuckled lowly and felt herself drifting from the Demerol the nurse had given her.

Al felt the bassinet and reached inside to touch his newborn son. "Hello there. I'm your dad." He felt how tightly the little baby was bundled and was a little disappointed he couldn't let the little guy grab his finger. "We have to tell you your name. Elaine?" When he didn't get a response, he talked softly to the baby. "Mommy and I decided that if you were a boy we would call you Christopher. I hope you like it. We're sure glad to meet you. You're going to like your two brothers. They are very excited to start playing with you." Al knew this was true but also wondered how the next several weeks with two active little boys and a newborn would unfold.

Jayne Kelly

Chapter VII: Bring It On

&hristophers first week at home gave Al and Elaine a deeper understanding of the family's new dynamic. Larry could not understand why his parents were not immediately available like they used to be. He began to make the connection with Chris and was not happy.

"I thought Albert would keep him distracted. He is always following him around and imitating whatever he does." I just pulled Larry off the changing table while I was diapering Chris. I put him into his crib thinking it would hold him for a few moments but he climbed out when I turned back to finish Chris." Al stood while rubbing the newborn's back.

"I'm just glad Mom is still living with us. You were right about needing a live-in babysitter." Upon hearing Elaine's voice Chris let out a loud cry. "Thank goodness she enjoys it." Al handed a freshly diapered Chris to Elaine.

"Where are the two tornadoes?" Al kept turning his head from side to side trying to listen for activity. "Larry took off the minute I lifted Chris off the table.

"I saw both boys run upstairs to visit grandma. They're quiet, so she must have fed them sweets or turned on cartoons. It's Bugs Bunny's half hour on channel seventeen." She started to feed Chris his bottle. "Chris eats like he's preparing for a tournament."

"He is. It's the tournament of life. At least we have him down to feeding every four hours during the night." Al yawned appreciatively. "Too bad Larry is waking up with him. I've been trying to figure out how to stop that."

"I think if the bedrooms were further apart he might not hear him."

Al knew a preface when he heard one. "How are we going to accomplish that?"

"Let's start thinking about doing a little construction downstairs. Chris will be sleeping through the night and the holidays will be over. I'll be starting nursing school. We can calculate our ability to handle the expense of a small rise in our utility bills. Mom helps out financially, but I would like to be in a position where she can live with us for free." Elaine decided that they were fast outgrowing 19 Lake Road, but knew they were not in a position to move. Al's cousin had expressed interest in purchasing the house and, after the spring flood of 1977, she thought they should give it serious consideration in the future.

Al agreed with Elaine, but for now all he could think about was getting through each day. "I'll talk to Mike tomorrow at the Baptism. I'm sure he and Laura are still interested." He paused for a moment as he remembered a detail. "Are Mike and Laura prepared for the ceremony? I don't think they were at Albert or Larry's Baptisms."

Elaine nodded her head. "I think they'll be okay. The Priest will give prompts if needed. Laura didn't realize the Baptism was done so soon after the birth. She thought we waited until the boys were six months old."

Al shook his head. "Are you sure you want to have them as Godparents? They seem to be staying away from the church."

Chris started to fuss and Elaine took a moment to lift him to her shoulder for burping. "They're not any different than we were before Albert was born.

Al thought back to their early years together before the boys and before the accident. They had both been raised

Catholic and were married in the Catholic church in a large, lovely ceremony with the usual reception following. It made him happy just to think back to that day with its joy and expectations.

After their return from a honeymoon in Jamaica, both he and Elaine jumped into work, always trying to put money away to get ahead. She worked two jobs and so did he. Going to Mass on Sunday was not a priority for either of them. The accident, its aftermath and the birth of the boys changed that.

Al breathed out deeply. "You're right and they're good people. That's what matters."

Christopher finally let out a small burp and then fussed for more of his bottle. "I don't know how people can go through troubles or even the day to day cares of life without their faith. Mike and Laura will probably come to the same conclusion once they have children."

Al was thoughtful for a moment. "I have my bible study thanks to Fred not giving up on me, but we should start taking the boys to Sunday school and/or Mass. Albert's old enough to start."

"I agree. It's time." She looked over at the pile of cards that had been mailed for both Christopher's birth and the upcoming Baptism. "It would have been nice to have a big party like we did for Albert's Baptism, but I just can't manage it. We have enough on our plates."

Al took her hand. "Please don't feel guilty. You're still recovering from giving birth while chasing two little boys around the house. A nice quiet dinner with the godparents and our immediate family is fine." He leaned closer. "By the way, I'm having it catered."

"Al, we can't afford that." A worried look crossed her face.

"It's a gift from Michael and Elizabeth." He squeezed her hand.

"Wow." Elaine had no other words. The generosity of the residents on Lake Road never ceased to amaze her.

"Our neighbors are wonderful." They were both quiet for a moment. "I'm going to miss the street." The statement hung in the air.

"I know Sweetheart. Our little family is growing and the flooding from the river is not something we want to continually deal with given our situation." They held hands. "My cousin will still be interested when we are financially able to move. They cannot afford a home without the price point we offered them."

Because the buyers were family, Al offered the cousins the original price they had been selling the house for when the accident happened. The cousin was not in a position to buy when Al and Elaine had accepted another offer right before the accident and gone under contract. After having to back out of the sale because of the accident, they promised the cousins they would ask them first if they ever were able to sell. The misfortune of Al and Elaine was the financial good fortune of their cousins. The house had increased in value since 1974, but Al's word was his bond and he did not want to seem unfair. They also did not want to list the house with a realtor and have strangers coming and going with three boys.

"The river is my main concern. I love the view, but I have a feeling that eventually these boys will find their way over the fence." Elaine paused as Al nodded in agreement. "The flooding is getting worse each season. Have you made that clear to your cousins?"

Al nodded again. "They know. It's different for them. Don can deal with it. They're getting a good deal and they realize that. It's the start they need and the incentive we need to move forward once the case is settled."

The year remainder of 1977 saw no advance in the progress of the case for either side. It was not a stalemate, it was drawn out stalling meant to delay the culmination of the facts and create an atmosphere that would lend itself to resignation on litigents side. The Pleviers continued to live their lives with as much normalcy as possible, celebrating the holidays and enjoying the children. After January 1978, the particulars of the case were dissected and Al's attorney narrowed the scope of their focus. The forward moment came to a grinding halt February 5 when a snow storm rolled into the northeast slamming Wayne.

Tuesday February 7th over two feet of snow was deposited on the northern New Jersey area where they lived. Albert and Larry watched the snow fall with excitement, having experienced a smaller storm several weeks earlier. The family had snuggled in for the forty-eight, hour ordeal with games, cookies and lots of hot chocolate to keep the boys happy. By Tuesday they were anxious to get outside and Al was anxious to start shoveling them out.

"Elaine, how bad is it?" Al sat in the official family rocking chair with Chris and wondering if he should go out and shovel at night after the snow stopped while his family slept.

"It's bad. The news stations said a woman in Wayne was having a heart attack and called for help, but they couldn't get to her. She died." Elaine stared out the window at the fading daylight and the ending storm. "It's just about over now but it's also getting dark."

Al walked over to her and felt a draft escape around the windows as the constant wind had only now begun to slow. "It doesn't matter to me if its dark out. I might as well get started shoveling out as soon as the storm passes."

"I'd rather you wait until tomorrow. I want to watch you and to be honest I'm exhausted. After we get these guys to bed, I want to sleep. I don't want to ask Mom to stay up. I haven't heard her moving around upstairs. She may already be asleep." Elaine pushed a towel she had on the window frame closer into the pane to try and control the draft.

"Whatever you want. I promised the boys that we would play outside too. I just thought I could get a head start on it." Al could feel Chris falling asleep on his shoulder. "One down, two to go."

Both he and Elaine were up at sunrise the next day before they heard the boys begin to stir. Al jumped out of bed and into his thermals, preparing his attack on the mounds of drifted snow that were everywhere.

"The snow shovel is inside the kitchen door, right?" Al was getting warm and wanted to get outside the bedroom and into his coat, gloves and hat.

"Yes. There's snow piled against the door. Maybe you should go out the front and work your way around." Elaine followed him in her robe and slippers.

"That sounds like a plan. Guide me on the lowest level of snow to start my route."

"There's only a couple inches against the front door. It blew out there. Most of it is built up in the driveway." She pulled her robe against her as Al opened the front door while he put on the rest of his snow clothing.

"It's going to be a long day but if I work steady today and tomorrow I should have us cleared out by late tomorrow morning." He slowly stepped out the door. "I don't think the plow guy will get to us." He felt around with his foot. "Honey, can you get me the shovel?"

The minute Al had the shovel in his hand the sound of little feet and excited babble could be heard behind Elaine. "Al, I'm shutting the storm door and locking it. The boys can watch you until they eat breakfast."

"Good. By then I should be to the driveway. Keep an eye on me so I make a straight path."

Busy with the boys, half an hour later Elaine realized she never looked to see what direction Al's shoveling had taken him. She also realized he hadn't banged on the door or come inside to take a break. It was twenty-five degrees outside and although he was dressed for it, she went into a small panic. Carrying Chris, she left the other two boys at the kitchen table eating their breakfasts.

She threw open the storm door and yelled. "Al?"

A voice from the other side of the house near the kitchen yelled back. "Hey!"

Elaine pulled the heavier oak door closed and headed for the kitchen. When she reached the back door, she pulled back the curtain and saw Al five feet away. She opened the door to talk to him and the mound of snow in front of it spilled inside. Both Larry and Albert squealed excitedly from their places at the table.

Al was still calling to where he thought she was at the front door. "Hey! Elaine? How did I do?"

"Sorry, Al. I had to come to the kitchen door. You're about five feet away, but you're about to hit a large wall of snow. It drifted. There's three feet in front of the door and the steps are completely covered." Chris shivered against her, and she pulled her sweater around them both. "Do you want to come in for a break?"

"No, I'm going to keep going. I'm fine." He filled the shovel and flipped the load to his right.

Elaine marveled at the cleared path. "You stayed right along the house line."

He stood straight and rubbed his hand along his lower back. "I know. Didn't you hear me smacking the house with the shovel?"

"No." She pulled Chris a little tighter against her. "I have to get Chris inside. The boys are almost done eating. What do you want for breakfast?"

"Food. Lots of food." He went back to shoveling steady.

She stepped back into the kitchen. "Alright. It will be ready." The door shut firmly.

The boys looked at Elaine pitifully when she shut the door. "Finish everything on your plates and your juice and then Mommy will put on your snow suits. Remember Daddy has to eat too."

Al was struggling by the time he cleared off the back steps a half hour later. He banged his boots noisily on the stairs before he came in and left the shovel outside the door. "I'm starving." He spoke out loud thinking Elaine was still waiting for him with breakfast.

Larry and Albert came running into the kitchen fully dressed in their snow garb and ready to go play.

"Daddy! Let's go!" Albert sped past him and threw open the back door. Larry, just two years old last month toddled in his over-stuffed snow suit, still managing to keep up.

Elaine came running behind the boys after she dropped Chris into his playpen. "Whoah! Daddy needs to eat." She turned to Al. "They ate all their breakfast and I thought you would be shoveling a while longer."

Al heard the excited boys and caved. "I'll take whatever you got handy to eat, Hon. Let me get these two outside while the three of us are still dressed. Throw some peanut butter on toast. That should hold me."

Albert had barreled down the cleared stairs with Larry right behind him. They were slick and they both slipped their way to the bottom giggling as they went.

Chris looked up from his view from inside the playpen and stared at the excitement. "Al, go after them." Elaine was trying desperately to get a glob of peanut butter on the toast for him and then shoved it into his hand.

"Relax. There's a five-foot wall encasing them on one side and the house on the other. I'll be right behind them." He walked outside and followed the sound of laughter that ended at the bottom of the stairs.

"Daddy let's build a fort with tunnels!" Albert started to dig with his mittens.

Al talked around a mouthful of peanut butter bread. "Don't you want to build a snowman first?"

"No. Fort!" Four-year old Albert had a clear mind on what he wanted at all times.

"Fine. A fort it is." He brought down the shovel and gently pushed the two boys back a few feet. "You two have to stay out of the way of the shovel. Dad will try to keep it low."

Both boys stepped back with Larry hiding behind Albert. "Daddy let's make it like Eskimos."

Al stopped what he was doing as the sound of a tractor reached him. "Boys, do you see lights?"

"Yes, Daddy."

"Everybody back up on the stairs, now!" Al turned and felt in front of him for both boys. He got a handful of each snowsuit and pushed them to the stairs.

"Daddy stop pushing! I don't want to go in!" Albert struggled a little but felt the firm grasp of his father not letting him loose.

"You're not going in. You're going to get to watch the snow plow man from the top of the steps." Al couldn't believe what he was hearing.

He knew it wasn't the man they had called to plow. That service had called this morning to say he wouldn't get to them for two days. Al suspected this was the nextdoor neighbor who had a tractor and attached a plow to it when he knew a storm was coming. An audible toot above the tractor sound greeted them and Al held his free hand up to wave.

Behind him Elaine had come to the door and now yelled to be heard. "I can't believe it. Frank is doing our driveway!"

Rose had come downstairs after hearing the tractor. "These neighbors are amazing." She stood behind Elaine and unfortunately was yelling in Elaine's right ear.

The sound of the tractor came closer until Al heard the motor shut off. "Hey Al!"

"Frank! I can't believe you're getting to us. You need to take care of your own yard." Al kept a hand hold on both boys.

"Are you kidding? I'm angling for your wife's great coffee." The good-natured man talked over a giant snow mound.

Elaine smiled. "Hi Frank! If you can get to the front door, I'll bring your coffee out in a thermos."

He held up his gloved hands. "Not yet. Let me clear this driveway up and give you a way to get your car out of the garage. It'll take me fifteen or twenty minutes."

She put a hand on Al's shoulder in front of her. "Whatever you say. I'll have breakfast waiting for you if you have time."

The kind man waved his hand again in her direction and

then to Al's mother who peaked her head around Elaine. "Al, I'm going to start up again. Do you want to get the boys inside until I'm done?"

"Absolutely. I'll let them watch from the door."

"Nooooo!" The two boys protested in unison as Al opened the door and shoved them inside.

Albert and little Larry pressed their noses to the door watching the plow go back and forth. Elaine was able to get their coats and gloves off, but they both refused to take off their snow jumpers. When Frank pushed the last pile off to the side he shut off the engine and the two boys ran for their coats yelling at Al.

"Daddy come on! He's done, he's done!"

Al sipped the last of his tea, and grabbed at his coat and gloves hanging next to his chair. "Alright. Let's do this. I bet there are huge snow piles we can carve forts into now. Don't forget to thank Mr. McCormick."

"Mommy, help! I can't get my coat on." A frustrated Albert was turning in circles as he tried to push his arm through.

Frank was coming in the back door as Al and the boys headed out. "Frank, I can't thank you enough." Al started to make conversation with him.

"Go, go before those two get away from you. I tried to make some mounds you can build forts in." He smirked as Al stopped dead in front of him. "Raised a couple of boys myself. Remember?" Frank's three boys were grown now and he had taken a special interest in trying to help this young couple when he had the opportunity.

Al laughed good naturedly. "You know what I'm up against then. Wish me luck."

Frank relaxed with Rose and Elaine as he ate a full breakfast and finished his coffee. "I think I'll go see how the men are doing with the piles I left for them." He stepped outside to the sight of Al patting snow onto the middle of a giant snow bear. "Didn't you ever hear of snowmen?"

Al stopped what he was doing to look toward Frank's voice. "Albert said bear, so we're building a bear."

"That thing has to be twelve feet high and ten feet around. How'd you sculpt it so fast and get the head up there?" It was then that he spotted a folding ladder jammed into the snow bank by the bear. "You have to be kidding me. You used a ladder?"

"Yup. I don't kid about snow bears." Al continued his work while he talked. "We just carved into this big mound. Albert is quite the artist."

Larry sat on a snow pile, bent his head back and pointed to the head. "Ears."

Frank stepped back and took a better look. "That thing has ears!"

"It's a gizzly bear, Mr. Cormack." Albert was so proud of his bear he didn't grasp what a huge deal it was that his father was able to make it recognizable to anyone besides them.

"I can see that. It's very scary." Frank came over to them and walked around the bear.

Al stood back with his arms crossed. "It's not done yet. I'm happy to hear you can tell what it is."

"Al, it looks exactly like a teddy bear!"

Albert immediately took offense. "It's not a teddy bear. It's a gizzly."

Larry sat licking snow off his gloves and then patting down around him. "We make a bear."

Frank looked at the little boy in the puffed snow suit. "Al, the little one is eating snow. Is that alright?"

"As long as Elaine doesn't know."

"Elaine doesn't know what?" She came around from the front door quietly. "Oh my, look at that bear!"

Al started to laugh. "It's official. The Plevier snow bear is born."

Everyone cheered together to the delight of Albert and Larry. The bear lasted almost until mid-March. The entire neighborhood came by at one time or another to take pictures of the giant creation that stood as evidence to the fact that anything is possible.

Chapter VIII: The Return

A couple of days after the roads were cleared, the icy conditions were still wreaking havoc over most of New Jersey. In the middle of the night Al was awakened by Elaine.

"Get up!" She tried not to panic at the sound of pounding on the front door, but couldn't help herself.

"Wha, what? What is it?" Al fumbled around.

"Someone is at the door." Now Elaine was pushing him up out of bed.

"Is it morning? I feel like I hardly slept." He rubbed the top of his head and reached for his glasses on the night stand.

"No. Its one o'clock. Someone is banging on the door." Larry woke up from the banging with a yell. "I'll get him." Elaine was up and going into the room he shared with Albert before Al was pushed back the covers.

He felt his feet slip into his slippers and groggily walked into the living room stumbling, as the knocking continued. "Hey! I'm coming." Before opening the door, he yelled out to whoever was on the other side. "Who is it?"

"Please, could you call the police? I slid off the road." The female voice sounded panicked.

Al figured he would go for broke as he heard his mother coming down the stairs. He opened the door. "Are you hurt?"

The woman standing in the opened door did not answer him immediately. "No. But I'm stuck. I need to be pulled out. It's freezing."

Al's mother reached his side. "I'm sorry. My son doesn't have sight. Please come in."

Al gave her a strange look. "What's my lack of sight have to do with anything?"

He heard the young girl giggle. "Thank you. I know it's the middle of the night but I'm alone and I got scared."

Why is this girl giggling? I hope she hasn't been drinking. I don't want her in my house if she's loaded.

Rose spoke sympathetically to the shivering young girl. "Come get warm and we'll call the police. Al, I have this. Why don't you see if Elaine needs help? I heard Chris crying with Larry."

What is going on? Why is she letting a stranger into our home in the middle of the night and sending me away? He headed back to the bedrooms to find Elaine.

"Al?" Elaine carried a fussing, angry Chris into the hall.

Al held up his hands for her to speak quietly. "It's a young girl who drove off the road. Mom is with her. They're calling the police. Something isn't right. Mom sent me away and took the girl into the kitchen."

"Al?" Elaine tried not to laugh.

"It's wierd. She's says she's alone, but she giggled when Mom let her in." He felt the side wall.

"Did you wonder why?" The hint of laughter had faded from her voice, sarcasm replaced it.

"Why she drove into the ditch? Maybe she's been drinking. I'll feel better when the cops get here." Al leaned heavily against the wall.

"Do me a favor." Elaine started to laugh.

Al made a face. "What is going on?"

"Put some shorts on before they get here. You're naked except for your Jobe shirt." Elaine covered her mouth so her laughter wouldn't wake up the little Plevier's sleeping that night. "Didn't the young girl scream? Probably thinks you're a pervert."

"Oh, geez." Al slid against the wall to their bedroom. "I hope she wasn't laughing at what she saw." Then a worse thought crossed him mind as Elaine laughed harder. "Oh, man. My mother saw me naked."

Elaine lost it as she laughed uncontrollably. "Forget it. She's seen you naked before."

"Whoa, I can't take any more. I'm too embarrassed to be around that girl. I'm going to bed and try to forget this night ever happened."

"I'm sure that young girl will try too. I better get in there before she calls the cops on you, forget about her car." Elaine walked into the kitchen to check on everyone.

Al talked to her back. "Yeah, that's just what I need more legal problems."

He sauntered back to bed and slipped between the covers trying to shake off the feeling of the legal battle's shadow always hovering behind the family. He had been anxious about finances more than usual lately. They knew that MTZW had still been using the private detective to follow them. Mr. Bayplaza discovered that the cost for the provate detective was over $100,000. Al found himself balancing his family's needs against the ramifications of the outcome of the legal case.

Dr. Leesville stopped worrying that the stress of the legal case would adversely affect Al's continuing recovery. The opportunity for a possible experimental camera implant to restore sight in his right eye was real. He believed his patient was one of those rare people who thrived on challenges of any kind and was goal oriented. As with any goal, there were obstacles that needed to be met and overcome. Dr. Leesville was confident his patient would meet and conquer them.

During a recent visit the optometrist's office, it was discovered that lesions had formed on Al's eyelids and they would require immediate attention. A week later Al showed up for the procedure with trepidation and his wife and children in tow.

Al sat in the examination chair as Dr. Leesville entered. "Good morning, Albert. I met your three boys. The nurse insisted." The doctor smiled.

"We decided to take the kids to visit the place where Lassie is supposed to be buried on our way home." Al could hear the kids even though he was in the examination room at the back of the office. "Now that I'm living without sight again, I'm not comfortable coming to your office alone. My neighbor offered to continue to drop me off while he was at work, but it's better to come in with Elaine."

Dr. Leesville washed his hands and put gloves on as the nurse prepared the instrument table. "I'm glad to hear that. There's no reason to take a chance of getting lost on your own while you wait for someone to pick you up. The children are not a problem, Albert. I think the staff is getting a kick out of the boys. Let me offer belated congratulations on the newest Plevier. My nurse tells me he's a real flirt."

The nurse stepped closer to Al strapping his arms to the chair. "He's a cutie. Never stops smiling."

Al did not try to stop the nurse from immobilizing him. "Is this necessary?"

The nurse patted his hand lightly. "Yes. We need you completely immobile. There will be a strap around your torso, both legs and of course your head will be held in place so the doctor can work."

"How bad is this going to be? You've never held my whole body down before." Al felt himself tense up.

Dr. Leesville tried to ease Al's fear. "We will numb the eyeball before we begin. You'll feel the pressure from the cutting of the lesions. We'll do one eye at a time." The nurse and the doctor exchanged looks. "Albert, we're ready to begin."

Al felt the nurse strap his torso down as Dr. Leesville placed his head in the proper position and anchored it. His eyelid on the right eye was opened wide and held there with clamps.

The nurse reached for the needle. "Mr. Plevier, I'm

about to anesthetize your eyeball."

Al felt the nurse lean over him and the next thing he knew a sharp unbearable pain was sticking him in the eye. "Shit!"

The nurse finished. "I know that was uncomfortable."

"Uncomfortable? You have to be kidding me." He felt himself shake. "Do you have to do that again?"

"Not right away. After we finish with this eye."

"Great. Something to look forward to." He wondered if he was going to get through this without screaming.

The doctor leaned over Al and began to cut the lesions from the between the eyeball and eyelid. He felt every tiny movement not as pain but as a pressure with the cutting sound to accompany it. The procedure seemed to last forever. Al was exhausted. He felt his left eyeball being held open as the right eyeball was released. Fluid was squirted into the right eye. He felt the fluid irritate and slightly burn the eye even though it was still anesthetized and then the second needle was inserted in the left eye.

He gripped the armrests almost tearing them off. "Enough!"

The nurse retracted the needle. "That's the last one."

He heard a stool being rolled across the floor and come near his left side. Dr. Leesville's cologne assaulted his senses this time as he leaned closer and began to cut. Al felt and heard the lesions being cut. This time there was an odd sense of being freed from something. Since he had no discomfort from the lesions, he didn't realize the absence of them would be noticeable.

Finally, he felt his right eye released and heard the stool wheel away. "Are you done?"

"Yes. It's over." The nurse and Dr. Leesville both worked to unstrap his torso and legs. "I want your head and arms strapped for a few more minutes. I don't want you to accidentally rub your eyes. Try to relax."

Al tried to climb inside his head, but found it impossible. He thought he heard the nurse still in the room so he began to talk, hoping someone would answer. "I told a friend of mine that blind people are the true minority. Once oxygen levels were corrected in incubators for newborns, incidents of blindness decreased dramatically leaving only the older folks, genetic abnormalities or poor buggers like me blinded through accidents."

Dr. Leesville responded. "That's true."

Al did not realize Dr. Leesville was still in the room. He thought he heard only one person moving about. "Since I joined the Lions Club, I'm finding that because it's mostly older people there are definite communication issues." The anesthetic had begun to wear off and an immediate headache from the surgery was growing. "These older people are set in their ways and when you try to teach them anything new they fuss or ignore you. Even a simple technique of using the face of a clock to tell you where your food is on a plate is a stubborn point for them. They refuse to accept that this is their new reality after having lived with sight until now."

Al thought about how he used to like to order steak out when he had sight but now it was almost impossible to eat cleanly and easily. As a rule, he no longer ate it at restaurants and unless he really had a craving for it, he wouldn't ask Elaine to cook it. He absolutely hated to have someone cut his food like a child. To be completely honest he didn't like the way Elaine cooked it at home so he accepted he would be eating steak very seldom.

"Hamburger or other sandwiches are the simplest when I am out to dinner." Without a response from the doctor, Al continued trying to talk his way around the building discomfort. "A lot of the older generation want to rely on the new touch pads that I find slow me down. How do I know what I'm touching? I prefer dials like I have on our microwave that I can mark with tape."

Dr. Leesville turned to Al. "Do you have a headache?"

"Yes, and it's building in intensity." He learned after the accident to be honest with the doctor treating him at any given time. "I was trying to talk my way through it. I have a long afternoon ahead of me. I didn't expect this pain after the procedure."

"I'll give you a prescription for the discomfort. It will only be for the next two days. You should be fine after that. If you are still in pain, please call the office." He stood. "You've adjusted well to living without sight again." He took off his own glasses and rubbed his eyes. "I want to continue to explore the potential of your receiving the new experimental surgery where they implant a camera into the eye. It isn't something to consider this year, but soon."

Al turned his head slowly toward the doctor's voice not wanting to aggravate his growing headache. "I wish it could be this year."

"We have to monitor your continued recovery process to see if you'll be a candidate." The doctor studied Al closely. "I don't want to give any patient false hope but, I'm confident in your ability to do what is asked of you in preparation. It's a relatively new option."

"I appreciate your honesty." He was thoughtful for a moment. "Should I mention that it is not a definite yet to my wife?"

"Yes. I'll have more information for you as I learn about the success or lack that there is in the field." He prepared to leave the room. "Take it easy today. No running around the park with the kids."

"Thanks Dr. Leesville." Al shifted slightly, hardly noticeable, against the hard examination chair.

The nurse stepped next to the chair to assist Al. "Sit up slowly. Don't stand until you're sure you have your equilibrium."

Al sat up and felt his head settle into recovery from the surgery. He knew he had a long afternoon ahead of him with the children and decided he and Elaine should have saved an outing with the kids for another day. He powered through the afternoon and when all three boys were asleep across the back seat for the ride home, he and Elaine had time alone before returning to the household chaos. Trying not to fall asleep himself, it seemed like the perfect time to talk.

"Elaine, the new procedure being tested may be an option for me instead of another corneal transplant, but it's not a certainty." He did not want to get his hopes or hers up too high. "Dr. Leesville does not have all the data on it and even if he did he said he needs to monitor my recovery progress to decide if I'll be a candidate. It's a longer and potentially permanent solution instead of a temporary fix."

Elaine looked over at him. "Al, you know I support any opportunity for you to have a chance at sight. Our goal is for our family to have as normal an existence as possible and we've achieved that with or without your sight."

Al's face became expressionless. "I want to see you guys again."

"I know. We'll follow up with him on this. We'll keep it as a long, term goal like the lawsuit." She felt a change of subject was in order. "We were so busy this week there wasn't time to talk about what the case status is. Do you want to catch up later or go over this now?

The last thing Al wanted to talk about was their legal issues. "Let's go over a brief update. I'm not up for a lengthy discussion about the details. My head is still pounding." He thought back to the last meeting he had with Mr. Bayplaza. It was disconcerting to Al, the lengths to which people without ethics would go. "I have another deposition coming up and I'm not looking forward to it. The attorney feels that the case is now beginning to come to a head. We're not discussing a settlement, as we both know, but it is building in intensity. I was worried that they were going to perceive us as a couple of 'breeders' trying to live off the system when they found out we were having Chris. Bayplaza said not to worry, those were only my thoughts. MTZW, the main target, is only concerned with the bottom line and what my level of disability is." Al snorted. "My level of disability? Can you believe that?" The pain in his eyes pulsated. "My scars itch, they bleed sometimes, they hurt and I can't see." He stopped himself short from building into a crescendo of anger and self-pity. "This deposition is not a trial. I have to answer questions from lawyers on both sides who will each have a team. My answers can only be used if I contradict myself." He was not looking forward to the deposition, and he knew it was apparent to Elaine. "Bayplaza can't object at the deposition. I have to answer all the questions asked, even the embarrassing ones and he suggests I use as few words as possible each time."

"When is the deposition?" Elaine pulled the car into their driveway.

"July. Bayplaza said it could be changed on the calendar. He postponed it from the earlier date so that the cornea would have failed already and I wasn't walking into the deposition with sight." Al was hoping this was enough conversation about the case for today. His headache was getting stronger the more he spoke instead of abating.

Elaine lowered her voice. "Al, how bad is your headache?"

He thought he had been hiding the growing discomfort from her. "I would really like to take one of the pills the doctor gave me and lie down. I'm sorry to dump the evening routine on you and Mom."

She heard Albert begin to stir in the back seat. "It's fine. We can handle it. I'll try to keep the boys as quiet as I can. I don't know how you remained so chipper through the afternoon with all of us."

Al started to get out of the car. "Any time I get to spend with all of you is worth it. Don't worry about keeping the boys quiet. Once I take the pill I won't hear a thing. I'm going to go in before they see me."

Elaine watched her husband walking carefully, not at his usual pace with the cane. She knew the afternoon with the boys had been more uncomfortable for him than he told her.

"Mommy?" A sleepy Albert sat up rubbing his eyes as he watched Al disappear behind the kitchen door.

"Hey, Pal. You want to have dinner and play with Grandma and me?" Elaine looked over her shoulder at the still sleeping figures of Larry and Chris.

Albert considered this as he opened the door. "No. I want to play with Daddy. He said we were going to take off the training wheels again."

"Daddy has to rest now. He's really tired from seeing the doctor today."

Albert climbed out of the car, slammed the door and yelled over his shoulder. "Okay. I'm going on the swing." The independent little boy didn't give a thought that he needed someone to watch over him.

The second the door slammed both Chris and Larry woke up with a jolt. Chris started to cry and Larry immediately saw Albert was gone. He slipped off the seat, away from his unhappy little brother and opened the door to chase after Albert.

Elaine climbed out of the front seat and Chris screamed loudly as he surmised he was being abandoned by the entire family. The second Elaine opened the back door to reach for him he jumped into her arms.

Elaine lifted him high on her shoulder. "Looks like you're going to get a little more sunshine before dinner."

Rose Plevier came out of the house and followed Elaine to the tree swing and play area. "Hi Elaine." She had a worried look on her face. "Al looked terrible. Is the glaucoma back?"

Elaine shook her head vigorously. "No, Mom. This was a procedure to cut the adhesions from the eyelid." She suddenly realized they hadn't told Rose what this doctor's appointment was for.

"Oh, good." A look of relief spread over her face because she didn't understand the severity of the procedure Al had just gone through. "He looked very pale."

Elaine handed a squirming Chris to Rose. "It was a painful procedure. The doctor gave him medication for tonight and tomorrow to help with the residual discomfort and headache." She looked over to the river on the other side of their fence. "Mom, you would think this was a simple legal case, wouldn't you? Al can't see and he continually has to endure medical procedures that are both painful and frustrating.

Instead we have private detectives watching us across the river from our home, invading our privacy and a couple weeks from now the actual case begins with, what I consider, an interrogation of Al. How much can he take?" She inclined her head toward the opposing river bank at an enemy she couldn't see.

Rose squared her shoulders. "How much can you both endure? You may not have been burned and blinded, Elaine, but you are enduring the aftermath with Al." She watched Elaine close and open her eyes.

Chris squirmed and whined until Rose lovingly placed his feet on the ground. The two women watched him toddle to his brothers.

"Somedays there are times, Mom, that I stop and think about where we are and what has happened and what will happen to us." Albert and Larry looked at their mom and grandmother to make sure they could continue playing.

Rose laughed and spoke loudly to the boys. "It's not dinner time yet. The pizza man hasn't arrived." At the mention of pizza, the boys smiled, cheered, and then went back to playing. Rose turned to Elaine. "Al knows you'll be home waiting after the 'interrogation' of the deposition. It will get him through it. Just like it carries you."

She smiled at her mother-in-law. "Thanks Mom." Rose looked over at the boys while Elaine studied her profile. "Mom, why don't you come to the shore with us. Mom and Dad rented the same house in Point Pleasant they rented two summers ago. I think you could use a mini vacation too."

Rose brightened. "I would love that. Helen and I can help take the boys on the kiddy rides. I think Point is much more family friendly than Seaside." Secretly Rose was not looking forward to being alone in the house while the family was at the shore next week. She was used to the constant noise and activity of the boys.

"Great! We scheduled today's procedure so Al would be healed in time to enjoy himself." Elaine relaxed at the thought of going back down the shore again. She pictured the last time they were there when Al had the corneal transplant and he saw the ocean again. She hoped he wouldn't be melancholy.

Elaine had nothing to worry about. Al's spirits rose as the discomfort from the latest procedure disappeared over several days. A week later he sat on a bench next to a total stranger making conversation as his father-in-law took Albert and Larry for ice cream. The sun shown down on his covered shoulders and felt comforting. The stranger had overheard the conversation between Albert, Mr. Hinds and the boys and did not make his presence known to Al until Mr. Hinds had left with the boys.

"Your kids are going to soak your dad for everything he's got." The stranger joked and laughed with Al.

"What?" Al was a little startled to hear a strange voice talking to him in familiar overtones.

"Sorry. I'm waiting for my wife to come back and I heard the conversation." The man talked quickly to cover the misstep he had just made.

Al thought the man must have listened very carefully to know those facts from the brief interchange he had with his father-in-law. "I think you might be right. That's my father-in-law. He is something else. Always right there when we need him. I can't ask for more than that." Al leaned back against the bench enjoying the feel of the sun on his face.

"I guess that's really important to know since you can't see." The man stood up to take pictures of the sea scape and included Al in the shots.

Al was a little surprised at how honest but rude the guy was. "I can do a lot for myself. It takes me four times as long as when I had sight, but I get it done."

"Really? That's interesting. I would have thought you had to permanently depend on other people for help." The man continued to take pictures.

Al became defensive. "Well, to some degree, sure. I help my wife with our kids. The last thing she needs is another kid to take care of instead of a spouse."

Mr. Hinds walked up with two ice cream dripping boys

in tow. "Hey, Al. We're back." The man abruptly walked away. "Who's your friend?" He handed Al an ice cream.

"No idea. Just some guy. Thanks for the cone." Al loved the orange and vanilla twist cones and ate it greedily.

"Do you realize he was taking pictures of you?" Mr. Hinds put a hand on Albert's head as he tried to escape.

Al held his cone mid air. "No. I heard the camera clicking, but I thought he was taking pictures of the ocean.

Mr. Hinds shook his head. "Son, I'm telling you he was taking pictures of you. Did he ask you any questions?"

Al thought back to the dialogue. "You know Dad it didn't dawn on me at the time but it was weird. Would the private detectives go as far as to follow us down here?"

"Yes." Mr. Hinds did not hesitate. "Remember to tell the lawyer about this. The companies you're up against will use anything they can. You have the depositions coming up in a couple weeks, correct?"

The smile faded from Al's face. "Yeah. I've been trying not to think about it."

"Well, you should be thinking about it. I can guarantee the lawyers for the other guys are." Mr. Hinds wiped ice cream from his chin.

"When will this end?" Al's mood change had nothing to do with depression from dealing with memories of the last time at the shore.

"It will end when the case is settled. This is business." Mr. Hinds loved Point Pleasant and looked around at the people walking up and down the boardwalk.

"It's draining. I know it's all necessary, but it's draining. To think that after everything we've been through they would actually hire someone to follow us on a family trip is insane." Al felt himself slipping into a melancholy that felt like a surrender to anger.

"Snap out of it, son. This isn't going to go on forever. It's just one more thing you need to survive."

Chapter IX: Normality

Several weeks later at 3:30 p.m. on a hot July day, in an antiseptically clean attorney's office, Al sat stoically in the chair next to his attorney as the opposing counsel conducted the deposition Al had been dreading. He had been in the chair since 9:30 that morning, taking breaks only when allowed to use the men's room.

It was during one of these bathroom breaks that Mr. Bayplaza took Al into a private bathroom to talk to him. "You have to regroup. You are giving answers that are too long."

"I'm starving. I'm starting to lose it." Al, who did not need to use the bathroom, leaned against the wall to which his attorney had guided him.

"I understand however, you have several more hours with these attorneys. This is the beginning. We don't want to lose the case before we even start. Pause before you answer if you need to, but keep the answers short."

Al and his attorney rejoined the group and he was led back to his chair. He sipped the water given him to assuage his growing hunger.

A female voice representing one of the defendants continued her questioning. "Sir, could you please state where on your body you have been burned."

"My face, neck, torso, arms, hands, legs and feet."

116

The female attorney representing MTZW, the main defendant, studied the medical file in front of her gazing at pictures the doctors had taken. "Mr. Plevier would you please remove your shirt and stand where we can view your entire body."

He kept in mind that Mr. Bayplaza had reminded him not to smart mouth the attorneys and to answer the questions with as short an answer as possible. He was told not to argue or ask why they were asking a particular question. The opposing attorneys could only utilize the answers at the deposition in court if he contradicted himself. Al had learned that you never have to remember what you said when it is the truth. Continually he tried to give only yes or no answers and to remember that his attorney could not object to any of their questions at the deposition, only in court.

Al dutifully began to unbutton his shirt and stood up. He pulled at the sleeves of the oxford as it clung to the Jobe shirt. Tossing it on the table he then began to pull at the Velcro strips holding the Jobe shirt in place. The shirt opened as he pealed each sleeve off slowly. The Jobe shirt was tossed on top of the oxford and Al stood before all the attorneys.

"Mr. Plevier do you wear the, what is it called, Jobe shirt all the time?", asked a male voice.

Al: "Yes."

Opposing Counsel: "Is it uncomfortable?"

Al: "No. I'm used to it."

Opposing Cousel: "Do you wear it at night while you sleep?"

Al: "Yes."

Opposing Counsel: "Is it eliminating your scarring?"

Al: "No."

Opposing Counsel: "Does it stop the itching and pain from the scarring?"

Al: "Not completely."

The opposing counsel from the three represented defending companies did not speak as Al stood in front of them for several minutes. Finally, a male voice that was not Mr. Bayplaza spoke.

Opposing Counsel: "Thank you Mr. Plevier. You can put your shirts back on."

As Al pulled and rolled the Jobe shirt sleeves onto his arms no one in the room spoke. He thought they must have been measuring his ability to dress himself and take care of his own needs. While buttoning up his oxford, the woman attorney spoke to him.

Opposing Cousel: "Please do not tuck in your shirt. Are you scarred below your waist at all?"

Al: "In several small spots."

Opposing Cousel: "We will need you to drop your pants next so that we can view the damage to your legs."

Al turned his head to his right to indicate to his attorney he needed advice. "Is she joking?"

"Mr. Plevier please do as they ask." His attorney was not happy with the question but could not object to it.

Al stood stock still, letting his arms fall to the sides and turned his head forward again to the group. "Can't you get the information you need from the files?"

The only response from the female attorney. "Please step back two paces from the edge of the table so we can see and then please also drop your underwear."

Al was shocked into sarcasm. "Sorry lady. You're gonna have to throw me some singles first. I don't do that for free." His arms still lay limply at his sides.

The room remained silent. The eight attorneys present, including his own, stared at him waiting for him to do as requested. Al stubbornly stood there in the silence until angrily grabbing at his pants and yanking down both his boxers and jeans in one swift movement.

His sarcasm and anger flowed freely without consideration to his lawyer's advice. "Let me know when you've had enough." This time he stood with his arms hugging his body as much as the Jobe shirt allowed. His lawyer cringed slightly at the small outburst from his client.

The woman attorney spoke in a flat emotionless manner. "Please turn around."

Al was mortified as he turned slowly and tried not to be tripped up by his pants around his ankles. "Let me know when you're done." Al spit the words at her.

A male attorney spoke next. "Thank you Mr. Plevier. You can redress now."

Al snorted slightly. "You're welcome." He couldn't contain the sarcasm in his voice.

For a moment, as he stood there zipping up his jeans, Al thought about the part MTZW played in the destruction of his body. In that moment, standing in the room where he was giving his deposition he relived the accident.

He felt again his fight to live as the concentrated sodium hydroxide forcefully blasted his unprotected body. He was again crawling backward through the onslaught as it burned and almost killed him. He was dragging his disintegrating body over the top and down the other side of the forklift truck to the relief of the safety shower he knew was waiting on the other side of the storage tank.

He did everything right that day and when he pulled the chain on the shower, it fell limply into his hands. The entire mechanism broke at exactly the moment it was supposed to work, October 1, 1974 at 4:45 p.m. on a clear, warm Indian summer day in northern New Jersey's notorious chemical industry at the end of his workday as the plant production manager.

Al couldn't help but wonder how much of his bodily damage would have been reduced had the emergency shower done exactly what it was designed to do. Standing there pulling up the jeans and boxers he couldn't see, he wondered if he would have been able to save his eyes. In his heart, he knew that if the shower had worked he would have opened his eyes under the flowing water and not moved as his clothes would have been torn off of him. Would he be able to see his children today?

He found out in recent weeks that the brass shower head been manufactured in 1954. The chain attached to the shower head designed to be pulled in an emergency was not made of brass because it was manufactured during the Korean War when the availability of brass was limited. If the shower head and chain had been made of the proper material, the mechanism would have lasted several decades ensuring its' successful operation on October 1, 1974.

The accident happened at work. Under New Jersey law, one of two states in the nation an employee cannot sue their employer or fellow employees. Sarcastically he thought to himself that his former employer, A&K Chemicals, had done everything right in the event of an emergency by relying on the products they purchased, like the safety shower, to work properly. The safety shower, the only safety measure that would have saved his eyes during the tragedy had failed.

His attorney had explained to him that if the defending company could prove Al was at least 51% responsible for the accident and the subsequent damage to his body he would receive nothing. Al was also warned that the monetary award he needed to continue with his life would in all likelihood not be as high as they were initially suing for. At the end of the fight it would be better to settle and that meant, in literal terms settling and accepting. His stomach churned at the thought.

"Mr. Plevier we are finishing up for today. Please have a seat."

Al felt his way back to the chair in front of him. He had inadvertently left his cane hanging on the table edge in his frustration. Swiping his hand from side to side he tried to hold his head up in as dignified a manner as possible and then decided it was more important to just sit down. He stumbled a bit and bumped into his attorney's chair.

"Sorry Art." Al apologized unapoligetically.

The attorney secretly thought the small stumble legitimized the 'show' the opposing counsel thought they might see or not see. They had a front row seat to a small part of what his client lived with on a minute by minute basis.

"No problem, Mr. Plevier." Al and Elaine were on a first name basis with Art Bayplaza, but in the public forum an air of professionalism needed to be maintained. In a louder than necessary private conversation, he followed up with a comment reflecting his own frustration. "I should have you out of here in the next thirty minutes."

Al nodded his head in the direction of his attorney and took his seat preparing himself for the next question. This time a voice spoke up from the right side of the table. It was the male voice he had heard twice in the morning.

Opposing Counsel: "Mr. Plevier, who is responsible for your daily hygiene?"

Al was stumped that they actually believed he needed a nurse to take care of him? "I am."

Opposing Counsel: "Do you shower alone?"

Several smart, ass answers went through his mind and he swore he could feel his attorney tense up next to him. "Yes."

Opposing Counsel: "Are you able to shave yourself?"

Al couldn't imagine what this guy was leading up to. "Yes."

Opposing Counsel: "Do you ask anyone how you look when you are finished?"

Al: "Yes."

Opposing Counsel: "Who?"

Al: "My wife."

Opposing Counsel: "Does she find the mustache you now have attractive?"

Al had decided to grow a Fu Manchu mustache over the winter. Elaine hated it. "No."

Opposing Counsel: "Had you been clean shaven before the accident?"

Al: "Yes."

Opposing Counsel: "Is it easier to let your facial hair grow now after having a burned face that has healed?"

Al: "No."

Opposing Counsel: "Is it easier to take care of?"

Al: "No."

Opposing Counsel: "Why do it?"

The truth was he was bored half of the time now that he didn't have visual stimulation or any projects to keep his mind off the recent corneal failing. This mustache was just another project to him. "I thought it would look good."

Opposing Counsel: "Was you face burned completely at the time of the accident?"

Al: "Yes."

Opposing Counsel: "How is it possible that you have no scarring on your face?"

Al held his hands open in front of him. "I don't know."

He remembered Elaine had described him as looking like a giant black pumpkin. A monster is one word that he never forgot.

Opposing Counsel: "Mr. Plevier how is your sex life?"

The blunt change of topic caught him off guard. Al couldn't believe his ears. All he could think was that these people had just viewed 'all of him'. Why did they need to ask? The question came from the only woman attorney. "Fine."

Opposing Counsel: "Can you elaborate?"

Al tensed up and tried to find a way to answer this in a shorter manner. "Normal."

The questions became rapid fire in intensity and duration.

Opposing Counsel: "Are you able to perform and maintain a sex life in your marriage?"

Al: "Yes."

Opposing Counsel: "How many children do you have?"

Al: "Three."

Opposing Counsel: "When were they born?"

Al: "1973, 1976 and 1977."

Opposing Counsel: "So, you are telling us two were born after the accident?"

"Yes." He was beginning to lose it. "You had a full view of my genetalia. As you can see, it's normal."

The lawyers were not deterred in the manner of their questions.

Opposing Counsel: "Are you planning any more?"

Al: "I don't know."

Opposing Counsel: "Yes or no?"

Al: "Yes."

Opposing Counsel: "How many?"

Al: "Don't know."

Opposing Counsel: "Most people plan how many children they want without a catastrophic accident. Surely you can answer this question."

Al: "One."

Opposing Counsel: "When?"

Al: "A couple years from now."

There was a pause of several seconds. "Mr. Plevier, do you play with your children?"

Al was ready for a quick sarcastic response but he remembered his lawyer's advice. "Yes."

Opposing Counsel: "In what capacity?"

Now he was confused. "I don't understand the question."

Opposing Counsel: "Let me rephrase the question. Do you play baseball with your boys?"

Al: "Well, I teach them to the best of my ability."

Opposing Counsel: "So, the answer is yes."

Al: "No."

Opposing Counsel: "Do you or do you not pitch a baseball to your boys?"

Al thought briefly about the 'deadly beeper ball' Elaine had picked up for him to use. "My wife bought a beeper ball from the blind association to allow me to pitch to my son." He felt his attorney tense up beside him. "Yes."

Opposing Counsel: "Is playing with your children something you value?"

Al: "Yes."

Opposing Counsel: "Has your time with them been compromised in any way? In other words, since you are no longer working, do you find yourself able to spend more time with your children especially since you are considering having more?"

Now he was stumped. How in God's name was he going to answer this question? "I cannot see my children. Every day I live with that."

Opposing Counsel: "Do you now have more time with your children than a father who has to go to work every day?"

Al seethed in anger. "I can't answer that. I would have to take a poll with all the working fathers. Some working fathers I suppose have quality time after work. Some unemployed fathers I suppose might ignore their children. If my lawyer is willing to take a poll I will get back to you on that."

Now the only woman in the room, who had been the attorney asking Al to take off his clothes, asked another question.

Opposing Counsel: "Mr. Plevier are you telling this room that after what you consider to be a life altering and life threatening accident, an accident that destroyed your finances and your ability to support your family in the manner to which you were accustomed you plan on continuing to have children even though you have three children?"

Al: "Yes."

Opposing Counsel: "Are you expecting other people to take care of your family through a settlement?"

Al: "No."

Opposing Counsel: "Are you counting on this settlement to finance your future?"

Al: "No."

Opposing Counsel: "Did you always plan to have more children?"

Al: "Yes."

Opposing Counsel: "Don't you think an accident of this proportion and the fact that you are now blind should have changed your plans?"

Al: "No. My wife was pregnant at the time of the accident."

Al could almost feel his lawyer tense as he elaborated on the answer.

Opposing Counsel: "Wait, that doesn't make sense. Your second child was born in 1976. The accident was in 1974. Are you confused, Sir?'

Al: "No."

Opposing Counsel: "Please elaborate."

Al: "The first time I came home from the hospital my wife miscarried our second child. That was six weeks after the accident. Her Obstetrician said it was from all the stress. Is there a monetary value you can put on my child's life as a secondary event after the fact?"

The room went silent. Al knew he was going to get a tongue lashing from his attorney on the car ride home. He also knew he deserved it. In his defense, he was on his last nerve of patience and he was starving. It was his assumption the opposing attorneys realized this and saved the worst of the questions for the end of the day. After several minutes, the rapid, fire questions started again this time from a male lawyer he had not heard from all day.

Opposing Counsel: "Do you have a TV in the back of your house, Sir?"

Al: "Yes."

Opposing Counsel: "Do you sit in a recliner in front of the TV with company?"

Al: "Yes."

Opposing Counsel: "When you are in the recliner is the TV directly in front of you?"

Al: "Yes."

Opposing Counsel: "Are there chairs to the left and right of you?"

Al: "No."

Opposing Counsel: "Do you watch TV in the evening with anyone else?"

Al: "Yes."

Opposing Counsel: "Who?"

Al: "My wife. I listen while she watches."

125

Al could feel his attorney tensing up next to him. He heard papers being shuffled. No one explained to him what was going on until they were finished.

Opposing Counsel: "Mr. Plevier I've laid out pictures for your attorney to view. They are pictures of you sitting on a bench in the beach resort town of Point Pleasant Beach. Did you recently take a vacation with your family?" The male attorney speaking to him sounded almost angry.

"Yes." Al answered in the recommended word answers by his lawyer. He was tired and becoming worn down by the entire proceedings.

Opposing Counsel: "Are you telling this room that you enjoy a normal life?"

Now Al paused. "As much as possible."

Opposing Counsel: "Can you elaborate?"

Al: "I can't see. Shut the lights out in your house and walk around or better yet, wear a blindfold and then you will understand. You never know who you are talking to or what that person might be doing." Al felt almost betrayed by the man on the bench who had made conversation with him.

"It is 4:00. Let's resume this tomorrow. Are we all in agreement?" Mr. Bayplaza was speedy with his question making sure all present knew that this was not a request but an absolute statement.

The attorneys present for the three different defendants looked at each other and nodded their heads in agreement. The woman spoke for everyone. "Yes. Tomorrow at 9:30 to resume. Thank you everyone for coming today."

All present in the room including Al and Mr. Bayplaza left unceremoniously and without comment.

Once they were in his attorney's car Al spoke bluntly. "That was the most embarrassing thing I have ever been put through and that includes my hospital stays. At least in the hospital I knew they were trying to heal me, not break me down. You could have at least warned me that it might happen and that I might have to strip. Are they kidding me? Didn't any of them look through my medical records? There were many pictures taken of my injuries by you and the doctors. I remember you coming to the hospital the first time I was in right after the accident in '74. You took pictures that day, right?"

"Yes, son, I did." Mr. Bayplaza understood the frustration he was watching Al display, but given all his client had been through he was surprised Al recalled that.

Al continued his rant. "And how did they know where I sit in the family room? We moved the TV when I opened the porch up to enlarge it. How could they know that unless they are still watching me? When they started watching me you couldn't see inside the house beyond the porch. Now they're seeing everything my family does. This is crazy. All they need to do is see my medical records. That's it! The records speak for themselves for crying out loud! The pictures are always kept current with the doctors. I know Elaine has given those to you. Do they just look at me with my clothes off? Even a little boy at McDonalds could see what happened to me."

Mr. Bayplaza let his client have his moment, knowing he desperately needed to vent after the hours he spent in the chair. Then he gave him a weird look. "What little boy at McDonalds?"

Al breathed out heavily. "Nothing. It's not important." Al leaned back in the car seat feeling the energy drain out of his body. "It's like I'm constantly reliving the accident over and over again. Coming back to the same place no matter how hard I try to leave it."

The attorney raised his eyebrows and shook his head slightly. "As you just said, they were trying to break you down. Psychologically playing with you so that you would contradict yourself by accident and damage your credibility." He glanced at his silent and angry client. "Let's get something to eat. It's my treat. There's a great Diner up ahead and they make an amazing hamburger."

At the offer of food Al calmed down. "I'll carry some food, you know, like a candy bar, in my pockets for tomorrow so that when I go to use the men's room I can sneak a bite. I can't last this long for two days in a row."

The car pulled into the Galaxy Diner and Al smelled burgers immediately. "You know I never thought I could eat hamburger again after I smelled my own skin cooking."

Mr. Bayplaza grimaced slightly knowing his client couldn't see his expression. "I can imagine."

"I'm over it now. When I eat out, hamburger is the easiest thing for me. Anything I have to cut up is a disaster and I don't want my wife cutting up my food like she does for the children." The second the car stopped Al was reaching for the handle, but he stopped abruptly when Mr. Bayplaza touched his arm.

"I didn't realize that. Was it hard for you when we went out for steak?" Mr. Bayplaza felt terrible and then remembered it was before the corneal transplant had failed.

Al's heart sunk in his chest. He went to extremes to make others comfortable. "No, no. I was still seeing shadows. That was the best steak I ever had. Now that my sight is completely gone again, I'm adjusting to my old routine when I'm out." He hoped the kind man could not tell he was lying.

"I'm glad you said something. This diner has the best chicken franchaise and I was going to suggest it to you." The two men jumped out of the car at the same time.

Al spoke over the hood of the car and hoped the attorney was still standing by his door. "There's something I have to tell you. Elaine is pregnant. We haven't told anyone else yet because we want to make sure everything goes well." Afraid of his lawyer's response Al began to speak quickly. "Elaine is still hoping for a girl, but as long as it's healthy we're both thrilled."

"I'm happy for both of you and I thank you for not mentioning it at the deposition. Since the private detectives are still following you, the defendants will find out eventually. Are you guys going to be alright financially? I thought Elaine was going to nursing school?" The attorney and Al stepped to the front of the car.

"She still is and she should be halfway through when the new baby is born. Moving is out of the question right now.

We're planning on that happening after the baby is born and I'm picking up some part time work here and there." The quicker he spoke the more obvious it was that he worried how the lawyer would process the good news.

The lawyer interrupted him. "I do not want to ever hear you talk about that." He took another step closer and met Al toe to toe at the hood. "Let's get you something to eat. We can talk about our strategy for tomorrow after dinner." He let Al put a hand on his shoulder to guide him and both men practically ran into the restaurant.

Once their stomachs were full Al felt he should divulge to the attorney the possibility of a camera implant that Dr. Leesville discussed with him. "I'm definitely going for this if he says it's possible. I want to see my boys and this new baby."

The attorney leaned back in the booth and had an expressionless face that Al could not see. "When is that going to take place?"

"We don't know if it is definite yet. It's just a possibility that I want you to be aware of."

"Do you want anything else? Coffee?" The lawyer's tone of voice had a distinct edge to it.

"No, I'm good. Elaine is probably wondering what happened to us." Al felt the air between the two men change. "I don't know how many of these depositions I can go through."

"You'll get used to them." The attorney was still absorbing the fact that his blind, broke and burned client was continuing to build his family.

Al whistled low as they continued the conversation on the journey back to his home. "The deposition today was a personal attack."

"It's getting serious now. I mean that in a sarcastic way, not flippant. We have narrowed the defendents down to three companies. MTZW does not want a precedent set for similar failures who may file suit. They would rather pay the private detective to follow you and take a chance than to admit fault." The car hit heavy traffic and both men quieted for a moment as a semi flew past them. "You do have the option of settling the case for a sealed amount before its goes to trial. It would save you the aggravation of a trial and the roll of the dice of whether you win or lose."

Al thought for a moment. "I want to fight. If we lose we can appeal, right?"

Mr. Bayplaza cared about the young couple and wanted, in his heart, what was best for them. "Yes, but it could drag on for years."

"For now, I want to fight. I'll talk to Elaine about this. We still have two more days of testimony." He leaned back into the seat to relax for the rest of the car ride.

After he was dropped off Al came in the house and found Elaine trying to wind the boys down for the evening. Christopher was giggling nonstop at his brother's antics and behavior. He never took his eyes off either Albert or Larry anxious for his turn to become part of the larger brood.

"Hey Sweetheart, how are you feeling?" Al found his way to her through the maze of toys and gave her a quick hug.

"How did the deposition go, Son?" Rose spoke up to let him know she was in the room.

"Hi Mom. It went fine." He figured he could fill Elaine in on the truth later.

"You look tired. That was a long day." Rose picked up Christopher and took him in for a bath.

"It was but I have a new strategy for tomorrow. I'm putting food in my pockets. They wouldn't let me take a lunch break so I'll eat during bathroom breaks.

Rose tickled the baby and started toward the bathroom. "I've got this one, Elaine. I'll give him his bath, and I'll let you know when he is tucked in."

"Thanks Mom." She waited for her mother-in-law to be out of listening range before confronting Al. "It was that bad?"

"Yes. Glad I don't have to lie to you." Al felt Larry grabbing at him, trying to get his attention. "They made me take off my clothes so they could see the damage."

"Didn't they look at the medical records and the pictures The attorneyand the doctors had taken?" She sat down on the couch and continued to fold miniature clothing.

"They had everything, but it didn't matter." He picked up Larry.

"I hope this was the worst. You still have two more days."

Al jostled Larry to entertain him. "I know. At least we have Saturday night out with the *Images Group*." Al tossed the little boy lightly in the air until he felt Albert crash into him with jealousy.

Elaine was glad for the subject change. "What are we going to see?" She stopped folding clothes and tried to get Albert's attention.

Al stopped tossing Larry and concentrated on the conversation with Elaine. "Karen Miller said it's a show called 'Puddle Jumpers'. Never heard of it. We tried to pick neutral shows that everyone would enjoy. I hope this is one of them." Albert gave up his attack on Al and climbed into Elaine's lap for attention.

She pulled Albert close for a hug and turned to Al. "Who is going?"

"Not sure. We have thirty people and about twenty are couples." Al made his way over to the couch with her.

She slipped closer to him. "We'll have a good time and it will help you forget the misery of today and the next two days."

Al became quiet. "It will help to get me through that." He hesitated to bring up the next point. "The attorney brought up the idea of settling the case before it goes to trial." The comment hung in the air. "I want to fight. He seems to feel that it would be easier on us and our family if we settled. I guess he is counting on the fact that we are very good with money and that we would not blow through a settlement." Elaine was not commenting. "What is your opinion?"

She hugged Albert into submission. "A solid known amount would go a long way to begin planning out our future finances again. The unknown is what makes me crazy. It's like winning the lottery if we go to trial."

"If we lose, we can appeal. If we win, they could appeal. It could go on for another decade." In his heart, Al did not care how long it took. He had always been a fighter.

"We don't have to decide in the next couple of months, do we?" Elaine wanted to have a peaceful pregnancy.

"No. We can revisit the idea after the new baby is born." Albert slid down, bored with the adult conversation and went to play with his workbench. "Elaine, I need a little time alone tonight. Would you mind if I went to the basement to play darts? I won't be down there all night. Just to regroup and blow off a little steam."

Holding his hand, she tried to convey her support. "Do whatever you need to. If you could wait a little while until the boys wind down it would help. They've all eaten dinner. I was getting ready to give them baths."

"I can help with that." Al answered with the gratitude of family contribution most men would turn up their nose at.

A few hours later Al made his way to the basement. It was early evening now and he wondered if the neighbors saw someone moving around their basement in the dark they would call the cops. He hoped not because he had no intention of playing darts.

Reaching to the left he found the BB gun he had hidden. It was fully loaded. He found the string he had tied to it and walked over to the target he hid behind the dart board. He used the same string and bell that he used for darts and took aim. The paper ripped the first, second and all the subsequent times he hit the target. When all the BB's were spent, he felt better for reasons he couldn't explain. He packed up and hid the empty BB gun high up in the cubby he discovered the first year they bought the house. He then found his way into the house and fell into a restless sleep.

The following three days of depositions seemed like an eternity to Al. Questioning by the attorneys did not reach the depth of the first day, but instead dealt with minutia that drew him once again to the conclusion that MTZW would look at every detail to find an opportunity to discredit him and his testimony. When the three days were over Friday evening, he and Elaine hurriedly gave the responsibility for the boys over to Rose, Ronnie and Mr. and Mrs. Hinds.

"I don't know what we would do without you guys." Elaine carried a light sweater over her arm in case the air conditioning in the theater was chilly. "I'm feeling so great with this pregnancy. I don't want to take a chance on catching a cold.

"We wouldn't be going out tonight without help from all of you that's for sure." Al waited for Elaine and when he heard her move away from him, he let his cane follow her to the back door. "You guys have the phone number of the theater if you need us. Good luck!"

"Thanks, Son." Mr. Hinds laughed but then looked over at the three boys and honestly felt a little intimidated.

Elaine and Al knew none of this as they rushed out the door and then to the theater. They met everyone outside and Elaine was happy to see that half of the people had sight. It was comforting for her to find people outside their family and immediate social circle who were also living with someone without sight. The couples tonight looked as happy as she and Al and the singles had family for company.

"Hello you two." Karen Miller's husband greeted them both.

"Hi Tom. Is everyone here?" Al turned his head from side to side in acknowledgement.

"Yes. Karen kept a list and has everyone checked off. The idea of *Images* was great, Al. You and Karen do a lot more for people without sight than you realize. I'm really proud of my wife and glad that it helps the two of you give back." Tom was genuine in his admiration of Al.

Typically, al resorted to sarcasm to deflect the compliments. "Hey, I'm just in it for the free stuff we get for having disabilities."

There was an announcement for ticket holders to take their seats. The group, with the help of their mates or companions, came down the center aisle together and found their seats. Everyone was seated when the youngest member of the blind group, a twenty-two-year-old who had been blind since birth, stood back up, lifted her dress, rearranged her underwear, and sat back down.

Al felt an elbow in his side. "Owww. What's the problem?"

Elaine's voice was ice cold. "The young lady with Sherri just stood up lifted her dress, rearranged her underwear and sat back down."

"Whaaaaaat?" Al was shocked and embarrassed for Elaine. "Who else saw?"

Elaine elbowed him again. "Everyone."

The lights went down at that moment and the show started. Al didn't even try to talk to Elaine until she told him it was intermission. She was still furious.

"Al, someone has to talk to that girl. Her sighted guide did nothing. She obviously has mental or emotional problems." Elaine kept her voice low.

"Maybe she doesn't care or just doesn't know any better." He decided it was time to bring humor to this. "She could have thought she was doing the world a favor."

"Al! This is your group. You and Karen are going to have to handle this. If you're going to continue to open the group to the general public something weird like this might happen." She looked around to see if there was anyone in the theater they knew.

"I'll talk to Karen and see how we should handle this." He shook his head and laughed softly. "I thought the sight of us at events was funny, but this takes the cake."

Elaine looked at him quizzically. "What are you talking about?

"When we go out we're like a whip or a chain gang. There are usually eight to ten blind people with sighted helpers. The people without sight have their hands on the shoulders of the person in front until we basically form a line. I'm usually at the end and eventually it acts like a whip. I'm always hitting someone." They both laughed. "We must be quite a sight.

Elaine started to laugh, releasing the tension and anger of several minutes ago. "That's hysterical. It sounds like a comedy skit."

"Yeah, and I'm the butt end of the joke." He lowered his voice. "We went out to eat last month after the square dancing class, which itself was a riot, and by the end of the night we went from one waitress to four with each person asking for separate checks. I don't think that restaurant will ever have us back."

"Why don't the sighted helpers do something?" Elaine was stunned that Al had been dealing with this type of behavior in the group.

"I think by the time they get to the end of the night they're worn down." Now he was laughing and didn't care if anyone heard. "We had a horseshoe contest a couple months ago, and we started off using real horseshoes. I was bent over moving one of the stakes and a shoe landed four inches from my head. No one bothered to tell the lady tossing the shoe that the game hadn't started yet." They were both laughing. "That's a quick way to get rid of me, Sweetheart."

"You, Karen and Carla must be all bruises after each outing." For the moment, she had forgotten about the young lady who had exposed herself to the entire audience.

"I'm not going to lie to you. It's a challenge. Carla and Karen work mostly with the music training for those interested. Carla's very talented. You can thank her personally for my attempt at the banjo." He relaxed when he realized she was probably over the embarrassment of the previous hour.

This time Elaine shook her head and smirked. "That was something to listen to. I had no idea where you came up with that. I just figured it was one of those things you always wanted to try."

"Nah. Karen and Carla are giving a talk about potential instruments for each group member and she didn't mention the banjo, so I did. They thought it was a joke so they called me on it and found one." He thought back to the first time he felt the strings and how cool he imagined he looked. "I thought my Fu Manchu mustache added to my mystique."

"If you say so. I got a picture of that for posterity." Elaine smirked satisfactorily.

Al leaned back in mock surprise. "Did you really? That's great."

"Yup. You're sitting on the porch with your feet up on the railing. It's a classic." She thought hard about where she put that picture and wondered if it was in the wrong album. "I haven't said anything up to now, but when are you planning on shaving that thing off?"

After what Al had put her through tonight, he felt like he owed it to her to shave off the thing that she hated so much. "Honey, if you really want me to, I will."

Now Elaine felt guilty. "I guess I can stand it. It just isn't you. I don't know how else to explain it to you. You were always a clean, shaven guy."

"I would have a regular mustache, but I can't grow a thick one. Never have been able to. This is the best I can do. I don't want to look like a guy from the twenties." He played with one end of the mustache as he talked.

She relented knowing that if he was in a work environment every day he would not be allowed to keep it. "Alright. If this is some kind of a secret wish you always had, enjoy. I'll deal with it until you give it up." Always surprised and happy to see her husband not giving up, Elaine wondered what he was working on next to keep himself busy and to prove his life was still moving forward. "What do you have planned next?"

Chapter X: Milestones

"*I'm* trying to figure out a way to play ball. The biggest challenge is finding sighted people to work with us that don't worry."

This was one subject Elaine was afraid to bring up, knowing how much the sport meant to him. "How's it going so far?"

"I get beat up pretty good most of the time, but it's worth it. The Pioneers from Bell Telephone are working with us on anything that might help, from the beeper balls that are manufactured now to clickers attached to our clothing." Al thought back to three weekends ago when a sighted helper offered to pitch.

The man was timid about throwing toward a man who couldn't see. After a half hour, Al was able to convince him to stop throwing underhand and really bring on the heat. The ball got him in the ribs when he leaned in. It took him the rest of the afternoon to quell the man's guilt.

Elaine was very proud of what her husband was doing for other people. It was a statement to his character that he tried to move outside his own circumstances. "*Images* is very lucky to have you."

"Truly, I don't know whos is helping who. I need to give back to the outside world. *Images* offers something for people to look forward to. It's really sad, Honey. Some of the members are either shut ins or don't have the money or helpers to leave their comfort zones. Fear holds people back with or without sight."

"You and Karen should run classes on social skills for individuals learning to live without sight."

"Sorry, Honey. That's the job of the New Jersey Commission for the Blind. Our Wayne *Images Group* is an offshoot of the blind group in Ridgewood. We wanted something closer for social outings. Members should already have basic social decorum." He didn't mean to sound uncaring, but he designed the club for a specific purpose. "We work with the Lions Club and Bell Telephone. I'm an engineer not a social worker. We just want to get out on our own, find people to help us find ways to do everything sighted people do and have fun." He thought he may have sounded heartless and tried to soften his response. "I'm aware of the circumstances the young lady at the theatre comes from. I don't think I'll get very far with her immediate circle. There's a reason for her behavior." He turned his head toward Elaine. "Living without sight is a pain in the ass not an excuse to act poorly in social settings."

She decided to turn the conversation. "Are you working with Bell on anything beside the baseball possibilities?"

"No inventions for me right now. I'm a little busy." He reached out and touched her still flat stomach. "I'll leave the brain trust to Bell Labs and satisfy myself with being the part of the population they use as a test rat." Al chuckled and moved his hand away. "They have all kinds of gadgets. Bowling is interesting."

"I can imagine." Elaine eased the car off the highway onto their exit.

"We tried to use the cricket the Pioneer Group invented for horseshoes for our bowling trips but it didn't work."

She had never heard this gadget mentioned before. "What's the cricket?"

Al was about to launch into a good bowling story about the blind, but answered her question first. "It's a beeping device with a volume control used to discern distance. It works great for horseshoes but not bowling." He felt he had built up a little anticipation for his story. "The best example was when I was keeping score, and we sent up a young blind girl with her helper. The helper turned to talk to us, and the girl decided she wanted to show how independent she was. She swung the bowling ball back and whacked her helper knocking him over. All I heard was a thud." He laughed hard at the memory. "Boy, did I get in trouble for laughing when they told we what the thud was. If we're going to teach life skills the first should be to have a sense of humor. It's life, we're not getting out alive so we might as well get over the weird stuff."

She glanced at her husband as they pulled behind her parents' car in the driveway. "Maybe we can get a game of cards going before my parents leave. I have some munchies I can throw together for snacks. Dad will want something even though they had dinner. The night is still young."

"So are we. Let's go have some fun."

The card game lasted late into the evening. The children all went down without fussing and the adults did not want the laughter and light heartedness to end. The night grew late when the cards were packed away and the ladies went into the kitchen to clean up. Al grabbed this opportunity to speak alone with Mr. Hinds.

"What's normal Dad?" Al turned his head toward his father-in-law and drummed his fingers on the table.

Momentarily stunned, Mr. Hinds understood the point of view the question came from. "Wherever you are standing, whatever your circumstance." Mr. Hinds, always grateful for food that he didn't have to prepare, finished off the finger food left behind during the table clearing.

"Albert's first day of Kindergarten is soon, and I can't see his little face as he either runs to the bus or is dragged to it." All week Al had been melancholy as they built up to this day for Albert, hoping preschool had prepared him for the moment.

The family had been talking about the new baby and Albert knew that meant there would be another little human demanding his parent's attention. He also knew it meant one more eventual playmate as Larry had proven to be. Even Chris had begun to walk this month. Already he was throwing toys. Albert's house was a fun and busy place.

"You'll have the entire army here to see the big man off. What a parade." Mr. Hinds raised his eyebrows as he spoke. He felt the women were going over the top with Albert's send off into the world of education. "That little boy has a huge group of people that love him. You asked me what's normal. Was it normal for you to not have a dad to see you go to school each September? It was your normal. This is Albert's." Mr. Hinds stopped for a moment to think. "He is a happy, healthy little boy surrounded by love. There are people in this world whose reality is not as wonderful and they work through it. To Albert, this is his normal, his reality. The kid is more than okay."

Al breathed out deeply, remembering the incident with the young woman. He hoped would never embarrass himself or his family. He knew it was always a top priority that his children never feel that they were lacking in respect to his abilities as a dad.

"Thanks, Dad." He thought ahead to Albert's first day of school. "Time passes so quickly. That is going to be one big day for the little guy."

Albert's first day of school became the family focus after his birthday party in July that was held outside under the shaded playground his dad had transformed their yard into. Balloons decorated the tree branches as they had done each birthday before. There was a difference this year. A milestone was approaching for not just Albert, but for the entire family.

The rest of the summer flew by. The half day practice session the school held for the Kindergarteners in August energized Albert's anticipation even more. He talked about the big yellow bus and all the new kids. When his official first day arrived so did the entire family, as promised.

"We're glad you're all here. Albert feels like the King today." Al was there when Elaine woke Albert up that morning and heard the little boy jump up and out of bed like a rocket. Al hoped the happiness carried him onto the bus and throughout his first day. It warmed Al's heart for Albert to have the whole family there that morning. "Dad did your boss give you or Mom a hard time?"

Mr. Hinds gave Al an incredulous look. "Are you kidding? He's lucky I haven't retired yet."

The sound of many feet running, stomping and just walking reached Al's ears. At the head of the entourage was Albert, five years old and proud with his backpack over both shoulders.

"Daddy? You coming to the bus stop?" Albert stood in front of Al's chair staring up into his face.

He bent down and hoped his head was facing Albert. "Of course. You don't think I would miss the biggest day of the year, do you?" He reached down and felt the back pack. "I see you're all ready to go. What do you have in there?"

"Teacher said we needed crayons, nap mat and a snack. Mommy's getting my snack." Albert marched over to where Elaine put his snack in a brown paper bag.

"Mommy what did you pack me?" Albert tried in vain to peak into the bag before Elaine popped it into the backpack.

"Cookies. Don't eat them on the bus. You'll want to keep them for milk time. The teacher will hand out the milk. Remember?" She knelt down to his level.

Albert scrunched up his face. "Mommy, I don't like milk."

Elaine felt her heart ache at the adorable sight of Albert's expression. "I know pal. It's going to be chocolate for your first day."

Albert looked at her disgruntled. "Okay."

Elaine stood up and rallied everyone. "Let's go outside. We have a couple minutes before the bus comes and I want to take more pictures."

Al grabbed his cane and followed the sound of footsteps toward the back door. "How many pictures did you take already?"

Elaine concentrated on the camera in her hand as she answered. "Not enough."

Albert dutifully led everyone to the mailbox. He knew from the practice bus ride in August that this is where he would climb aboard. The steps were so high he had to use the grab bar to pull himself up the first step that day. This had only made him feel more grown up.

Once he reached the mailbox he turned to make sure everyone was behind him. "Come on Mommy. Come on!"

Mrs. Hinds held Christopher's hand as he toddled along while Larry was permitted to run to his brother. Chris tried to pull out of his grandmother's grip to catch up to the boys, but she held tight. Even at one he was finding his place among his brothers.

"Everyone gather around Albert so we can get a group shot before the bus arrives." Elaine waved her free hand for encouragement.

Her Dad interrupted. "Ronnie, take a shot of Elaine and Al with Albert first."

Pictures were taken with every family member present in at least one shot. Al did as he was told as he tried to swallow the lump growing in his throat. Time was passing very quickly. So much had happened since he first laid eyes on Albert the day he was born.

"Daddy, Daddy! Here comes the bus!" Albert began to jump up and down.

Elaine swallowed deeply and leaned in close to Al. "I guess we didn't have to worry about separation anxiety."

"Are you kidding? That one is the leader of the pack. He's looking for more groups to conquer." It was a relief to know Albert was an independent child, no matter how much it hurt to watch him stretch his family cords.

The bus pulled up, Albert gave a wave, smiled and climbed aboard. Mrs. Shinn, the patient and kind bus driver, waited until Albert had dutifully waved goodbye to everyone from his front seat before pulling away. The group seemed mesmerized watching the bus grow smaller as it moved down the country road.

"Can we go back in now?" Al had a feeling he knew why no one was talking or moving.

"Sorry Al." Elaine stood next to him and then reached down to pick up Christopher who pointed after the bus. "Does anyone want coffee?"

Ronnie spoke up first. "I have to get to work. I'm already late. See you guys this weekend. You can let me know how his first day goes." She rushed to her car and carefully pulled around the group, beeping her horn goodbye.

Mrs. Hinds was next. "We should really get going too. Dad and I both called out for the morning, but they are expecting us at work by noon. I need to go earlier and catch up on yesterday's inventory lists. Do you need help cleaning up before we go hon? Dad and I took separate cars to get to work so he could stay longer."

"No Mom. You go ahead. Rose and I can get the house back together. Dad and Al can keep the little guys busy this morning."

Rose reached down and grabbed Larry's hand to keep him focused on going back inside on the beautiful September day. Al's mom had been pretty quiet this morning. Even after living with her son and his family for over a year, she still felt as if she were intruding. She helped out all the time, thinking how overwhelmed Elaine must be.

Rose turned to her friend. "Helen we'll be fine. The house will get pulled back together before Albert comes home and then we can get all the boys outside after nap time."

Elaine had been very tired lately with the new pregnancy and was grateful for her mother-in-law's additional help. "Thanks, Mom. I'll probably grab a nap with the boys."

Al spoke up. "Dad you take Larry." He reached toward Elaine for Christopher. "Instead of going inside let's take these two for a walk in the direction the bus went. It will keep them looking for Albert."

Mr. Hinds took Larry's hand from his wife and followed Al to the double stroller sitting outside the back door. "Sounds good. Helen, I'll see you at home later. Don't let them work you too hard."

"Bye everyone." Helen walked to her car and pulled out waving to the little boys.

The men wrestled the two little boys into the carriage and headed down the driveway. Al pushed and Mr. Hinds walked on the left, guarding the cargo from passing cars. The boys began to entertain each other and left Al and Mr. Hinds free to talk.

"Dad, you were right. Normal is wherever you happen to be standing. You have to work within your own normality." They reached the end of the driveway and turned in the direction the bus went. The two passengers in the carriage immediately started to babble and point down the road. "I had a meeting with our attorney last week and he gave me a severe talk about the new baby, again. His thoughts were that the outside world would not understand how a couple that went through our trauma could consider managing a growing family. The jury in our case would think that we were looking for a free ride, or worse, we have no common sense. That would lend itself to the possibility that I was responsible for what happened to me." He snorted in disgust. "The fact that determining what was happening that day in the back of the production area was my job would be lost under the guise of portraying us as poor white trash looking to suck off the system by a frivolous law suit." Al took his hands off the carriage for a second and did air quotes around the word frivolous.

"He's just doing his job. If he didn't say those things to you I would wonder about him." He reached out to steer the carriage that was heading right toward the woods.

Distracted by his thoughts, Al continued to vent and did not concentrate on where he was pushing the stroller. "First I get hurt for doing my job by trying to save the men who created the mess and then the rest of the world thinks it has the right to tell me how to live my life? Not one of those men involved ever came to even apologize to me. Not one. They were safe from any lawsuit involvement. They were under my supervision in the plant. It would have given me and my wife a little comfort in the early days. Now, it's too late."

Mr. Hinds shrugged his shoulder slightly. "It's never too late."

Al stopped the carriage short. "No Dad. You don't understand. Charlie dropped dead from a heart attack two months ago. I just found out." Al spread his hands in front of him as he explained. "He was in his fifties."

Mr. Hinds raised his eyebrows. "Hmmmm. Maybe the guilt got to him."

Al snorted again derisively before returning to pushing the carriage. "Maybe he ate wrong, drank too much and never exercised. Personally, I don't think they ever gave me or my family a second thought." Al thought he was past any anger he felt toward the men, but knowledge of the one man's death brought it all back. He knew now that any hope was gone that one or all three of the men who under his supervision and without his permission built the contraption that nearly killed him would show up at his door one day to apologize.

Mr. Hinds could feel his son-in-law's justified anger rising. "You're alive, he's not. These feelings of anger are going to come up. Don't think just because you accept your life as it is that you're over what happened to you. When the anger comes up, let it come. These guys screwed up, you did your job, and you paid the price." He peeked over at the two boys still babbling to each other.

Al walked quietly for a couple moments. "Dad I will see the new baby."

Mr. Hinds shook his head in agreement. "Yes, you will. Patience is something you've always had and if this camera implant Dr. Leesville offered is going to work, you have to let him do his job and do what he tells you to do."

"Of, course." Al felt the rise of determination inside him driven by hope. "I'm going to be dealing with Dr. Leesville and another doctor named Elbac. I haven't seen him yet. According to Leesville, Elbac wants to leave the left eye as a spare and implant the camera in the right eye."

The older man nodded his head in agreement. "That makes sense."

"They both feel I'm several years out from the ability to do this." They reached the stop sign.

Mr. Hinds tapped Al on the shoulder. "Let's turn around. We're at the end of the street. I should probably head to work early myself."

Al dutifully turned the carriage around and the two men walked back to the house with the babbling of the children as background. Al left his father-in-law at his car as Rose helped get both children into the house. The backdoor shut and he turned to put the carriage away as he heard another car pull into the driveway.

Several female voices shouted together cheerily from the convertible they drove. "Hi, Al!"

Al recognized the voices immediately. "Hi ladies. Is it that time already?"

"It sure is." The two young girls practically jumped out of the convertible with enthusiasm.

Unknown to Al or the two women, Sue from two houses down was pushing her son in his carriage just as the women pulled into the driveway. She couldn't believe what she saw. Thinking Elaine wasn't at home, she walked quickly back to her house both embarrassed and ashamed for Elaine.

"So, what are we covering today?" Al felt an arm slip through his.

"Chemistry. We aren't sure we want to learn it anymore. Could you teach us how to cheat?" The two girls giggled in unison as the back door opened.

"Hi girls." Elaine leaned against the door frame smirking.

"Hi Alaine. We were just kidding about the cheating thing." All the girls from nursing school adopted a new pronunciation for Elaine that had begun to take hold outside the classroom, but they did not include Al in this.

The small group started into the kitchen and past an eye rolling Elaine. "I know. Al wouldn't let you cheat anyway."

"Unfortunately, I guess we have to learn and understand this stuff even though for the life of me I can't see how it pertains to nursing." The girls each handed Al money.

"Thank you for the extra work girls. I'm expanding to high school kids this school year. I've had parents already asking Elaine." Al shoved the money into his pocket as Elaine headed out the back door.

"Al, I have to run an errand. I'll be back in an hour." She left quickly.

Al escorted the girls into the dining room where he had set up his tutoring. The minute Larry spotted the girls he jumped away from his grandmother and ran for a hug.

"Oh, this one is so cute!" Exclaimed the blond. "I mean, all the boys are cute, but this one is coming home with me."

In spite of the constant interruption from Larry, Al managed to cover all the tutoring needs of the women in the hour they paid him for. The girls were gathering up their books as Elaine came in the back door laughing.

"What's so funny?" Al stayed seated and waited to hear what he missed.

"You are not going to believe this. I was on my way to the post office when Sue from down the street waves at me with both her arms over her head with a scared look on her face. I thought something terrible had happened so I pulled into her driveway. She walks right up to me, very upset, with her baby on her hip and tells me she has something I need to hear." Elaine stopped in the middle of her story to laugh again. "I'm thinking her marriage is breaking up or something like that, but it turns out she is worried about mine." She starts to laugh uncontrollably again.

Al stood up. "What is so funny about our marriage?"

"There's a one liner if ever I heard one." Carol, the younger of the two women could not resist the opening.

"She saw the girls coming in the convertible for their tutoring session and apparently didn't hear all of the conversation only the flirty part." Elaine started to laugh. "She thinks you're sneaking around behind my back with young girls."

Now all three women were laughing.

Al held both hands up in defense. "Whoah, hey, what's so funny about that? I still got it." He jutted his chin out with a smirk.

Elaine suddenly felt bad, as she thought Al might think she was laughing at him. "That's not what I was laughing at. You absolutely still have it, but if you try to use it, I'll kill you. Everyone knows that."

The two younger women made a low noise together. "She's not kidding. No one messes with Alaine or her stuff."

He felt Elaine stand next to him. "Now I'm stuff'?" He scratched his head. "I feel like a piece of meat." Al slipped an arm around Elaine's waist. "I guess that's not such a bad thing."

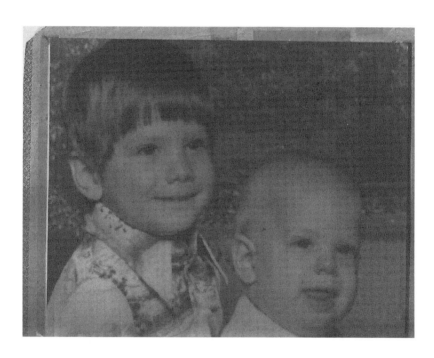

Albert Jr. and Lawrence Plevier: 1976

Jayne Kelly

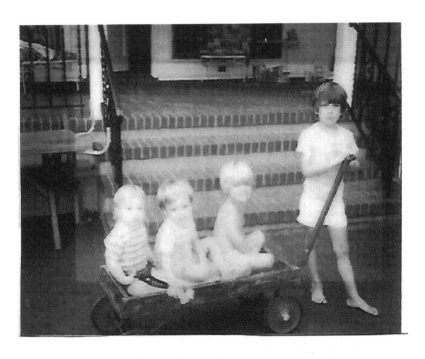

Nicholas, Christopher, Lawrence and Albert Jr. 1979

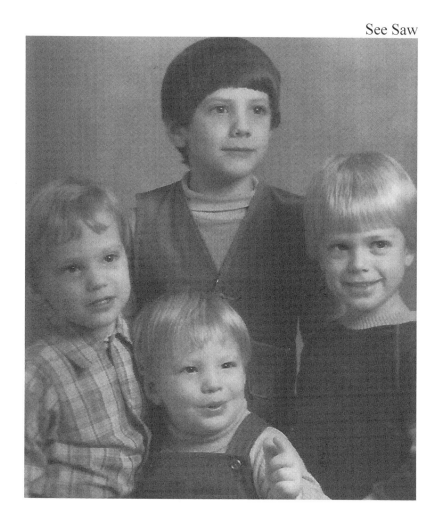

Clockwise from top: Albert Jr., Lawrence, Nicholas and Christopher Plevier 1979

Jayne Kelly

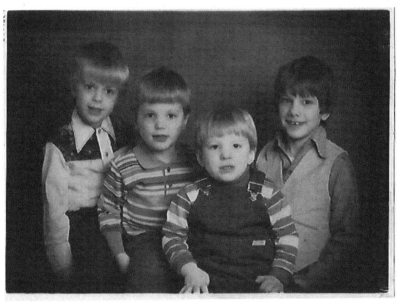

Left to Right: Lawrence, Christopher, Nicholas and Albert Plevier circa 1980: Ridgeview Terrace NJ

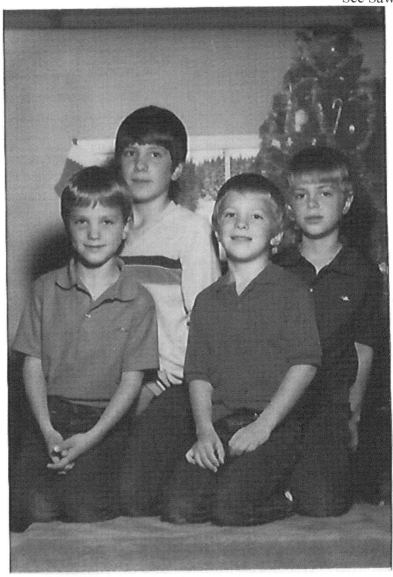

Left to Right: Christopher, Albert Jr. Nicholas and Lawrence Plevier: 1984: Audonbon Parway, NJ

Chapter XI: Outside

Super Bowl XIII was going well for Al. The half-time show featuring Caribbean bands took the field in Miami and he turned down the radio to go to the fridge. A Jets fan at heart, he had to make a choice between the two teams that made it to the Super Bowl and he had bet twenty dollars on the Steelers only for geographic reasons. Texas seemed too far away.

Elaine came into the kitchen with one hand on her back and one arm over her expanded middle. "Call Dad. I need a ride to the hospital. It's time."

Al went on high alert. "Where's Mom?"

Elaine tried to breathe and relax herself into the contractions. "She's going to stay with the boys. Call Dad."

Al made his way over to the phone and pushed the buttons, remembering how quickly Christopher had been born. Mr. Hinds picked up on the third ring. "Dad, it's time. We need a ride to the hospital."

Mr. Hinds turned away from his TV. "I'm on my way. Hey, how bout that last play?"

Al's thoughts about the game had vanished. "Yeah, yeah, we'll talk in the car." Al hung up the phone and turned to Elaine. "Are we going to make it or should I call for an ambulance?"

"We're good. Call Ronnie and Fenna to help mom with the boys. I hope Fenna will bring her two kids so Mom will

154

have all her grandchildren running around like tornadoes for a couple hours. That will make the boys happy." She closed her eyes as another pain washed over her. "Maybe I was wrong. We need to get a move on, please. This one is not going to wait."

But the fourth Plevier child did wait. After Elaine arrived at the hospital what she thought were contractions stopped. Al and his father-in-law caught the highlights from the Super Bowl on the car radio driving home late that night with a tired Elaine in the back seat.

She looked sheepishly at the back of her father and Al's heads. "How mad are you guys?"

"Shhhh." Al leaned into the speakers as Mr. Hinds stared transfixed through the windshield.

Elaine breathed out heavily. "Let nothing get in the way of sports in this household." She looked dejectedly out the window at the darkness when neither acknowledged her statement.

Not realizing how rude he was, Al continued his conversation with Mr. Hinds. "Dad, I have to tell you, listening to football and baseball on the radio is better than being at the games with or without sight." Al inclined his head toward the older man.

"You don't mind having a conversation with him, but I'm interrupting the announcer when I try to talk." Again, she was ignored.

"I know what you mean, Son. I used to love going to the games when I was a kid. Not anymore." He glanced over at Al with guilt. "I hate to tell you, but when I took you to the Yankee game over the summer, I was bored to tears."

Al laughed good naturedly. "Don't worry about it. I fell asleep on the guy next to me when you were in the john. He started to yell and then realized I couldn't see. He thought the sunglasses were actually for the sun." The two men laughed together as Al continued. "Hockey is the worst. I don't have any interest in going to a live game for any sport without sight. The radio announcers give you me a great summary from all the angles."

Mr. Hinds continued to stare out the windshield. "With or without sight I think listening to the announcers is the best way. I can get up and do jobs around the house as long as I have the TV up loud." He thought back to November when his wife came into the room and turned down the TV. They had the biggest fight of their marriage.

Al was still oblivious to how both men were ignoring Elaine in the back seat as the conversation turned inevitable to coaching. "The structure of baseball is going to enable me to coach the boys effectively. I could never do it with basketball. Football would be the next best alternative but not as good as baseball. Baseball's a slow game. There are rules and I can slow it down further when needed." Al played out in his head several scenarios he wanted to utilize to help teach Albert the game this spring when he starts T-ball.

Mr. Hinds was mulling over the outcome of the Super Bowl and half listening to Al. "We talked about your focus on coaching the boys in baseball. I know you'll do it, but I think you're going to need a head coach to buddy up with. You'll need a set of eyes on the field with you."

Al swallowed his pride before he spoke. "I know there's no way around that. I'll find a coach to prove it's possible." He realized his father-in-law was distracted. "Dad, how was the point spread for you? I never asked."

"It was good. I did fine." He left the answer hanging in the air. "I told you before I have no doubts you can coach. The people you're going to have to convince are the powers that run the league. Make friends with those parents ahead of time. That will not only help, it will allow it to happen." Mr. Hinds relaxed into the driver's seat as the clear night sky reflected on the windshield.

Elaine spoke up from the backseat. "You'll need me to pave the road for you, Al. You're a great guy, but sometimes you're like a bull in a china shop getting to know people. You always have been." Elaine was tired of the two men ignoring her.

"Thanks, Dear. I love you too." Al turned around in the seat, very aware that they had been so caught up with sports he overlooked his very pregnant wife. "I'm sorry, Sweetheart."

A sullen, hormonal Elaine began to let her anger show. "Sorry I messed up your plans for the evening. I happen to be exhausted and starving. Who is going to make me something to eat when we get home?"

Al smiled at her. "Me. I'm sorry again. The Super Bowl was a good game this year and we just got caught up in it."

She answered him sarcastically. "It's fine."

Al's smile faded. "No. This little one is as important as its three brothers. I guess when we knew this wasn't the real moment, we relaxed."

Elaine started to feel guilty, knowing it was her hunger and the night's events making her cranky. "I'm sure when the real time comes we will all be on board with the urgency and importance of the moment.

Two weeks later on February 5 she felt contractions again, but this time Elaine was less anxious and took several hours to set up the three boys at home. Her mother drove them to the hospital and while Mrs. Hinds helped Al fill out the paperwork, a nurse came up to them.

"Mr. Plevier?" Directly by Elaine that her husband didn't have sight, the nurse approached the only blind man in the reception area.

"Yes?" Al dropped his hand from Mrs. Hinds shoulder.

Mrs. Hinds looked at the nurse with concerned look. "Has the doctor arrived?"

The nurse smiled broadly shaking her head. "No. He hasn't arrived yet, but your new baby has." She laughed good naturedly.

"Whoah. That was fast." Al had a look of shock.

"Would you like to come with me? Your wife is amazing." The proud nurse beamed at her accomplishment of delivering the baby alone and the young family in front of her. "I'm so happy for you." The nurse smiled to Mrs. Hinds. "She said she was here a couple weeks ago with a false alarm. This little one must be a practical joker. I hope you're prepared." The jovial nurse walked next to Mrs. Hinds. "Congratulations again. There is a shift nurse with Elaine working on getting her room ready. I'm directing you to the delivery area and then I'm going to leave you. I have two other ladies that have just come in. It's a busy day here."

Al was speechless and thrilled. Mrs. Hinds spoke for both of them. "Thank you so much for bringing the baby into the world safely. I do believe my daughter thought it was a false alarm again. Her contractions were five minutes apart at the closest and then they would stop."

The nurse nodded in agreement. "Your wife said this was the fourth baby. Every delivery is different. You just never know."

Al and Mrs. Hinds were brought to an open area separated by drawn curtains. Elaine was in the room with four other women.

Crying babies was all Al heard. "Listen to that, Mom."

"Al?" Elaine was in the bed immediately in front of the drawn curtains. The nurse pulled other curtains around her bed to give the family privacy.

"Hi, Sweetheart. How are you?" He found the edge of the bed and leaned to where he had heard her voice and realized one of the crying infants was with Elaine.

She kissed him lightly. "It's another boy. I told you we were building the baseball team you always wanted." Elaine cradled her newborn safely to her.

"Wow. This is amazing. He sounds healthy and strong." Al stood straight up. "Did they give you a bassinet yet? You must be too tired to hold him."

"I'm fine. Honestly, this one came so fast it hardly drained my energy." She cuddled the baby. "I love holding him. Al, give me your hand."

He hung his cane on the side of the bed and lifted

158

his right hand to her. Elaine guided his hand until he felt his forefinger poking a little fist that wrapped itself around it.

"Wow." The moment settled in for all three of them as Mrs. Hinds looked on silently. "We need a name for this little guy."

Elaine looked thoughtfully at the newborn who answered her gaze with wide eyes. "If we had a little girl she would have been Nicole, so let's go with Nicholas."

Al felt the baby grip his finger tighter each time he cried out. "I think little Nicholas is hungry. Being born takes a lot out of a guy."

Elaine looked at the baby intently. "You're probably right." She watched Al's expression. "Nicholas, you have a very special place in our family. You're going to be the youngest."

Al heard the finality of Elaine's tone and was aware his mother-in-law was still standing in the room. "Four is a nice even number. I like even numbers. This little power house rounds out our family. Welcome little one. You've got three brothers at home waiting for you."

Once the new baby was home, it became clear to Elaine and Al that the time had come to give serious consideration to settling the lawsuit and moving on with their lives. The size of the Lake Road home alone gave them the incentive to move before the four boys got older. The monetary judgement, if any, would help them recoup the financial losses that occurred at the time of the accident and allow them to begin to rebuild their future.

A cozy winter evening after the Albert, Larry and Chris had been put to bed, Al held a sleeping Nick as he and Elaine discussed the case. "I'd prefer to keep fighting, Sweetheart."

Elaine sipped her tea and weighed her words. "I understand that." They were both quiet before she spoke again. "We both found out how short life can be and that it can change in an instant." She paused again. "I'd like to move past the legal issues and focus on our family. If we don't settle the case, the associated issues will be a constant distraction." Her thoughts went immediately to Al's mood after the depositions. "You stayed down in the basement for hours after the depositions trying to move past how upset it made you."

"I remember. That humiliating experience is one of the reasons I'd like to continue to fight." Pride and revenge were rising inside him again and then he felt Nick stir in his arms. "Elaine, you five come first. I thought fighting to the bitter end would benefit all of us, but maybe I'm wrong. I can admit that."

She watched the infant settle into his bundling. "I believe you are wrong on this point. We have four children to raise and I don't want to miss a second of that time with unnecessary distractions. If the attorney feels that we can settle with a reasonable offer, then we should take it."

Al thought back to the conversation he had with Mr. Bayplaza several weeks before Nick's birth. "There is a number that the attorney mentioned as a target to begin negotiations." Al had felt deflated that day, sitting in the attorney's office. "The beginning dollar amount he mentioned may not be where we end up but it is the place to start." He wanted to go to trial even as he and Elaine logically worked through the practicality of settling.

This was the first discussion Al had with her about the conversation he had with the attorney concerning a actual possible settlement amount instead of a trial. "How does it work? Will you be in the office to agree or disagree when they begin negotiations?" He felt an unspoken decision had been made that they were going to settle. "No. According to Mr. Bayplaza I cannot be in the room which doesn't make sense to me."

His frustration was obvious to Elaine, but she wanted to keep him focused on settling. "We have to trust him and the fact that he has won many cases. I know he has our best interests prioritized." She knew they were working as a team and believed there was an end in sight to the case.

"Elaine, remember that we have to pay back the Worker's Compensation I have been paid so far. That comes right off the top of any settlement money. After the settlement, I will no longer collect from Worker's Compensation. I will collect from Social Security." Al wanted all the terms of their financial future regurgitated and clear when they made the final decision.

"I remember most of this from the initial conversations with the attorney. Collecting from two federally funded agencies is not possible. What I have a hard time making sense of is paying back the Worker's Compensation. You paid into that every paycheck. You also had the private insurance policy. They made us choose between the two and the private insurance would not have had to be paid back. That bothers me." Elaine looked at the tired, stoney expression on Al's face.

"We have no recourse for that. The focus has to be on getting the largest amount possible to cover the lawyer's fee and still have enough for us to move forward with our lives." Al and one of the younger attorneys at Mr. Bayplaza's firm felt they would have a better chance at a larger settlement if they set a precedent, but he was not in this fight alone. Setting a precedent would mean dragging on the court case and pulling his family with him. He knew that was no longer an option.

"Call the attorney tomorrow and find out if we are in the position of negotiating a settlement. In the best scenario, I would like to be out of this house before the spring flooding season but that can't happen without the settlement money. After paying off the mortgage we won't be able to buy anything else if we sell this house before the settlement." Elaine reiterated facts they both knew.

Al's cousin was ready to purchase the home and did not have concerns about the flooding. He and his wife felt the below market rate they were going to pay for the house would compensate for any inconvenieces. Elaine and Al had to consider that the potential for continual flooding was unmanageable for them with their current life circumstances. Last year the river rose high enough to swamp the property.

"Elaine, I don't want to be here this year for flood season either. The river was such an issue last year that I believe it's more than we should be handling with our little tribe." Al handed Nick to Elaine as he began to fuss for his bottle.

"I agree. We have enough to deal with." She stepped over toys as she walked with a fussing Nicholas.

"I'll call the attorney's office tomorrow. Through him I'll get an idea if we can proceed with settlement discussions without showing our hand. I was hoping MTZW would present something first. I don't want to look desperate and negatively affect an offer." Al played poker in college at a regular game night and knew the value of a good bluff.

Unfortunately for the Plevier family, MTZW was fully aware of the birth of the fourth baby boy and their financial constraints and considerations. However, the company was also aware of how the plight of a blind man with a wife and his four babies may look to a jury. All sides were becoming anxious to settle.

If the case did not settle, a trial would mean more public displays. Al's scars would never heal and this time it would be his attorney that would request Al to disrobe for the jury so that they would see the full impact of what he dealt with daily. The initial fury Al had felt after disrobing for the deposition, has dissipated and he was now more than willing to make the other side appear heartless and callous.

A returned phone call from his attorney, on a blustery, rainy late winter morning solidified their trajectory. "Al, I think you and Elaine are wise to set the ball rolling in this direction. Even if you and your wife won a trial settlement, the company appeals could last another decade or more. You have growing boys." Mr. Bayplaza had been hoping the young couple would embrace the reality of their situation.

"When this started, I was naïve enough to believe the companies would have been intimidated to settle early. I did not know that accidents of the proportions I experienced have been happening regularly in the industry for many years. Hospital's and doctor's waiting rooms confirmed that for me."

"It's a sad commentary on your former industry." He

paused. "To be completely honest negligence cases are wide spread." The attorney gazed over at a stack of files.

"Based on what I've seen and heard in the last five years, I believe you." The sound of a baby fussing and little boys chatter carried to him from the bedroom hallway. "What is the next step?"

"I'll reach out to the other side today and get a meeting date. What's your availability?" He pulled out his datebook from under one of the Plevier files.

Al snorted sarcastically. "Whatever works for you. My mother is living with us so we have backup if Elaine needs to drive me."

A wave of compassion and genuine caring flooded the attorney. "I'll pick you up. You have a new baby at home."

"Are we going to a courtroom to mediate the discussions?" A sense of dread washed over him.

"Yes. There will be a court reporter present. I'll try to have a private room for you to relax in." Strategy, a familiar subject for the seasoned attorney, was being set in motion.

The little Plevier tribe traveled as one unit into the family room. Rose Plevier walked heavily down the stairs to greet everyone. Al heard them getting louder and his heart warmed.

"Let's do this. Call me with the date." Both Al and the attorney hung up without pleasantries. "Hey Elaine. I'm taking on the attributes of a lawyer. Rude, brash and to the point. Maybe I should go back to school."

She came into the room with Christopher toddling after her. "You and I have learned enough to consider our experience a crash course in the legal, medical and establishment systems I hardly knew existed."

Al was pensive. "Here we go, Sweetheart."

Their attorney phoned back two hours later. "Al, the other side is anxious to settle this. They were looking for an opening. You need to be available on Friday."

"Friday? Why would they choose the last day of a work week?" The logic of a lawyer never ceased to amaze him.

"To get inside your head over the weekend. This will not be finalized on Friday. Be clear on that. Above all do not let it ruin your weekend or think about the outcome until we are in the next meeting. It's just part of the game." The attorney was energized for the fight. His attack positioning was the attribute that made him successful.

Game. This is a game to them. Maybe they wouldn't feel that way if they had to dip the tips of their fingers in concentrated sodium hydroxide for five full seconds.

"Al? Are you there?" The attorney was expecting Al to be as excited as he was.

"Yeah, sorry. I was lost in my thoughts for a moment." He shook himself to stay with the conversation and Elaine saw the movement. "What time are you picking me up on Friday?"

"Eight a.m. The meeting starts at ten am and I want you relaxed. See you then." For the second time that day he hung up without courtesies.

Al replaced the receiver slowly. "It's happening faster than we thought. I don't know if that's good or bad."

Elaine picked up Christopher. "It is what it is."

Friday morning Al found himself seated on a bench in the hallway of the courthouse. Al was already uncomfortable in an unforgiving hard wood bench alone. There would be no one for him to talk to except when Mr. Bayplaza came to discuss each offer presented.

"Al, don't expect this to be settled today. You have to be here so please make yourself comfortable. There a glass of water next to you and I can bring in anything else you might want when I come in to present offers to you." The anxious attorney was pacing.

"This day would go quicker if you let me inside the negotiation room." Al knew he would probably fall asleep within the first fifteen minutes of being left alone despite his seating accommodations.

"No. The principles of MTZW will not be present either. Today only the attorneys will be at the table negotiating." His attorney looked up as the door across the hall opened and a young woman stuck her head out.

"Mr. Bayplaza, they're ready." She left immediately.

The lawyer spoke quickly. "There is a men's bathroom down the hall on the right. I brought you a bagel from the shop across the street. Raisin with butter. Would you like coffee?"

"No coffee for the moment, thank you." Al wanted to be able to maneuver alone as much as possible for the day. "Thank you for setting me up. I hope this isn't as long as you think it will be."

The lawyer spoke low and serious. "It will be. Settle in." The attorney looked. "Here we go."

Al made himself comfortable and being alone helped. He drifted off with his head resting against the wall behind him not sure where he was or what day it was when he felt someone tap him on the arm.

"Jack? Mary? Elaine?" He groggily began to come around when a male voice greeted him.

"Al, it's Art Bayplaza. Wake up." The attorney stood across from Al staring down at him.

He sat up straight and tried to shake off the grogginess. "Oh, sorry. Fell asleep."

"We have a number." The attorney held a paper in front of him. "We are also breaking for lunch. It's noon."

Al sat up straight and cleared his head. "I'm ready."

"Four hundred thousand before my fee and pay back to Worker's Compensation." The lawyer deadpanned the amount.

"No." Al didn't hesitate.

"Good. Remember my job is to present all offers. I'm countering with $750,000." The electricity emanating from the negotiating attorney was felt by Al.

"Go higher. Counter at an even million and see what happens."

The lawyer did not answer. "Want to take a walk with me and get lunch?"

After the break for lunch Al did not have to wait too long for an answer to their counter. He was beginning to drift off again in the chair when Art came in and foregoing any polite entries, jumped into speaking mid sentence. "$500,000. They countered at half a million."

Al sat up again. "Counter at $900,000. We can do this all day and then next week."

Art left the room unceremoniously. Al was alone for another hour as Friday afternoon wound down.

The attorney walked in with hard steps. Al was not impressed by this blatant play on the serious nature of the negotiations. He didn't even ask if Al was awake before he started to talk.

"They came back at $780,000, firm. No further negotiations." Mr. Bayplaza walked around and then took a seat next to Al, sitting tall, that gave presentation and authentication to his position. The fact that his client could not see the gesture did not matter to him.

Al did a mental calculation in his mind at what he and Elaine would net after the attorney's fee and paying back Worker's Compensation. "That leaves Elaine and I with $365000."

"Yes. That's better than I hoped for. Victims hurt on the job usually get next to nothing due to the Worker's Compensation Laws." The attorney leaned back.

"Have they left?" Al was not feeling grateful and did not appreciate the lesson in gratitude the attorney was approaching him with.

"Yes. They wanted to give you something to think about over the weekend. I discussed with you that they would use this tactic." He looked at the stubborn expression on his client's face.

"Can you drive me home now? If you're busy I can call my father-in-law." Al would not make a final decision on anything without discussing the topic with Elaine.

"I'll drive you home. This was my only appointment today. We can talk on the ride." Both the attorney and Al rose at the same time. "Keep in mind the story of the Postal Service car accident that was proven to be the fault of the Postal Driver.

The victim was injured permanently, the case dragged on for fifteen years and the victim received nothing."

"Art, I'm aware of the facts against us. I need time to discuss this with my wife." Al occassionally referred to his attorney by his first name and it was usually indicative of stress. "Before you bring it up, I haven't forgotten about the man who lost both his hands in the pipe cutting accident either. The case was left to the bench to decide and the victim was determined to be sixty percent responsible for a machine override the manager installed." He was cranky and the attorney did not shrink away from an attitude he dealt with every day from different clients.

The car ride back to Lake Road seemed to take forever. Art continuously went over percentages, case studies, and options available to Al and Elaine. Within the options, he mentioned were the long, term goals of the family in regard to their future and their children's future.

When the car pulled into the circular driveway Al knew without sight that he was home. "Art, thank you for everything. I will have an answer for you first thing Monday morning. I guess these guys succeeded in getting inside my head for the weekend." This time it was him who exited unceremoniously.

Elaine was upstairs and had seen the car pull in. She left her mother-in-laws tiny one room living quarters without comment. Rose Plevier knew what was at stake and worried incessantly about her son and his family. She did not follow Elaine downstairs. Blind hope kept her upstairs entertaining Albert and Larry with new army men she bought for them. Chris and Nick slept side by side on her double bed, taking a nap that they had fought all afternoon. Looking at the two boys, she knew it would be a long evening.

Al was already at the kitchen counter leaning heavily on it. "Hi Al. How are you?"

"Busted. That's the only way to describe it." He felt around the counter for something to nibble on.

"I can make dinner early if you want. The boys are getting pizza because it's Friday." She looked at the lines on his face which understood intuitively were from anger and fatigue.

"Naw. I can wait. All I'm looking for is something to nibble on. Art took me out to lunch." The usage of the attorney's first name was noted silently by Elaine.

Instinctively she felt the frustration and helplessness Al was exhibiting. "Do you want to talk about this while Mom has the boys upstairs or do you want to wait until tonight when we're alone?"

"It will take at least an hour to go through this with you. Do we have that kind of time?" Al found a half eaten peanut butter and jelly sandwich. "What do I have in my hand?" He held the sandwich up to Elaine.

"The remainder of Christopher's lunch. Peanut butter and jelly. The bread is probably hard. It's been sitting out for a couple of hours." She watched Al shove the lunch scrap into his mouth.

He swallowed hard and walked wordlessly to the fridge for milk. Feeling the marked container, he drank straight from the fresh bottle and emptied it. He dropped the bottle hard on the counter and walked back his seat.

She followed him to a seat at the breakfast bar. "What's our move?"

He took a deep breath. "The last offer was $780,000." She was silent. "After the lawyer, paying back Workman's Compensation, and refunding the law firm for the expert testimonies that were needed, we net $365,000." She was still silent. "Art said that was their final offer. If we reject it, we move forward with a trial."

"Do you think they're bluffing?" She played nervously with a magazine.

"Maybe. It's hard to tell. He was very serious and pushy about this offer. If we don't take this, it might be ten years before we receive money if we do win. I feel that we would win, otherwise they would not want to settle at all. It is going to take a long time. I would have to schedule work around court dates, not the other way around." They were both quiet. "We have to think about the boys."

Elaine grabbed a pen and started to write on the back of the magazine. "How much was the expert testimony?"

Al shook his head. "I have no idea of the total but they were all $1500 per hour. Even when the court date was canceled, we still had to pay them for the time."

She continued to write down figures. "With that balance, we would have enough to buy a house outright, a new car, some furniture with cash, and invest the balance in stocks or keep it in the bank. We could reinvest the interest if we are able to live off of my nursing work, your woodworking, telemarketing, and the Social Security."

He turned to her. "You're considering accepting the offer?"

"I think we should spend the weekend giving it serious consideration." She stared at the numbers she had calculated.

"That is exactly what Art said they would want, to be inside our heads for the weekend. That's why they called for a Friday meeting. Looks like their strategy worked." He heard little feet on the stairs. "Looks like we didn't get our hour."

"We have something to mull over. Over the rest of the weekend we can discuss details." Chris came up to her dragging a blanket. "We've always done well with real estate, Al. I'm confident we can invest the money properly and have it grow."

Al believed Elaine had made her decision. "I knew this was never going to be a windfall that carried us into a mansion, but it is enough to get us back on our feet."

Elaine picked up Chris who then laid placidly in her arms. "I don't want to roll the dice. We need to have a solid understanding of the parameters of our finances."

More feet were heard on the stairs. Rose came down carrying Nick. Walking behind her, Albert and Larry carried fistfuls of little, plastic, green army men. The two boys landed on the shag carpet immediately dumping and intermingling their inventory.

Jayne Kelly

"Mommy when can we have pizza?" Albert spoke to his mom but did not take his gaze off his brother or their shared toys.

Elaine readjusted Chris to her shoulder and turned to face Albert. "Say hi to Daddy."

Chris lifted his head and answered for his brothers. "Hi Daddy." He saw what his brothers were doing and squirmed out of Elaine's arms.

Albert still did not look up from his toys. "Hi Daddy. You weren't at the bus stop today. It's Friday."

"Teacher taught you the days of the week?" Al thought all his children were sponges.

Albert looked down at the line Larry had built with his men. "I know lots, Daddy."

"I believe you. Do you know what kind of pizza you want?" The banter with his children dissolved the angst he had developed all day.

Albert and Larry's head both shot up and they spoke together. "Cheese. No peppies."

His children learned early to avoid the little round circles that were their dad's favorite topping. "How about one cheese and one with pepperoni?"

The two looked at Al cautiously as Chris ambled over to them still clinging to his blanket. Both boys nodded at him. "Good."

"I'll take that as a yes. Mom? Does that work for you?" He heard Elaine pushing the buttons on the phone.

Rose looked carefully at her son. "That's perfect." She held Nick over her shoulder and rubbed his back. "You look tired, Son."

"It was a long afternoon. I caught a couple naps while the lords were negotiating my family's future. They should have let me into the room while they were negotiating."

Elaine watched him and listened as she ordered the pies. "Yes, one cheese and one pepperoni both large. Thank you." She hung up. "Boys, the pizza will be here in a little while."

The boys lost interest in the tone of their dad's voice. Elaine leaned in close. "Al, let's talk about this later."

"I'm sorry Elaine. I brought it up. He looks worn down. I didn't mean to stir a bad subject." Rose Plevier always supported Elaine.

"It's okay, Mom. Al did have a difficult day. We've started working through the offer. It's a lot to absorb." Elaine tried not to disclose how nervous she was to either Al or Rose.

Rose was protective of both Al and Elaine. They both had insisted she come live with them when, after she purchased a small home on Shore Road, someone had tried to break in. At her advanced age, the event had shaken her. In all the years' she had lived in Patterson, before and after her husband died, she had always felt safe. She had never been a victim of a violent or non-violent crime. They would not allow her to help them financially either. When her own home sold, she offered to buy into theirs, but they said no. It was enough to have her with them and they joked that all the free babysitting she offered more than paid her way in the house.

The family was busy for the rest of the weekend only allowing time in the evening for Al and Elaine to review the settlement parameters. The lawsuit started with nine companies named in 1975. In January of this year, the attorney had informed him that they were down to three and the two small companies were settling. The smaller settlements with the two other companies were only a negotiation tactic to pit those companies against MTZW and create leverage needed for the main target company that created the failed shower head.

Sunday night Al sat beside Elaine on the couch after the boys went to bed. "I still wonder how much damage could have been halted if the shower head hadn't failed. OSHA had just been in the plant two weeks before the accident. They gave it a passing grade. No one tested the shower. If it had worked that day, I would not have left the shower stall until all the chemicals were off my body. They would have had to drag me out of the shower."

Elaine looked at his worn and tired expression. "Al, this is why we have to put this behind us. I don't want you to relive the accident over and over again. You are alive. You survived. You have moved past it and the lawsuit by necessity requires you to go over and over every detail. I'm more convinced than ever that we must agree to a settlement." She leaned her head onto his shoulder. "You have the possibility of an experimental surgery in the future. You don't need a legal proceeding adding to your stress. I'm adamant Al. It's time."

He knew she was right. They still had a life to live. "I agree. The fighter in me may have to be reconvinced."

"Pick up one of your sons. Hold him tight and dream of the surgery being successful. That will be all the convincing you need." She relaxed against him. "I'm grateful all the medical bills and hospital stays were covered. That would have bankrupted us. The first stay immediately after the accident was $28,000. I'm grateful that Dad stepped up to force us to talk to the attorney. I was so naïve. I thought it was a good thing to just have the medical bills paid in full. I wasn't thinking about our future. We were concentrating on your survival and quality of life in your recovery. God Bless Dad and our families for watching out for us."

He nodded in acknowledgement. "We will be able to be there for them with the settlement money." Al's thoughts went to utilization of the settlement and in that moment, he knew he was completely ready to settle. "I want to take the boys to Disney when their older. We could bring the extended family."

She smiled and snuggled closer. "Moving forward."

Monday, after Albert was on the bus for school, Al and Elaine called the attorney. "Art, we're accepting the $780,000 offer to settle. We ran the numbers after you, Worker's Compensation, and the expert witnesses are paid and the we still came up with a final number of $365,000. Do you agree with that?"

The attorney nodded his head in agreement while alone in his office. "Before I call the opposing counsel I will have my paralegal finalize all the expenses. I will make it her first job today. The office will call you with the final accounting and then you can reaffirm your acceptance of the offer." The attorney pulled the top file off the Plevier stack on his desk.

"Thank you, Mr. Bayplaza, for everything." Relief spread throughout Al's body.

"I'm glad I could be a part of moving your family past this terrible event. We'll be in touch by this afternoon." He hung up the phone without saying good-bye.

Al breathed deeply. His mind was already planning out the wisest investments.

Chapter XII: Love

"Have Mike and Nettie write up the contract tomorrow. I trust them. They're family." Al paused while he did a mental calculation. "We bought the house for $23,000, so I feel we're doing okay by selling it to Mike and Nattie for $45,000. I know it's worth $70,000 in this market, but we have the settlement money to invest. They can't afford $70,000 and after how wonderful they were to us when we almost lost everything, I'm not looking back. Did you like any of the houses we saw last weekend?" He sat down on the floor with Christopher and tried to entertain the little boy to no avail. Christopher wanted to be outside on this rainy day.

"Al, are they confident that they can handle spring rains and the subsequent flooding? I'm starting to worry about that, not the loss we are taking financially." She slipped a bottle into Nicholas' mouth and all the boys seemed to quiet down along with him. "I liked 50 Ridgeview Terrace. Albert won't have to switch schools, it's a bit larger than this house and it has a finished basement. We can throw all the toys down there." She looked over the entire brood. "We'll be moving before summer so the boys will be able to enjoy the pool."

"If you like that one, why don't we make an offer? I'm good with whatever you choose as long as it's within the budget." Al ripped open a small bag of peanuts he had in his pocket and tossed them into his mouth. "To be completely honest, I gave Mike and Nettie that price point when we thought we would be settling quicker and we would have the ability to buy something nicer. It isn't fair to stick it to them because the case moved slower and we just settled this year. Our family needs more space, and we can afford to give the boys a large yard that doesn't get flooded."

Elaine studied the baby as he ate. "Al, this one is going to grow as quickly as his brothers. He eats like a linebacker."

"He should. He was almost born on Super Bowl Sunday." Al thought he would make Elaine laugh. "I'm going to turn the next yard into a park like I did for this one. If the house has an inground pool then that is a big bonus."

She didn't laugh. "Life is different now that we are working on our budget instead of trying to create a budget out of thin air and the goodwill of those who love us." Elaine was lost in thought for a brief moment. "Ridgeview Terrace it is. 1979 is shaping up to be a great year for the Plevier family. Don't you agree, Nick?"

Three months later the family relaxed in their new home amid full and empty boxes repurposed as forts and moved into the basement by Albert and Larry. Nick and Chris shared a room and the only negative of the home they could discern was the absence of Grandma Rose. Al's mother had decided not to go with them and instead moved in with her daughter, Fenna, and her family. She lived only two miles from the new house, but it was an adjustment for everyone.

It was early June and the rainy day had forced the family inside. Elaine loved looking out the window, enjoying the falling rain and not being nervous about flooding or a leaking roof. The boys were not complaining about being stuck inside and continued to take over the basement. Al had surprised Elaine with a player piano a woman at the *Images Group* wanted to get rid of. It was an upright and built around the turn of the century. Just the kind of antique she revered even though

Al was still working on trying to get it to play correctly. He was working at the back of the piano when the doorbell rang.

"I got it Al. Keep working on the piano. I'm hoping you'll have it running tonight. The family is coming." She dropped a quick kiss on his head as she passed.

"You're already have company coming?" He finished what he was doing and pushed the piano against the wall.

"The boys will love it and it's easier than packing them up to go to the house of a relative. Mom and Fenna will probably help with the food." She opened the door without looking through the peephole the new house came with and the neighborhood didn't warrant.

Standing in front of her was Bob Kaye an old High School friend of both Al and Elaine. "Hi Elaine. I hope it's okay that I dropped by like this." He held out a plant as a house warming gift."

Elaine opened the door to hug. There was no screen door. It wasn't the type of neighborhood that coveted front storm doors.

"Bob it's so good to see you. Come in and check out the new place. We're settling in nicely." Elaine led him over to Al.

Al always took several seconds to place a voice to a face and now he realized it was Bob. "Hey Bob. How are you?" Al sat on the piano bench letting his fingers run across the keys as the music played.

"You finally learned to play an instrument. That's great. People expect that from blind guys." Bob was always sarcastically prodding his good friend.

Al remembered the plant Bob placed on his chest during his first hospital stay after the accident. "My mother made me take lessons as a kid. It's been years." He continued to let his fingers run freely across the keys. "I'm getting good."

"I hear that. Are you taking requests?" Bob made himself at home on the couch.

The music sheet from the piano finished and a new piece started. Al got up from the bench without missing a beat.

"What's new?"

"Nothing." Bob stopped short and gave his friend a sarcastic look. "Nicely done."

"All blind guys can play the piano or at least they can fix them." Al extended his hand toward Bob for the conciliatory shake.

Bob acquiesced. "I ran into your mom yesterday and she told me about the new house. I gave Elaine a plant from me and Kerry. I hope she likes it." Bob leaned back on the familiar red sofa. "Al, you could make extra money playing at some of the piano bars when you get bored. I could give you a ride. It'll be boy's night out. What do you think?"

He laughed at his friend's attempt at humor. "I'll keep it in mind." Al paused with something he wanted to ask Bob. "Do you and Kerry live closer to this house than the Lake Road house?"

Bob got excited thinking Al was seriously considering a boys' night out with him. "Yeah, I'm a half mile from here."

"The boy's night out sounds good. Elaine could use some time away from me." He hated to ask for rides from anyone even an old friend and he knew this was an opportunity for a boys' night without begging for a ride.

"You should have called me sooner. I miss hanging out with you. Between our two families we never get to see the old crew unless we're doing something with our wives and kids." Bob sounded as if he was as anxious to spend time out of the house as much as Al.

"You want anything to eat? Totally forgot to offer you something." In the past, before either of them were married, they would just help themselves to their parent's respective fridge. Bob was constantly dodging Al's Grandma Padula-a short, spunky Italian immigrant who believed in keeping young men in line.

"No, I just wanted to see how you're doing. Rose told me there might be another eye surgery on the horizon. That's great, man." Bob always felt his friend got a raw deal.

"I hope so. The doctor is just starting to discuss it with us. I'm trying not to count on it yet." Al heard a commotion in the basement. "Here we go. Sorry, Bob. The boys are really coming into their own. You can see why a night out would be refreshing. I spend more time policing and refereeing than on my wood working." He and Bob both mumbled in agreement. The commotion downstairs momentarily stopped. "Elaine mentioned you wanted to pick out a gift for Kerry from my projects. I should have my inventory unpacked in the next couple of months. I won't have a workroom set up for a while, but we can see if you like the stuff I still have from Lake Road."

"I'm sure there will be something for her." It got very quiet in the house. "Sounds like they worked it out down there."

Al listened carefully. "Quiet is not good. My apologies in advance if we have to cut our visit short."

Bob laughed good naturedly. "I have three myself. There's always a drama to work through. Don't know what I would do without it."

Yelling from the basement reignited at the same time Nick awoke from a nap. "That's no coincidence. It's a coin toss where to go first. Believe it or not we are getting a dog for the boys. I think we're nuts, but we all want a family pet."

"You get to it, Dad. I'll head out." Both men got up at the same time.

"Bob, I'll have Elaine call Kerry to get together as a couple, but let's not forget about a boys' night out. Maybe we could take in a game." Al knew going to a game would be a distraction in case their conversation became stilted after all these changes over the years. He walked smoothly through the room to the door.

"Good. Hey, I see you have the place mapped out already. You're looking good boss." The cacophony from the children grew.

"I had the schematic of the house in my head after the first week." Al stopped at the door. "Bob, thanks again. I have to get in the basement before they kill each other."

Al and Bob did not get their boys' night out. Instead

Elaine and Kerry decided on a couples' evening in the city with tickets to "Cats" the new musical sensation taking Broadway by storm. Elaine had brought the musical up several times and he had gently suggested she go with her sister or mother. Without sight theatre, movies and baseball games were just events he had to endure and try very hard not to fall asleep at.

"This is wonderful. Kerry and I have so much to catch up on. She has been wanting to see this show as much as I have." Elaine checked her hair and makeup in the mirror as they waited for Bob and Kerry to pick them up.

"Why didn't you and Kerry go into the city by yourselves? Bob and I could have gone out for a beer." Al could not summon a good disposition since he dreaded the night's events ahead of him.

"Because both of you are part of a couple and this is what couples do. We are not going to be the married people I see who do things separately. That is not a marriage." She got up from her vanity to storm into the living room to check on her mom with the boys.

When he thought she was out of hearing range he spoke out loud. "I bet those couples are happy."

She stopped dead in her tracks. "You're going to be happy too, whether you like it or not."

Bob greeted Al next to the car with the same enthusiasm. "We're married, buddy. This is it. Have a seat."

At the theatre in Manhattan, the men could not sit next to each other if they wanted peace. Elaine and Kerry talked continually until the lights went and down the show started. "Cats" was an interactive show with the actors coming into the audience to engage them. The two couples had splurged and purchased front row seats to the very visual production. Immediately before the start of the show, one actor rubbed against Al's leg and purred. The Patterson ingrained reaction was immediate and automatic: he kicked at the actor, hard.

The actor yelled and jumped back as Al's foot caught him in the side. "Ouch!"

Al sat straight up and rigid in the theatre seat. "Oh, sorry. What was that?"

Elaine elbowed him hard. "Shh. That was an actor. Everyone is staring at us."

Al could hear Bob snickering three seats away. Al assumed he was elbowed also and decided it might be better to slip into a nap. Relaxing into his seat he was jolted awake again, but this time it was to his right. He knew Elaine was on his left so confusion set in momentarily.

"Huh? What?" He turned his head from side to side and heard Bob snickering once more.

"Shh!" Elaine got very close to his ear. "The actors are right in front of us. Be quiet! You just fell asleep on a young girl's shoulder. She's looking at you like you're a pervert." Elaine sat stiffly in her chair until intermission.

Most if not all of the patrons had forgotten about the two small disturbances in Act I from Al with the exception of Elaine. As soon as the theatre began to empty out for intermission, she jumped on him.

"Are you kidding me? Do you know how much these seats cost? I have been waiting months to see this. We are able to do activities like this once again and I want to enjoy it." She crossed her arms for effect on everyone except the focus of her anger.

"You should have left me home." Al heard Bob giving a low whistle.

"Al, I'm going to the bar. Can I bring you back something? A stiff drink?" Bob laughed all the way up the aisle.

"Elaine, I'm trying my hardest to stay awake, I swear." He turned toward her.

"Don't talk to me." She turned hard in her seat and then got up and walked to the lobby with everyone else.

A few minutes later Bob returned. "Boss, she is pissed. We're switching seats." He placed a drink in Al's hand. "Rum and coke."

"Great. I'll be out before the next act starts." He took

a long sip of the drink.

"That's why I'm here.   You can fall to your left and land on my shoulder this time." Bob laughed uncontrollably.

"This just got weird." Al deadpanned.

Bob wiped tears from his eyes. "The show is actually very good."

"Glad you're enjoying yourself." He finished the drink in one more swallow. "Let me know when its' over."

"I think for you this show is going to go on for a long time." Bob laughed again as Elaine and Kerry walked up to their seats stone faced.

"Cats" remained an ongoing event for four more days in their household. Ronnie was hysterical when she heard what happened which only infuriated Elaine more. She did not speak to Al for almost a week. The only creature comfort he received was from his two new dogs who felt his sadness and jumped into his lap at every opportunity. He was eternally grateful that they had given in and adopted the brother and sister beagle mixes instead of only one dog they thought they had committed to. The dogs kept him busy and comforted until Elaine's anger had dissipated.

In hindsight when they could both laugh about it, Elaine agreed that Al was never a fan of Broadway shows even when he had sight. "Cats" was the last Broadway show they saw together.

During their make up session he pulled her close. "I think you believe you have me trapped now and I have to agree with whatever you say."

She nodded. "Yeah, that pretty much covers it."

"I guess you could call "Cats" your reminder of who you married, with or without sight." She kissed him.

Leaning her head back she looked hard at his face. "You fell asleep at other shows before the accident?"

He went still. "I refuse to answer that on the grounds that you might kill me or at least not talk to me again for another week." He became very serious. "Not speaking to me never happened before in our marriage. I don't like it. Yell at me, take a swing if you really feel the need, but don't shut me out."

She kissed him back passionately. "Agreed. We can't live like this. The kids will take over. We're at their mercy unless we are a united front. Separately, forget about it. We're toast."

"Agreed. These little ones are getting big and smart at the same time. I was trying to spank Albert yesterday, and he evaded me for an hour." He turned his head to tune in on the arguing coming from the living room. "I miss Mom living with us to run interference with those monsters."

"Me too but she was right. It was time for us to manage on our own and to figure out how to stay ahead of them." A look of impending battle crossed her face as she too listened to the escalating mini voices. "Let's get to it."

A month later at seven o'clock on a Friday evening in their new home chaos reigned. Suddenly the absence of Rose was deeply felt as both Al and Elaine tried to establish some form of control.

"This is it, Al. We're on our own." She held Nick as Albert and Larry built perimeter walls around their respective toy nests.

"When are Ronnie and Peter getting here? We need backup." He corralled Chris and tried to keep him away from the complaining voices of his two older brothers.

"Daddy, Chris wrecks everything. Keep him 'way from my fort." Albert continued to add anything that would not fall off onto his cardboard wall.

"Yeah, Daddy." Larry agreed with whatever his brother said, trying hard to keep up his own fort.

"Alright you two, enough. Include your brother and don't beat him up." Al heard noise overhead and knew Ronnie and her boyfriend, Peter, had come in the front door. "Elaine, I think they're here."

She had already started toward the basement stairs and yelled upward. "Hey, come on down."

Peter and Ronnie came down the stairs carrying two pizzas. "Thought we would break in the new house. Let's see how much sauce ends up on the carpet." Ronnie smirked in Elaine's direction.

Peter plopped down on the couch across from Al's chair. "How ya doing buddy?"

Al had a fondness for Peter since the moment he met him last year. "Enjoying the new house. This basement is a Godsend. We throw all the toys down here."

"Big boy toys too. I see the dart board. When are you setting up the pool table?" Peter glanced over at the table covered with boxes and household items.

"Soon, I hope. I want to get back to designing how to line up my shots. Elaine said I was doing better right before we left Lake Road." He had been working diligently at figuring out how to play pool again without the aid of his wife. Pool was his game and before the accident he used to decompress by playing pool and drinking a rum and coke on stressful days.

Elaine perched Nick on her shoulder, took one of the pizza boxes back from Ronnie and headed up the stairs. "If anyone wants pizza they can come up to the kitchen."

Chris looked up at his Aunt Ronnie and pointed to the one box in her hands. "Follow me shorty. I'll get you a piece."

Al felt Chris slip out of his arms and off the chair. "Ronnie, are you going to watch him? Elaine is busy with Nick."

"No. I'm going to open the front door and let him go." She turned on her heel looking over her shoulder and keeping an eye on the running toddler.

Once she was up the stairs Al and Peter snickered to one another. "We'll go up in a minute when these two decide they're hungry. I'm surprised they didn't chase after Elaine and Ronnie." Al turned his head to the noise he heard the two boys making behind the couch Peter sat on.

Albert and Larry, having heard the men talking, had their eyes glued to the dartboard their Uncle Peter pointed out. Not a kid's toy, Al had always made sure the darts were packed away, high out of the reach of children or completely hidden from access. Unfortunately, the move had all their belongings scattered in the room and not yet placed where they belonged. The two boys had spotted the darts earlier in the day and hidden them in their respective forts. Now, both ran to see who could get to their stash the quickest. Albert was first.

Peter and Al could hear the two boys giggling. "We'll know when their hungry. Little feet will scurry up the stairs."

"Yeah. I think we have a few minutes. Owww!!" Peter jumped off the couch and grabbed at the back of his head where a dart was limply hanging, still stuck in his skin. "What the hell?"

"What? What's going on?" Al turned his head sharply.

Peter pulled the dart out of his head and held it in his hand. Blood was dripping down his neck. He jerked himself around to face the two, suddenly still and frightened boys. "Hey! You boys put down those darts right now!"

Albert and Larry dropped the darts and ran for the stairs.

Peter did not chase after the boys. He was still stunned and touched the back of his neck. "Come back here and tell your dad what you just did!" Neither boy stopped. "Al, I just got hit with a dart!"

"On purpose?" Al didn't know what else to do until he could get to the boys and spank them.

Peter, still a little stunned, didn't immediately respond. "Umm. I don't think so."

Al tried not to laugh and secretly thanked God the boys didn't hit their soon to be uncle in the temple, eye or hard enough to penetrate his skull. "That's good. At least we know they're not targeting you."

He gave Al a scared look and touched the blood dripping down his neck. "Shit, I'm bleeding."

Al stood up and remained calm. "Another good thing." He reached out and pulled at Peter's arm. "Let's get you upstairs and have one of the girls fix that or see if we have to get you to the hospital." He had a feeling it was a superficial wound, but he didn't want the scared man to think he wasn't concerned.

Peter stopped at the bottom of the stairs as Al tried to

keep propelling him forward. "Al, you don't think those boys hate me, do ya?"

Al was trying to hold it together. "Nah. I'm sure it's just a passing thing."

Peter didn't know what to think. He was young and single. "Are kids this crazy?"

Al guided his arm in the direction of the stairs. "Not always."

When they reached the top of the stairs Elaine saw the blood smeared on Peter's neck and hands. "What happened?" She rushed over pulling him away from Al.

Dead silence enveloped the room as Albert and Larry ducked their heads and chewed their pizza slices. When they had come rushing up the stairs several minutes ago, Elaine had assumed they were hungry.

Peter touched the back of his head. "Your kids are trying to kill me."

This time Al couldn't hold back a snicker. Elaine turned on him. "Al, what did you allow to happen down there?"

He held his hands, palms up, in supplication. "I didn't do anything. I'm trying to save him."

Ronnie sat still in her chair, eating and trying not to look at Peter for fear she would burst out laughing.

Elaine turned to Albert and Larry. "Both of you drop the pizza and get into your time out chairs. Now!"

The boys jumped up and ran to their rooms where the time out chairs sat permanently. Al followed dutifully after them.

"You both better be in those chairs when I get there or your spankings will be worse." Al was looking to escape Elaine as much as the boys were.

She looked after his retreating figure and then turned to Peter. "He's not going to tell me what happened, so maybe you can."

Peter shook his head. "Those kids hit me with a dart. I thought you guys kept those things hidden."

Elaine stopped what she was doing and looked at him

defensively. "We're still unpacking."

Peter let Elaine lead him to the sink and wash his neck. "We were sitting on the couch talking and the next thing I know I'm pulling a dart out of my neck."

Elaine put the wet towel in his palm and marched out of the room toward the bedrooms. Peter stood there for a second and then turned to Ronnie.

He held the wet bloodied towel to Ronnie. "A little help here?"

She looked up from eating her pizza with one hand and holding a bottle for Nick in the other hand. "You look okay. I think the bleeding stopped."

In the background, they could hear Elaine talking loudly to the boys, smacking of bottoms and astonishingly no tears. Several minutes later Al came from the room.

"Peter, can you help me go on dart patrol? I've been directed to get down there and box those things up before I'm allowed to eat." He started down the stairs.

"This is one tough family." He saw that his bleeding had completely stopped, wiped his hands on the wet towel and followed Al to the basement.

Peter found Albert, Larry, Chris and Nick to be a crash course in parenthood. He and Ronnie were not yet expecting, but by the time Peter Jr. was born over a year later, his four cousins were all fully mobile taking on the world by storm in a different home.

After only three months in their new home, warning signs began to appear concerning their neighborhood choice. Neighbors did not show up at their door to welcome them and inquire about the family. Al and Elaine had been bombarded with care, attention and fun, loving people on Lake Road. This chilly reception gave them pause as they tried to blend in and find joy in the park-like atmosphere Al had started to create in the large yard.

Al and Elaine determined that as much as they loved their new house and yard, the neighborhood and neighbors were not conducive to the energy of four active boys all under the age of eight. They had lived on Ridgeview Terrace for eight months, but it was a long eight months for both Al and Elaine.

One particular morning left him with that unmistakable impression that his family was not completely welcome in their new neighborhood. Al was taking his morning walk with the two beagle basset hound mixes when he heard the mail truck coming, with its distinctive sound. He raised the hand holding the dual leash in salutation, his other hand holding his cane, and wearing dark sunglasses on the overcast day. The dogs, naturally went crazy barking. The familiar toot of the mail truck horn he was used to from Lake Road did not greet him here. Dejected, he stopped at their mailbox at the end of his walk. Reaching in, he pulled out the mail and felt something slip from his hands.

"Dammit." Crawling around on all fours he kept feeling for the lost piece as the dogs circled nervously around him. He heard his neighbor in the next driveway pulling out and continue past him, very close, without stopping or greeting him. Finally, he was just about to give up when he heard another car slow down.

"Excuse me." A man's voice greeted Al.

"Yes. Can I help you?" Al didn't recognize the voice as he tried to be hear over the barking dogs.

"Are you new?" The man's tone and delivery were both rude.

"Well, not exactly. We've been here for eight months." Al paused expecting a response or a laugh from the man but all he got was silence. "I'm Al."

"I live behind you." The male voice didn't even bother to introduce himself.

"Oh, really. I guess our houses are kind of far apart." Al knew this was partially true, but the rudeness of the man was reaching the end of Al's tolerance.

"Do you like it here?" The man still refused to say his name.

"It's quiet." Al couldn't bring himself to lie and say he liked the neighborhood.

"We want to keep it that way." The man pulled away without saying goodbye.

You gotta be kidding me.

Al went inside and blurted out his feelings on the matter. "Elaine, we need to move."

She snorted derisively and shook her head in agreement. "No kidding. Yesterday I tried to be nice and take a delivery package for Ann next door."

Al opened his mouth wide. "Oh, is that her name. Eight months and I haven't met her. They think I can't tell when they pull out of the driveway when I walk the dogs. She or her husband don't even toot the horn. Maybe they're related to the mailman."

Elaine continued where she left off. "I didn't want to tell you about it. I thought maybe I was being too sensitive, but when I handed her the package, she said 'Oh' and slammed the door in my face. She left me standing there." Manners are what Elaine felt separated humans from the animals. "Not even a polite exit. She just slammed the door." She felt the dam of frustration over the last eight months breaking. Over and over again they had tried to be friendly and engaging with all the neighbors and anyone associated with the neighborhood only to feel shunned or disrespected.

"This is a beautiful yard but when my children can't enjoy sledding on the terraces we have paid for, what's the purpose? I could stand people being rude to me if they are kind to my children but they don't even try to pretend. The looks they gave our boys that snow day were not just ridiculous but mean. The boys weren't doing anything except sledding with us and building snowmen. I felt like teaching Albert to throw snowballs at cars." Elaine finished her rant.

"You never told me about that. I would have been happy to go over to their house and give them a piece of my mind. We are a nice family. You don't deserve that." Al was always protective of Elaine.

"I knew it would upset you after the way they acted every time we tried to enjoy our pool last summer. We were so excited to be able to provide the boys with an inground pool. Listening to the nextdoor neighbors talk loudly about how loud our children were, was not just disheartening, it was cruel. I had to try to make sure the boys were out of hearing range. They're just little boys." Memories of last summer and how Elaine could not believe how childish and passive aggressive her new neighbors were came flooding back to her. "I shouldn't have tolerated the behavior, but after the barbecue incident, I was feeling guilty." They both burst out laughing now over the moment last summer when they actually felt embarrassed by their dogs.

It was a beautiful day and the nextdoor neighbors were hosting a catered barbecue. Al had let the dogs out in their fenced yard as he usually did without a leash or attaching them to a runner. The dogs never went beyond the border until that day. Al called and called and could not imagine where they went until he heard the neighbors screaming. Elaine came running to the back door to see what the commotion was when the dogs came to greet her with hot dogs fresh off the grill hanging from their mouths. Elaine knew in an instant that someone had left the garage door open.

Knowing they were planning to move, Al and Elaine laughed harder at the reaction of the neighbors. "Oh man. I never heard anybody so mad over a hot dog." Al was doubled over at the silliness of that moment.

"That man was dressed in his preppy shirt and dock shoes chasing after Mikki like he was a thief and yelling obscenities at you and me." Elaine, relieved with the knowledge that their exit from the neighborhood was iminent, let herself go with Al.

With or without sight, from the first, time Al met Elaine he did not allow anyone to disrespect her. "Time to go. This place is a little farther out of the way for people offering me rides anyway." Al was reaching for the phone.

She was surprised at his instant reaction. "What are you doing?"

He stopped for a moment to answer her. "What do you

think I'm doing? I'm calling the realtor. If you find a house you like right away, we're not waiting to sell this one. We will take a mortgage on a new house against this one since this one is paid in full, and we'll rent it out. I don't want my family spending more time here than necessary. We will find a house to stay in the same school district for Albert, but I want to go back to the Riverview community and live with normal people. There are plenty of houses not bordering the river. We will stay out of the flooding areas." Al kept talking as the ringing number he dialed finally went to the agent's answering machine. "There were several other people interested in this house when we bought it so there shouldn't be too much trouble for the agent to move it, but if there is, renting should teach the neighbors a lesson. The challenge is going to be finding another house you like." The machine beeped for his message. "Lou, it's Al Plevier. We are interested in moving. Call me as soon as you get this." He hung up the phone and turned to Elaine, still ranting on about the move. "You're finished with nursing school. Let's get a new house before you start a job."

Elaine knew an opportunity when she saw it. "Al, I think part of the problem is your mustache."

Al fell off the counter he was leaning on. "Huh?"

"You don't fit in here." She kept going. "It's important that we fit in wherever we live for the boys' sake. You look like, well, unkempt."

"I get what you're doing. You're not pinning this on me, but I'll acquiesce for you." He drew out the verb he used, pretending to impress her with a big word. "Fine. You can have your way on this one. It's starting to bug me anyway after all this time." Al shoved the stool back. "You want to watch the grand shaving?"

She smiled broadly. "I think we should all watch. It can be the sacrifice you're making for the new neighborhood we move to."

He gave her a sarcastic look. "Albert's too smart to buy that line of boloney."

Elaine called to the boys. "Albert, Larry, Chris? Come

in here."

Al tried quieting her. "Not too loud, you'll wake Nick."

Now she gave him a sarcastic look. "Are you kidding? That one sleeps through thunder, fireworks and his brothers running around his crib."

The three boys came into the room. Chris, fast approaching his second birthday, was already keeping pace with his brothers.

"Mommy, what'd you want?" Albert was the leader of the pack.

She looked lovingly at the three little men as they lined up in front of her. "Daddy's going to shave off his mustache. Do you boys want to watch?"

Larry looked to Albert for the answer. "Why?" Asked Albert.

She raised her eyebrows at him. "Because we thought you would want to see what he was going to look like."

Albert shrugged his shoulders. "Can't we see at dinner?"

Al laughed lightly and gave up Elaine's fight for her. "Go back to playing." The boys left the room and Elaine and Al headed for the bathroom. "It's just you and me, Sweetie."

Al stood at the sink feeling for his razor and cream. Elaine pushed it into his hand making an exaggerated scraping on the counter.

"I get it, I get it. I promise not to change my mind. I wouldn't want to deny you the privilege of watching what you've waited over a year for." He started to lather up his face. "Take a good long look. I'm not growing it back."

She looked at him relieved. "I'm done looking."

Al started a painstaking, exaggerated and slow process of removing his Fu Manchu mustache. He was ready to have a clean, shaven face for the New Year and a new start in a new house.

He was halfway done. "What do you think?"

"Keep going." Elaine said with a wicked smile.

Al finished, wiped his face and stepped back. "Now what do you think."

She stepped up and kissed him. "I think I have the man I married back."

"I'd like to say I did this strictly to make you happy, but I told you a long time ago that I would never lie to you." He squeezed her tighter. "I wanted to get the hair off my face for Christmas and before the lumpectomy next winter."

She kept running her hand over his cheeks. "Are you going to have it done?"

"I have to. Dr. Leesville and Dr. Elbac won't move forward with planning the camera implant until I do." Al ran his hands over his clean face touching hers. "I really don't want to go back under the knife again unless it's to regain my sight, but I have no choice. They want to make sure the lump isn't cancerous."

"So do I." Elaine couldn't imagine losing Al to a disease after everything he had survived.

He slipped his arm around her. "It'll be fine. I know it in my heart. All I want to do is get past that surgery and concentrate on getting the approval and commitment from the doctors for the camera implant."

Elaine looked pensively at their reflection in the mirror. "I'm wondering if I should put off getting a job until this surgery and our next move are over. It's all we can do to keep up with the four boys. Add moving and preparing for your next surgery and it's more than enough." She opened the bathroom door wide out of consideration for all the times Al had walked into half opened doors. "Besides, I can work full time after the camera implant is successful. I know it will be. After that we can handle anything from the outside world."

At that moment, a loud bang and crash could be heard from the living room. Elaine and Al waited for the inevitable scream or cry that never came, but the sound of running little feet was audible.

Elaine yelled first creating a harsh biting tone that bounced off the bathroom walls. "Boys! What happened?"

She marched out of the room still yelling. "Where are you?"

Al finished wiping down the bathroom sink and followed her down the hallway. "Hey, where are you boys and what happened?! Elaine?"

"I'm over here Al. They were climbing on the kitchen counter getting glasses out of the upper cabinets. We lost three juice glasses but I don't see any blood. Looks like they all walked away in one piece." She spoke now in an exaggerated louder voice. "It seems like they all disappeared. They better not have gone outside without permission or they will be in worse trouble."

It was Al's turn to talk loud. "Somebody better step up and take responsibility for this. Your spankings will be less if I don't have to find you." He turned to Elaine. "Do you have a broom and pan? I can do it for you."

"It's in the basement. Stay out of the kitchen until I clean this up. We're a blood free household at the moment." Elaine did an exaggerate stomping out the back door. "You boys better answer your father."

"Whose idea was this?" Silence greeted Al. He heard movement to his right as Larry slipped out from behind a door and crawled on his hands and knees around his dad. Al swatted at the air around him. "Hey! You're all in trouble now."

Al started to walk down the length of the room running his hand along the wall. Albert saw his dad too late as he was trying to dash to the bedrooms and laid flat against the wall while Al's hand ran over his head. The second he was out of arm length Albert ran with Larry to the bedrooms. Chris stayed under the coffee table where Elaine had pretended not to see him. He was concentrating so hard on watching his father's feet that he never heard Elaine come back in. She grabbed him as he was backing out and gave his legs a gentle pull.

"Gotcha!" The startled little boy tried to force out a few tears. "Not a chance. I saw you smiling while your dad was searching for you." Chris bit his lip, this time trying not to laugh. "Let's go little one. You need to have a chat with your Dad and I once we get your brothers.

Al was standing stock still in the hallway off the bedrooms listening for any movement. He heard something behind him and reached grabbing a body. Albert laughed with delight.

"Albert, this is not funny. All three of you are in double trouble. First for climbing on the counters and breaking things and second for running and hiding." Holding Albert tightly he started his search for Larry. "Elaine? I got one."

"Me too. I pulled Chris out from under the coffee table." She gave Albert a long scowl and he dropped his head trying not to laugh and make things worse for himself. "What were you doing? Why didn't you ask daddy or me for help?"

Albert's head shot up. "It was Larry's idea."

Al stopped and directed his face at Albert. "If you're going to lie then you're in triple trouble. I know you know what that means."

Albert dropped his head again as his dad caught and held him in a gentle headlock. "You're all in trouble."

Larry came out and stood in the doorway of his room. "I'm here Daddy. Can you spank Albert first? I wanna see what we're gettin'."

It took everything Al and Elaine had not to burst out laughing. "Why don't we have you boys draw straws?"

The three boys looked at each. "Daddy, we can color instead of spankings?" Larry looked at Albert with hope.

Now Elaine did laugh. "No, you're getting spanked, mostly for hiding from us. We might have just yelled at you first."

Albert made a face. "No way. You were going to spank us first. That's why we hided."

Al couldn't argue with logic. "Okay. Maybe. But you boys could have gotten very hurt. If you want a glass mommy or I will get it for you until you're bigger, like my size."

Albert made a face. "Are we gonna have to stay in our rooms?"

Al shook his head at the minimal attention span of children. They were quick, honest and logical.

"Mommy will say how long you guys have to stay in your rooms." Al took the hand Larry offered to him and set Albert on his feet.

"Thanks, Al." Elaine lined Chris up with his brothers.

"I have to do the spanking you can doll out the sentencing." Al swatted Albert's bottom first.

Larry brightened right up. "Me next."

"I'm not done with your brother yet." Al was done but he thought a scare would do all of them some good.

Larry's face dropped. "Okay."

"Albert, you do that again and I will swat you harder and more times. Now go to your room and wait for Mommy." Albert dashed out of reach.

Larry stepped up. "Daddy, here I am."

Al almost felt guilty as the little boy stepped up like a grown man. He swatted him lighter than Albert and sent him to his room as Elaine pushed Chris into position. Al felt the squishy diaper under the tap he gave the giggling Chris.

"Oh, man. Elaine?"

"Really? You're giving the changing job to me?"

"I had to do the swatting. I'm the bad guy. Can't you change him while you're lecturing?"

Elaine walked Chris into his room and the other two boys peaked out of their bedrooms watching where their dad went. "I hear you two. You better get into your rooms before Mommy comes." The sound of running feet could be heard right before two giggling boys landed on their beds with the accompanying squeaking mattresses.

Al walked into Chris' room on his way to the master bathroom. "It would be great if we could get him out of diapers."

"He's almost ready. Our newest arrival has set things back a little. Let him tell us when he's ready. It won't be long." Elaine looked at the smiling toddler. "They get over things quickly."

Al laughed. "Kids are pretty resilient. I hope we are just as tough. I'm starting to think life inside our own walls is going to be more challenging than the outside. And maybe a little scarier."

The Plevier family left behind the unpleasantness and disappointment of 50 Ridgeview Terrace and settled into a new home at 55 Audobon Parkway. Lou, the realtor they had used for decades found the perfect tenant for the Ridgeview Terrace home that afforded the Plevier's three times the average rent for that area. Fortune appeared to be turning for the young family as The Cosmos Soccer team lead forward, a Holland National, rented the home for his family. The rental gave the realtor more time to sell the house at a price that was indicative of the area.

The wonderful neighbors from the 19 Lake Road home in Wayne had set a precedent that the family aspired to whenever they were considering a move. It broke both of their hearts to leave behind the closed knit community of Lake Road, but the flooding river, and most importantly, the size of their family dictated that they find a more suitable home. Leaving the Ridgeview Terrace home meant they lost the full finished basement they loved, but they gained new neighbors on Audobon Parkway that were as wonderful as the friends they left behind on Lake Road. As inconvenient as moving was to a family of their size and with the consideration of Al's readjustment to new environments, a neighborhood with inclusivity was more important for their family than logistics. They were now in a neighborhood the boys could grow into with a large yard, a street to ride their bikes on and the size of the family room made up for the loss of the basement.

One night, Al and Elaine pulled up to the house from a dinner alone to a darkened fortress. "What's wrong, Elaine?"

"The house is dark." She looked guiltily over at him. "Mom forgot your birthday. When I told her why we were going out to dinner she felt horrible. This is the big 3-0 after all." They climbed out of the station wagon. "I wish she had left on a light or two."

"I'll prepare myself for the cake and screaming kids when they come through the door later." Al secretly loved the attention for any celebration including his own birthday.

"She would have remembered on her own next week." She held her keys out. "Did you like the dinner?"

"It was great." He tucked his cane under his arm and offered her his elbow. "Thank you. We needed time just the two of us."

Elaine put the key in the door and pushed it open. "You first birthday boy."

"Surprise!" Forty friends and family members screamed in unison as the lights turned on.

Al stood shocked for a moment as he was hit with toilet paper, crepe paper, silly string, streamers and anything else the excited kids could throw at him. A chorus of Happy Birthday to you followed as Al stood at the door feeling dumb. Someone handed him a drink and to his joy it was a rum and coke.

"Hey old man. It's all downhill from here." Bob's voice boomed and drew a collective laugh.

Elaine slipped off her coat as her mom came to her side. She leaned close to Helen's ear. "Mom, why did you shut out the lights? I couldn't see anything walking up."

"It was for the boys."

"Mom? Is that you?" Al turned to the two women.

"It is, Al. Happy Birthday. Your mom, Fenna and Elaine did all the work and covert operations. It's tough to keep four little boys quiet when they see cake and banners going up."

"When did this take place?" Al was honestly perplexed at how they pulled off the preparations in secret.

"All day around you. It was a lot of fun. The only thing we couldn't bring in were the people or the food. You would have smelled that."

"Yeah, I would have smelled the people, that's for sure." Al smiled broadly to deflect how humbling the moment was for him.

Lee Petereson walked over to Al and gave him a hit on the arm. "Happy Birthday, Al."

Al hadn't seen Lee in several years. "Lee is that you?"

"The one and only. You didn't think I'd miss out on a good party?"

"How've you been?"

"Fine. I hear you're doing great. Elaine told me there might be a new surgery on the horizon."

"Possibly." Al was starting to feel like a statue as he stood in the same place. "It's cutting edge experimental so it's perfect for me." He took a long swallow from his drink.

Elaine cut in. "Al, go get settled. There's a spot on the couch for you in the middle where the boys can tackle you and everyone can come up to say hi."

Ronnie came over and gave him a quick kiss on the cheek. "Happy Birthday old timer."

"Oh geez. Elaine, I hope you realize I'm putting you through this same torture in December."

"Can't wait. I'll design my own party. It will be a food festival." She walked away to give Al his independence.

He walked toward the couch and greeted everyone.

Fred found an opening in the crowd and slapped Al good naturedly on the arm. "Happy Birthday young man. You are blessed."

Al smiled widely. "What do you think of the new house? It's a much friendlier neighborhood. A great way to start my thirties."

"Absolutely. You deserve the best." Fred parted to give the next person their chance to say hello to Al.

The boys were busy blowing the party horns Rose had given them. The sweet family party noise of horns, loud conversations, children laughter, birthday wishes and music resonated in Al's ears long after the party ended reminding him that Fred's statement was a fact.

Chapter XIII: Spring Fever

Spring officially began the third week of life in their new home. Al's thoughts turned to the T-ball season ahead for Albert. One month from his seventh birthday the first grader had already been swinging bats at balls tossed by his dad for two years. Today Al carried a bag of baseballs, a bat tucked under his arm and a couple bottles of soda. There was no free hand for his cane. He was still learning to navigate the new property when his foot hit the steps into the kitchen on the pathway from the detached four car garage. The clatter of everything he had been holding hitting the floor through the door he had left opened resonated through the first floor.

Al found himself splayed over the threshold, his hands flat against the cold tile. "Shit," he exclaimed softly. The only thought that came to mind.

Used to the sound, Elaine did not rush to Al's aid, but walked in casually picking up a still rolling baseball.

"You want some help or do you have this?" She grabbed at a couple of loose rolling balls.

Al straightened up. "I hate not being able to walk normally. When I'm carrying anything outside, I have to think my route out ahead. When I don't," he waved his arms around, "this happens."

Elaine looked at Al without sympathy which is the only practical way to be when living with someone with a disability. "You do just fine. We pick up after each other. When I need help, you're the first person in my life to be there, always."

He breathed out deeply and leaned against the door frame. "I know and I hate to whine. It's just that I would like to walk and not have to be touching in front of me or to the side. Even when I'm carrying things I just want to walk like a normal person. I can't always walk backwards like I do in the house when I'm carrying stuff."

"You've never been normal with or without sight," Elaine deadpanned.

Al smiled. "Remember how it was when I first started teaching Albert to play ball after the corneal transplant?"

Now Elaine was the one to smile. "It was amazing.

"With sight, I could actually see the expression of concentration on his face. It was glorious, for me. When my sight was fading and he was becoming a blurred image, it nearly broke my heart. I went from seeing his confidence grow in his eyes to only knowing it was happening from the way the ball flew past my head." Al felt the doorframe and seated himself inside.

Elaine squeezed next to him. "I can tell you this. When Albert looks at you it is with absolute hero worship. He wouldn't look at you that way if he knew you could see him. He would be shy, like any little boy. He would want to impress you with what a little man his is." She stopped to see how Al accepted this. "I know it's a small consolation, but it is real. His confidence is building slowly because you started with him by rolling a ball on the floor. You have his back and even at the tender age of six, he knows."

He let his hand find her knee. "I started baseball right around his age. I was eight. It was the basis of my confidence. Nobody taught me. Dad was dead by then. All I had was the stickball games we played in the street. I can still see Mickey at my door telling me to hurry up 'cause we were all going to the fields. Me and him joined up with six other kids hanging on the chain link fence waiting for our turns to try out."

Elaine was comforted when she heard Al slip into the regional dialect from his old neighborhood. It usually signified that he had worked through whatever was irritating him at that moment.

Al laughed out loud. "I'm glad Albert won't have to go through that. All that coach Eddie Burns said was if we made it to base, we were on the team. Heck of a way to hold a try out. I learned by watching the other kids. The coach only did so much. We didn't even have uniforms, but we had fun. It gave me the confidence to get better and try out for other sports. CYO kept me busy in the winter with basketball. I never would have tried out for that if I hadn't learned baseball."

She covered his hand with hers. "I wonder which sports our boys will zero in on."

He laughed. "Who knows. I want them to try them all." He tossed a ball he still had in his hand. "I can still see Grandmom Padula's face when I told her I was playing ball. She started shaking her finger right at me and kept telling me that work comes first. For crying out loud I was eight years old! I already had my own paper route." He paused for a minute. "I had to quit sports when I got to High School because of work...and you." He smiled at her. "Fortunately, I picked it back up in College. I had a car at that point and you and I had broken up for a little while so I had free time." He was silent for a moment thinking and Elaine misunderstood.

Elaine elbowed him a little too enthusiastically. "Sorry I held you back."

Al laughed good naturedly. "Yeah, it was a real sacrifice." He kissed her on the cheek. "Do you remember that car? It was a 1954 Chevy that I bought for $200 when I was seventeen. What a great car."

"How could I forget. You loved that car more than me." She elbowed him.

His vacant eyes looked out into the nothingness that greeted him. "I really miss driving. We had so much fun cruising in that car. Remember Cape Cod?" Al was beginning to forget all about baseball.

She smiled. "How could I forget that weekend. It was our last hurrah for the summer before my teaching started."

Al had a look of concentration. "Yes, we went there in August. I remember because that trip we visited the Knolls. Bill and I raced into the ocean when we saw other people in there and the water was something like fifty degrees. No polar bear charity events for me, thank you very much."

Elaine stared back in time at the beachfront home. "Their house was so pretty on the cliffs. We haven't seen them since then. I wonder if they heard about your accident?"

Albert came running into the kitchen. "Daddy, come on. What are you doing?"

"Sorry pal. Mom and I started talking."

Elaine watched Albert drop his head and stomp out of the room. "I think you better get moving. I'll keep Larry in the house if you want."

Al shook his head. "No, let me him come out. He already tosses the ball to me and swats at it with the plastic bat when Albert throws at him. Albert has been really good about talking to him the same way I've been teaching him. These boys will be playing and teaching each other as the years' pass." He stood up and started to gather up the equipment again. "What do you think about taking the boys up to Cooperstown next month?"

Elaine brightened at the thought of a family weekend getaway. "We could also go to the Catskill game farm and Howe Cavern."

Al knew when he was beat. He never argued with Elaine when it came to what was best for the boys. Although he only wanted to go to Cooperstown, he agreed to the other side trips. "That sounds great. Albert's last day of school is June 20. We could leave the next day." He inclined his head over his shoulder. "I have to get this garage organized before school lets out. It's going to make a great work room. I feel like we've finally arrived now that we have a heated four car garage. I'll be able to work all winter in my half."

"Make sure you stay in your half. The boys and I need two of the bays for toys and my car." Elaine's tone was flat.

"I promise, Honey." Al knew he only needed one of the car bays but he was taking two.

From the other room came the high pitch complaints of Albert and Larry. "Daddy!"

"I gotta go. The troops are calling. You have two months to plan that outing. Let me know where and when to show up." Al left the doorway smoothly walking through the kitchen to where both boys waited.

Albert was progressing steadily with his skills in baseball. T-ball was starting in two weeks and he was excited. This was his second season playing. Last year Albert had more fun looking for shamrocks amid the clover in the outfield even though he was able to make contact with pitched balls. This year he was all about the game.

He stood about twenty feet away from Al who prepared to pitch a slow underhand. "Daddy, they don't do that all the time. Pitch it right ways."

Al stopped what he was doing. "Where's your brother? I don't want him to get hit in the head."

"He's okay. He's behind me." Albert took the stance Al had taught him.

"Albert, is he far enough away from your swing? You could hit him." Al heard Larry trying to talk over the both of them in his preschool voice.

Albert turned to his little brother. "Larry, move there." He pointed to his right.

Larry still did just about everything Albert asked. He looked to the spot Albert pointed at and dropping his head despondently, shuffled to the place.

"Alright, Daddy. He moved. Come on!" Albert set himself up again.

Al pitched a light overhand to Albert who swung and missed. "I didn't hear you connect. Was the pitch high or low?"

"Down the middle. I just missed." Albert set himself up again, unswayed by the missed ball.

Al walked toward him. "Let me see how you're standing." Without hesitation, Al found Albert and stood behind him correcting his stance and then how he held the bat. "Let's see if that helps."

Walking back to their designated pitchers mound, he heard little feet and then Albert's voice. "Larry! Go back to your spot. Daddy won't pitch if you stand by me."

"Thank you, Albert. Larry, listen to your brother." Al heard the little feet shuffle away from his line of pitching and then he did another soft overhand. Al heard the crack of the bat against the ball and felt it fly by his face. "That was good." *"Too good", he thought to himself. I gotta come up with another plan."* "You're getting better every day. Remember when we used to use the back of the garage on Lake Road?"

Albert kicked at the dirt around him. "Yeah, that's boring now."

Al laughed inwardly at the logic of a child. "You're doing so good you can help teach Larry the way you and I played."

Albert stopped, let the top of the bat he held fall to the ground and looked over at Larry. "Daddy he'll slow me down."

Larry knew he was being talked about and looked wide eyed at his brother and then turned to Al. "I'm good Daddy. I'm good."

"Yes, Larry. You are doing very well." Al walked toward Larry.

"Daddy, what are you doing?" Albert threw the bat down in frustration and Al heared the clink it made against the ground.

"Albert, pick up that bat and bring it over here. You're going to help me teach Larry how to stand.

This was the last thing Albert wanted to hear. "But Daddy, I want to hit!"

"You will hit, but if you want Larry to keep up with you, you'll have to help him." Albert guided Larry to the batting spot. "Larry, stand here like this." Al turned the little boy sideways and handed him the bat that was too big for him. "Your hands can be like this and swing like this." Al spaced the little boy's hands and wrapped his arms around him swinging the bat with him. "You get three swings because Albert said something mean, but then you have to let Albert have his turn."

"Okay, Daddy." Larry smiled all the way up to his eyes.

"Albert can teach you what he learns later. Albert you're going to get even better while helping your brother. How do you think Coach is able to teach you? He taught his brothers a long time ago or his brothers taught him." Al felt like he was losing the argument when he heard Albert obviously stomping dirt.

"I'm going to walk over here and pitch the ball." Al walked a couple feet away and lightly tossed the ball. To his surprise, Larry giggled when he missed.

"Daddy, I'm good. Let's practice baseball with me and you. No Albert." He made a face and stuck out his tongue at Albert, knowing his dad wouldn't see.

"Hey!" Suddenly Albert saw how this might not work out for him. "All three of us. Don't teach him without me. That's not fair!"

Big tears started in Larry's eyes and he made a move toward his brother just as Elaine came around the corner with Chris. "Al, there's a call for you." She looked from one boy to another. They had both stopped when they saw her and were now staring each other down. "What's going on?"

Al gave a serious look in the direction of the boys. "Just the beginning of a rumble. I got it under control. Who's on the phone?"

"Dr. Grove's office." Chris ran to Al and the bag of balls.

"Albert, toss some balls to Larry." Al walked toward the house. "Elaine, make sure Albert tosses to both his brothers while I'm gone. Chris likes swinging the plastic bat." He started to walk to the house. "When are we going to get a new cordless phone? Most of the people in *Images* have them in their homes. They say it's the greatest invention for people without sight, as long as you remember where you put the phone the last time you used it."

Elaine set the boys up to continue practice. "If they live alone, do they carry it with them all the time?"

Al laughed. "That would be too simple." He was at the corner of the house when he gave a parting comment. "I guess in this house we might lose the phones a lot."

"Daddy! What about me?" Albert had the beginnings of a full temper tantrum.

"Pal, I'll be back. Now is a chance for you to prove to Mommy and I how grown up you are. Bigger guys get bigger toys."

"Al." Elaine was not a fan of bribery.

Al continued toward the kitchen. "He has to learn how to teach others. That's part of the game."

Elaine picked up a ball. "I got this. Boys, line up. Albert first."

"Mommy, you don't throw like Daddy." Albert was losing all enthusiasm.

"Albert, help me with your brothers. You're the coach while Daddy's on the phone. I'm your assistant coach like Mr. Armenick." She walked to the spot to pitch and began to line up with the boys.

At this suggestion, Albert lit up and turned to his brothers like a general. "You guys stand over there." He pointed to a place several feet away. "That's the dugout. You gotta stay there until your turn. I go first."

Both Larry and Chris turned to their mother and began to whine simultaneously. "Boys, Albert's the coach. He's going to help you hit."

Larry and Chris looked at each other suspiciously and then to the place Albert told them. Elaine pitch a slow over hand to Albert who swung and missed.

Larry chimed in immediately. "Haha, Mr. Bossy."

Elaine held the next ball in her hand. "Nobody makes fun of anyone here. Understand, Larry?"

Larry dropped his head and kicked dirt. "Yeah."

She tossed the ball lightly preparing for her next pitch. "Albert gets an extra turn because you did that."

Forgetting for the moment that he was with someone who could see, Albert stuck his tongue at Larry.

Elaine stood tall. "You just lost your extra turn. Everybody knock off the fighting. At least until your Daddy gets back." She gave a light overhand to Albert's stubborn face and he made contact, sending the ball over her head. "Wow! Two more pitches and then it's Larry's turn."

Albert finished his turn and was lining up Larry and giving him hitting advice when Al rejoined them. "How's it going back here?"

"Albert is coaching Larry now. We're the assistants." Elaine looked over at Chris who watched everything his two brothers were doing. Chris stepped back as his dad joined them knowing he didn't know where he was.

"Where's Chris?"

"Here, Daddy." Al turned to the little voice behind him.

At almost three years old, Chris had walked, talked and picked up a baseball bat earlier than his brothers by watching their example. He knew how important the ball and bat were to his family. Al started teaching him with the same techniques he used with Albert when he could catch him, but Chris preferred to run with Larry and Albert and do whatever they were involved with at that moment.

Elaine watched Albert correct how Larry held the bat. "Are you ready Larry?"

Larry concentrated hard on the ball in his Mom's hand. "Go 'head."

Albert stood away from him. "Daddy, you better stand

over there with Chris. Larry's gonna hit."

Larry connected with the first overhand pitch Elaine tossed at him. "Got it Mommy!

Al smiled broadly as he kept a hand on Chris head. "Nice. Elaine. I think you pitch better than I do."

"Are you surprised? I've been keeping up with you and Albert since the first ball was rolled to him." She pitched another ball and Larry connected again. "Good job buddy. You're going to be ready for T-ball next year."

"Looks like you're doing a great job coaching, Albert." Al hoped the encouragement would redirect Albert's natural jealousy of his younger brothers.

"I'm good so he's good, Daddy." Albert stood with his arms crossed just like Al and his t-ball coach did.

Both Al and Elaine tried to hold back their smiles for different reasons. "You can teach Chris too."

Albert look patiently at his little brother, like a good coach would. "Yeah, he's next. He's already been hitting, but I'll make him better."

Elaine held the next baseball. "Al, did you hear Nick stir at all? He's been down for a half hour."

"Not a peep. Since the phone didn't wake him, he's probably good for a while longer." Al ruffled Chris' hair. "I'll go check on him now. You have these guys under control."

"Hey, wait." She still held the ball. Both Larry and Albert started to shuffle their feet in annoyance, just like their dad. "What did Dr. Grove's office say?"

"Just confirming the check up for next week before the lumpectomy. I should be out of the hospital in three days. I won't be able to pitch to the boys but that will be toward the end of the T-ball season and Albert will get lots of practice on the field." He turned to go in the house and then stopped short, whispering to her. "I reminded him that I wanted them to try and keep the nipple. Man, I don't want to look like I'm winking at somebody once I don't have to wear the Jobe shirt."

Elaine rolled her eyes and talked softely. "Seriously, Paul Newman? You were willing to climb on the roof without sight, but you're worried about cosmetics? If it's cancerous, it's coming out, nipple and all." She laughed lightly trying to contain herself.

Al hung his head and smirked. "Gimme a break."

Elaine called after him. "And lots of practice with me. I'm not too bad as a replacement. Just like the majors."

Al kept going. "I'll say you are. Now we really have a team."

Al was around the corner when Larry called to her. "Mommy, what's a lumptomy?"

Elaine gave him a second to set up and then tossed the overhand low. He missed, but didn't care as he waited for a response to his question. "Just something the doctor needs to do for Daddy. How much did you hear?"

Albert started to walk toward Larry as he waved Chris to come over. "For his eyes?"

Elaine watched three of her men gathered together and secretly said a prayer of thanks before answering. "Sort of. Daddy needs a big check-up before the camera goes in his eye."

Larry reluctantly stepped off the spot for hitting. "Can he take pictures of us with his eyeball?"

"No, honey. He'll be able to see us with one of his eyes." Elaine thought this had settled everything for the moment as she watched Albert seriously tell Chris where to stand and hold the bat.

Larry stopped and looked at her. "Boy, Daddy's gonna get shots."

Elaine didn't quite know how to respond. "I suppose he will, Buddy."

Chris stood waiting for Elaine to pitch. "Mommy. Throw."

Elaine tossed the ball underhand and Chris swung hard missing the ball but smiling broadly. Albert and Larry cheered him.

"How we doing out here? Sounds good." Al returned carrying a sleepy Nick. "Looks like you guys haven't missed me at all."

Jayne Kelly

Elaine looked at her five men and smiled. "Don't be so sure."

Al deposited Nick on the ground and he immediately picked up a discarded ball and tossed it. "Al, Nick already has a good arm." Elaine watched the toddler with wide eyes.

He gave her a sarcastic look. "He's only seventeen months old."

"Are you doubting me?" She knelt down as Nick came over to her and the other three boys started to tussle with each other in frustration and boredom.

Albert spoke up first as he stared at his new tire swing across the yard. "Mommy are we done?"

"No, Daddy's here. We can play together." She rolled a ball away from the boys with the bats for Nick to chase after.

Albert put both hands on his hips. "Can we please play now?" Albert was becoming more outspoken lately, no longer the little boy who was the leader of their little pack. He was starting to test his boundaries.

"Albert, don't sass your mother or you're going in the house for the rest of the day." Al lined himself up in front of the boys where Elaine stood. "Albert, are you the next one I'm pitching to?"

"Yes Daddy." A sullen Albert set himself up for the pitch.

Al looked toward Albert. "Where are your brothers?"

Albert looked at his brothers. "They're away by the house. I'm ready."

Al pitched a nice overhand to Albert who missed the ball but swung levelly. "Very good!" Elaine exclaimed and was surprised on how much progress he was making.

"I'm done now if Larry wants to go." Albert eyed his new tire swing again.

Larry, suspecting his brother had something better in mind mimicked Albert. "I'm done too Daddy if Chris wants to go."

"You guys can play in a couple more minutes. Larry let's do three pitches and tomorrow I'll let you set up a game with Mom and me." He reached around for the bag of balls as Elaine handed him two. "Thanks sweetie."

"We're a team, right? This means I get to hit tomorrow too, boys." Elaine knew the boys were glad for anyone extra to build the team.

Nick found another ball and threw it toward Larry who looked surprised at his brother. "Hey, hs doin' it Daddy."

Al turned his head from side to side. "Do you mean Nick? How was his aim, Larry?"

Not completely sure what his dad meant, Larry was still happy Nick threw the ball because it meant he wouldn't slow them down when Al and Elaine forced them to play together. "He threw it right."

Al smiled. "He's been watching you guys. You're all coaches like me now as long as you keep helping each other. Someday each of you boys will be helping the other players. That's what being on a team is all about." Al hoped his lesson was getting through.

"When do we get to have fun?" Larry was serious.

Al stood still listening to his sons doing what little boys do. "Everyday."

Chapter XIV: Ours

*A*nother medical procedure was behind them as the lumpectomy to remove the non-cancerous cyst on Al's left breast area was performed in late June of 1980. This procedure and a clean bill of health after it had to be completed before any consideration or hope would be given for the camera implant in his right eye.

He was in the recovery period from the lumpectomy when Albert finished his school year and Elaine decided the perfect chance for the trip they had planned to Cooperstown would be in late July. Al was actually hoping they could put the trip until they found out if the camera implant surgery could take place. Selfishly he wanted to wait until he could see these places that he never had a chance to see before the accident as a working man with his own resources or as a child growing up in Paterson. The boys were so young that he thought there would be time regardless of what the prognosis would be for the surgery.

Bandaged and recovering from the latest surgery, he tried to rationalize why Elaine's suggestion that they go this summer was reasonable. *There is still a chance I won't be able to have the surgery and even if I do, it may not be successful. She wants to take these family outings when the moment is upon us. We can't plan based on my sight returning. I get it, But unfortunately, I'm just a babysitter. I can't see the pictures and enjoy Cooperstown, a place I wanted to see since I was a kid.* Al continued the internal rant as he listened to Elaine make reservations on the phone for their upcoming trip. This was going to be the first time the boys would be in a hotel together and they were very excited.

"Thank you. Yes, we will need two rooms. There will be four adults and four children. The children will be dispersed between the two room. I need them to be next to each other." Elaine's face lit up as she planned the upcoming trip. She really needed the mini vacation before she started her new job. "How are you doing Al? Do you need anything while I'm in the kitchen?"

"No, no, I'm good. You do what you have to." Al wanted to sit and play quietly with Nick who seemed satisfied to build towers with whatever he had in his hands, giving his dad pieces to hold.

Several minutes later she hung up the phone. "We are all set. A couple weeks from now we will be looking over the heroes of baseball."

Great. "The family needs a vacation." He hoped there was no sarcasm in his voice. "This will be good for everyone." Al wondered if he was going to be able to hide his depression as the weekend drew closer and when they actually experienced the trip.

A month later he sat in the front seat of the station wagon holding Nick and trying to ignore Larry, Albert and Chris fighting in the back seat.

I still remember my dad talking to me about Cooperstown when I was five. He was supposed to take me when I got older.

The thought of his dad dying in front of him right before his fifth birthday flashed into his mind further depressing him. He tried to focus on the fact that this was a trip for the boys and bolstered himself up knowing he was able to do this for them.

He knew he would have the chance to share the Baseball Hall of Fame with his children even if he couldn't see it.

Well, I'm here at lease, I guess. I won't be able to see their faces or look at the player memorabilia but I am here. That's something.

Elaine had been concentrating so hard on driving that she was able to block out the kids fighting. She just noticed how quiet Al was. "Are you turning their yelling into white noise also?"

For a second, Al didn't realize she was talking to him. "What?"

"You're so quiet. I asked you if you were turning the boys' fighting into white noise like I am." Elaine returned to concentrating on driving, her least favorite activity she had taken over after Al's accident.

Al gathered his thoughts. He was going to try to hide his depression from her as long as he could. "Yeah. Sometimes it's better to let them work it out for themselves." Al went back into his head and Elaine let him stay there for the remaining hour of the drive.

When the family got out of the station wagon at Cooperstown, the three boys practically leaped from the back seat. Elaine had parked in front of a grassy area and they took full advantage of their freedom. Well aware of the theme for the day, the boys threw the balls they brought with them at each other while Chris dragged his plastic bat.

"Boys, you can play for a couple of minutes and then we're going inside." Elaine watched Al slowly get out of the car with a squirming Nick looking to get free and play with his brothers.

"Al, are you feeling okay?" She walked over to him as he let Nick loose on the grass.

"I'm fine," Al said a little too sharply.

She looked at him and decided he was irritated from the car ride. "Alright. I hope there are some interactive things for the boys inside. Albert just took a dash to the bronze statue he spied with the boys following closely on his heels. We have to hurry." Elaine put Al's hand on her shoulder.

He pulled his hand back. "I have my cane. Just keep an eye on me." He spoke a little too sharp and Elaine heard him.

"Al, my parents are about ten minutes behind us. We have to catch those four before we get thrown out of here. Once my parents get here you and I will have some breathing room." This time she grabbed his hand and put it firmly on her shoulder.

Al wordlessly accepted her lead. Elaine's parents were farther behind them than she thought. For the next half hour, the boys climbed over the brass statues and spent the energy they had saved up on the car ride. Mr. and Mrs. Hinds walked into a scene they were getting more used to as the months passed and the boys got older.

Mr. Hinds looked over at Al who now sat on a bench to the side of the activity. "Elaine is Al feeling okay?"

Elaine, already worn out from chasing the boys shrugged her shoulders. "I don't know, Dad. He said he's fine but something is wrong. He was quiet for most of the car ride."

Mrs. Hinds held Nick's hand as he looked over his shoulder at his brothers and laughed. "How do you think this tour is going to go?"

Elaine caught Chris. "I think the boys will enjoy the motel pool and the Catskill game farm better." Chris fought against her control but finally gave in to her tight hold. "I still want Albert and Larry to see everything. We'll bring them all back again when they're older." She looked over at Al. "Al, we're going to go inside now. Boys! Come over here. Larry, stay with Grandpop."

Albert strutted over to the group like the true leader of the pack that he was. "Mommy, when do I get to see the guy from the picture?" Albert referred to the picture his parents had shown him of Babe Ruth standing in front of the mantel of their Lake Road house when it was a hunting lodge.

Elaine suddenly realized that Albert expected to meet Babe Ruth. "Honey, you're not going to meet Mr. Ruth, you're going to see more pictures of him and his uniform."

Albert thought about this for a moment. "I guess that's okay. Is it all statues in there?"

Al had walked over and caught the end of the conversation. "No, there's lots of other stuff for you to see like the uniforms, mitts and balls that the famous baseball players actually touched. Not a lot of kids get to see that stuff up close." Al felt a sharp pain in his stomach. This was the exact description his own father gave him when he was four and they were planning the trip. He couldn't believe he remembered it.

"Daddy, did you see this when you were my age?" Albert stared at his father with an innocent face.

The stomach pain hit him again. "No, but it was open then. This museum was here since 1937."

Albert's face grew large. "That's a long time ago." The little boy watched the sad expression his daddy could no longer hide. "Daddy, it's okay. I'll tell you what I'm looking at. Mommy can read the words I don't know." He took Al's hand. "Come on. Mommy said after we finish the baseball museum, we are going to lunch and then the animal place. You'll like that. You can pet the animals with me."

The simple kindness and understanding Albert offered humbled Al. He took the cue that the boys wanted to finish with the museum as quickly as possible. "Thanks, Pal. I think there's some souvenirs for all four of you guys if you behave yourselves. Larry, did you hear me?"

Larry scrunched up his face. All he wanted to do was play outside. "Yes Daddy. Can we have candy when the museum is done?"

Holding Albert's hand, the troops started inside. "Maybe. You have to be good and listen to Mommy and me. Then we'll see."

Albert stood tall again like a leader and turned to his younger brother. "Yeah. You gotta listen to Mommy and Daddy. I want stuff at the end."

Al squeezed Albert's hand softly. "Easy, big guy. Mommy and I have this under control." He swung his cane lightly from side to side not trusting his oldest child completely. "I'm sure glad we're here to show you guys this place."

Albert distractedly looked at the first pictures he saw inside the open front doors. "Me too, Daddy. There's lots of pictures of baseball players."

Mr. Hinds walked immediately behind Al and Albert. "How you doing, Boss?" He looked at Al's face as he watched Albert staring at the pictures.

"I'm good Dad, but I need to make a stop. Albert, Daddy needs to go the lavatory when we get inside. You can come or you can stay with Mommy and the boys." Al and Albert kept pace as the group move forward and Mr. Hinds jumped to the front.

"I'll stay with Mommy. I don't have to go." Al and Albert waited with everyone for only a few moments until the group moved inside. Elaine's dad had paid for the group and they walked in without delay.

"Elaine, is there a men's room nearby?" Al held tightly to Albert.

She looked around them. "Yes, to your left. Albert, take Daddy to that door over there." She pointed to a door, five or six feet away. "Pop pop will bring Larry to stand with you while you wait for Daddy."

Albert, with souvenirs still dangling in his mind, readily agreed. "Okay, Mommy. C'mon Pop Pop. Daddy has to go." Albert began to drag Al to the door.

Once in front of the door reaching for the handle Al came to the same conclusion he always had. "When will someone put braille schematics next to the door of every bathroom in America? The plaque with 'Men's Room' spelled out is not enough. I need to know what I'm walking into."

"Al, I'll take a peek and tell you." Mr. Hinds caught up with Al, anxious to get the group moving as he watched Albert and Laryy immediately start to smile broadly and tussle with each other. "Okay, it's a one toilet closet. The bigger john is down the hall. The toilet is against the right wall. No urinal. Sink dead ahead."

"Thanks, Dad. I'll be quick." He went inside and pulled the door tight behind him without locking it. If he got into trouble he knew he would need to be rescued.

He found the bowl with his cane. Public restrooms were the dirtiest places on earth as far he was concerned and he was certain he didn't help. He aimed, heard water and figured he did alright. After washing his hands, he couldn't find the towels or a dryer and did not want to spend any more time feeling around. He exited the bathroom and walked right into Albert who reached for his hand.

"Daddy your hand is still wet, yuck." He let go and wiped his hand on his pants.

"It's just water. Daddy couldn't find the towels." He wiped his hand on his own pants before reaching down and feeling for the little boy's hand again. "Let's go everybody."

The afternoon at the museum passed quicker than Elaine thought it would. She was so busy keeping all four boys happy she was surprised when they were at the exit sign. By rote the family piled back into the station wagon and were heading for the animal farm when she decided on an alternate plan.

"Boys, I have a surprise for you." The car went silent. "We are going directly to the hotel. We'll do the animal farm tomorrow."

A collective little boy cheer went up from the back seat. Nick clapped his hands as he sat on Al's lap.

Albert stopped banging his blowup baseball bat against the back of Al's seat. "Daddy can we go swimming first?"

Relieved to have an activity they didn't have to chase the boys around at, Al quickly agreed. "Yes. You boys all ate your lunches so I think Mommy would agree that you can swim after you change."

Another collective cheer went up. Elaine breathed out. She knew she had her parents to help keep an eye on the boys and she wanted to relax tonight. A swim would wear down the boys and pizza in the rooms tonight for dinner would be a nice end.

Elaine was right. All four boys were exhausted by early evening. They piled into one bed passed out from the day's activities as Elaine and Al relaxed in front of the TV.

"Al, I bet Mom and Dad fell asleep before these boys did. I'm glad we didn't do the animal farm today." She looked over at the still body of her husband. "Al?"

"I'm awake. Just dozing." He had been doing a good job of both hiding his depression and pulling himself out of it, but now all he wanted to do was sleep and not think too hard about tomorrow.

"Do you want me to turn down the TV?" Elaine was actually hoping he wanted to talk. She needed adult conversation after the day with the boys.

Al let out an exaggerated yawn. "If you don't mind that would be wonderful. You're about to lose me."

Elaine lowered the volume on the TV and then found herself slipping into a sad mood. The weekend getaway was unexpectedly wearing on her as much as it was on Al. She wondered what the rest of the weekend would bring.

Al spent the next day pretending to be in a chipper mood. The first thought he had when he awoke was that this was for his family and he would do anything to make it a great experience for them for the remainder if their weekend.

"Are we going to the animal farm or Howe Caverns first?" Al worked to get Nick ready.

"I think the animal farm first. The boys can run around in the morning before lunch. Nick might sleep through the caverns tour in the afternoon." She finished drinking her coffee as Albert and Larry started to roll on the bed wrestling. "Al, the troops are getting restless. We need to move this army along quicker."

Even with the help of her parents, Elaine and Al were so busy chasing the four boys that the morning passed quickly. Immediately following lunch, they went on a walking tour of Howe Caverns with each adult in charge of a child. Al carried a tired Chris who leaned his head comfortably on his dad's shoulder when the tour guide shut off the lights. Immediately the crowd 'oohed' and 'aahed' as the luminescent colors came to life. Even Chris rose up from his near sleeping state. For Al, his stomach turned into a knot of frustration and he returned to an internal moodiness he tried to hide from the family. The rest of the afternoon dragged on terminally for him.

They drove home to the Audobon Parkway house that evening as the sun was setting. The boys crashed in front of the TV and Al counted the minutes until they could drag them to bed.

"Elaine, I'm going to mess around with the pool table." Al walked away from Elaine as they stood together in the hall outside the boys' bedrooms without giving her a chance to respond.

He made his way down the hall clumsily, not the usual confident stride he maintained inside his home. Even in a new home Al usually had the layout imprinted on his brain by the second or third day of occupancy and did not need his cane. Tonight, he was off balance both figuratively and literally. He needed to clear his mind and reground himself. Al knew moving forward that he no longer felt bad about what he thought he was missing when the weekend started. He also knew that he could care less where they went. Any trips or traveling was going to be for Elaine and the kids. He would always go because family stayed together in activities but this was for his wife and he knew coaching the boys in baseball was for him.

He felt the edge of the pool table and ran his hand along the edge until he felt the ball rack fully loaded. He found his favorite stick in the holder on the wall behind where he stood and grabbed at it knocking down several others.

"Shit." He bent and picked up the loose sticks.

Elaine had come in quietly and stood leaning against the door frame watching him. Before the accident, a night like this with Al trying to blow off the day at their pool table would have involved the addition of black russians. With the kids around, he only had a drink now at social gatherings.

Al found what he knew had to be the cue ball at the far

end of the table. He felt the middle of the table at a point he knew would hit the balls exactly where he wanted and took the shot. He heard several balls hit the sides but none went into poackets.

At least none bounced off the table and onto the floor. I should talk to the Pioneer group from Bell Telephone and start to motivate them to work on a pool table. Setting up two different types of beeper sounds for solids and stripes might work. Sound mechanisms for each pocket, all different from one another might work too. Lining up the shots I don't know about yet, but it has to be doable.

He felt on the table carefully, found a ball and took a shot at anything. He heard drop into a pocket with a soft plop.

This isn't bad. When I don't have rules, I make good shots. I really miss the days when the pool table was my way of dealing with life. Now I put on the radio or the stereo headphones to block out or forget life at the end of the day. I remember after we bought the house I would wait until Elaine was asleep and I would rack up the balls, set myself up with black Russians and play pool until I passed out. It worked for me. I can live without the booze now. Blind and hung over is not a picture I want my kids to see.

He smiled and laughed quietly out loud to himself then he felt another ball, was careful not to move it, and took another shot. This time no balls went in.

Can't win every time.

Al continued until he thought most of the balls may have gone in. It took several hours. He walked around the pockets and counted how many were there. There were two still on the table. He found both, line up a shot and pocketed one. Then he re-racked the balls.

Al kept messing around with the pool table until he felt the emotions of the weekend dissipate completely. He put everything back in the exact place he found it so that he would be set up for the next time. The cue ball didn't matter to him. One ball was just like the others. For him, the game was all that mattered.

221

Chapter XV: Shifting

"*I* guess the real question is how do you prepare to see again." The man in the chair next to him leaned back, ruffled his newspaper to straighten the page and settled back in.

Al couldn't believe what he was hearing. *What's wrong with this guy? I feel sorry for his wife.*

"Al, I'm done with the paperwork. Are you ready?" Elaine folded the newest papers for her medical file and put them in her purse.

Al stood up without hesitation. "Absolutely."

The man reading the paper looked up absentmindedly and without enthusiasm. "Good luck, Buddy."

"Hey, thanks. Best of luck to you and your wife." Al walked away, looping his arm through Elaine's practically dragging her with him.

When they were in the elevator and the doors closed, Elaine squeezed close to him. "I'm so happy for you, Sweetheart. You're so brave to go through this. No wonder you're anxious to get the clearance today."

Al whistled low. "Actually, my real bravery was spending two minutes next to that guy in the waiting room. I couldn't get away from him fast enough."

Elaine rolled her eyes. "You're preparing to have major surgery sometime within the next twelve months with the chance to see again and you let some stranger distract you?"

"Hey, I was just sitting there. He started talking about his poor wife, but he made it clear that he was the real victim. She's having a corneal transplant and all he could do was complain that it's only lasting six months and then he has to 'take care of her again' when it fails. She really picked a winner with that guy. I tried to change the subject and tell him about the camera implant surgery. He didn't ask questions about it for his wife or congratulate us, all he could say was that the real question was how do you prepare to see. Is he kidding?" The doors opened.

Elaine led Al down the long hallway with offices the entire length on both sides. "Who knows what some people are thinking." Elaine and Al were practically bouncing as they walked. "I can't believe this is actually coming together."

"Me either. If this works, and according to Dr. Elbac it should, I'll see you guys again. I hope this is going to take place this year." Al was striding down the hallway.

Elaine squeezed her eyes tight for a moment. "That's what he'e leading us to believe."

They reached the door with Dr. Elbac's name plate emblazoned on the door. There was no receptionist here as there was in his regular office. Elaine knocked softly.

"Come in," answered a male voice.

Al and Elaine walked in as the doctor in his hospital coat stood up to greet them. "Good afternoon Doctor." Elaine entered ahead of Al and held out her hand.

Al practically bounded through the doorway. "Hi Doctor Elbac. I can honestly say I'm glad to have the smell of the hospital assaulting my senses today." Al held out his hand and waited for the doctor to shake it.

The doctor smiled. "I'll try to get you folks out of here as quickly as possible. I talked to Doctor Grove and have looked over your records so I am very pleased about how you've healed and recovered from the lumpectomy." He sat back down behind his desk. "As you are aware you are still a strong candidate for the camera implant surgery. This is no longer considered experimental. Camera implants have been successful and offered patients sight for several years. I've been honest with both of you when I've told you that this is not a permanent solution. The camera will not last for your entire lifetime, but you will get an extended period of sight in your right eye that will be 20/30."

Al almost jumped out of his seat. "That works for me."

The doctor nodded and looked at Elaine. "I understand. We are probably a year away from the surgery as long as your health remains as good as it is now. I don't want you to have another surgery so close to your lumpectomy unless it is an emergency. Any surgery is challenging for the body to recover. As important as the camera implant is, it is an elective surgery. I want your body prepared for the recovery and to have every chance for success." He paused to see if he would get a reaction. "The camera will serve as a lens and will be connected to the optic nerve. You will have to wear protective glasses and you will resemble C3PO from the Star Wars movie. I know that when the movie was released your corneal transplant had already failed, but that will give your wife an idea of what I am speaking about. It looks like we will not have your camera transplant ready for you to see "The Empire Strikes Back".

"I'm getting the impression you're a big fan." Al thought about how excited Albert was with his Star Wars toys even if they hadn't taken him to the movies.

The doctor looked a little embarrassed. "Yes. I've seen each movie four times. The ticket takers now know my face. I hope the analogy didn't bother you."

Al laughed. "Not at all. I believe all four of my boys are going to be thrilled to have a part robot for a Daddy."

The doctor laughed modestly. "Good. It will be exactly like that because your eye cannot contract or expand like a normal pupil. This will not harm the optic nerve but you will not be able to adjust to sunlight or lack of sun. Your sunglasses will be necessary, not cosmetic."

Al couldn't help interrupting the doctor. "I don't care what I have to do or endure as long as I can see my family again."

The doctor watched Al and Elaine closely. "I completely understand, but the purpose of today's visit is not just a medical evaluation, it is to make the entire process clear to you. Information is power, and you absolutely need to know what will happen long before we decide to move forward with this option."

Al nodded in agreement. "I understand."

"As both of you are aware, a corneal transplant is no longer an option for your right eye. I know you thought that you would be able to do one every couple of years, but a misconception like that is what I want to avoid in the future." He watched them both nod wordlessly in agreement. "First let's go back over why the corneal transplant is not an option. When you attach a donor cornea to the eye it must be attached to a remaining part of the damaged cornea in order for the fluid to flow to the new cornea. The fluid does not flow properly and eventually the cornea will cloud up. We can only do one or two transplants to an eye because the remaining damaged cornea does not last. In your case, we could do only one. It may be a possibility for the left eye, but for now we are concerned with the right. Let me be clear that you can never have another corneal transplant to the right eye and since your left eye was more seriously damaged by the chemical, we will continue to monitor viability of the left eye. We will still consider it your 'spare tire." He paused for emphasis. "This brings us to the camera implant surgery."

Elaine watched the direction the doctor moved in. "I used to get squeamish when I realized what my husband was enduring. I think I'm becoming anesthetized."

Al jumped to her defense. "I think four childbirths will do that to a woman. What you go through is much harder than this."

Dr. Elbac smiled at the sweetness of the exchange as he moved from behind the desk to a cork board and white board combination on the right side of the room. He pointed to the diagram of an eyeball and jumped right into his explanation. "We are going to remove the entire front of your eye." He began to pull off clear sheets that held each part as he described. "We will remove the cornea, lens, pupil and iris. All that will be left is the eyeball and optic nerve. Your eyeball will be completely white. The new camera implant will not have an iris or pupil. An eyeball is not strong enough to support a camera so a method had to be devised to hold it in place and not be rejected by the immune system. In order to facilitate this, we will take a piece of your shin bone. You will be having two surgeries at once since we need to place the bone immediately."

"Ouch," was the only comment Al could think of.

The doctor nodded. "Yes. There will also be a time period of healing for your shin. We utilize the shin bone because it is the closest in shape to the eye. A tiny hole will be drilled into the center of the bone for the placement of the camera lens." He moved to the white board and began to sketch. "A piece of skin graft will be stitched over the entire piece of shin bone and the camera which will be screwed into place. The skin will then be stitched to the eyeball and surrounding socket. This skin will become part of the eyeball as it heals into place."

As interesting as he found the description, it also scared him. Al needed to add levity to the situation. "Make sure you line everything up correctly. I don't want to be walking around looking at people's shoes."

Now Elaine jumped to Al's defense when she saw the look on the doctor's face. "Al, you need to start having a little fashion sense."

Not expecting that, both men gave a quick nervous laugh. "I'll be careful, I promise. The skin covering the lens hole will fall back, but if it doesn't we will cut a slit that will scab and heal over. The process of the skin pulling away from the lens should take a week. During that time, you will have sight but it will be behind a screen. This will give you time to adjust."

"Time to adjust to what? I want to see right away. Can't you just cut the hole while I'm in surgery?" Al felt himself moving to the edge of the chair he sat in.

"No, Albert. That is not how this will work. You don't want to get an infection before the skin has a chance to heal in place. Then we will have to remove the camera and maybe the eyeball itself." He pointed to the graphic picture on the board for Elaine. "This is a successful camera implant procedure. Once healed, this man had 20/25 vision and so should Albert. You will spend at least a week in the hospital recovering if everything goes well. I don't want you overdoing it once you go home. I understand that you are a very involved father, but if you want this to work, you are going to have to follow my recommendations as we progress. I have to have that guarantee from both of you before we proceed."

Elaine jumped in. "Doctor Elbac, we have a very strong support system in place with our extended family. I will start setting the ground work now to make sure Al will have every opportunity to heal properly. I've started back to work in the nursing field, but I will be able to take time off when required. He deserves the chance to see again."

Al felt the familiar pride and love he had for Elaine that reminded him she was no longer the naïve, young bride of their early marriage. The capable strong woman sitting next to him was not just arm candy that an outsider might perceive. He dared anyone to challenge her when the love and safety of her family was in question.

Dr. Elbac met Elaine's look. "I agree Mrs. Plevier, and I'll trust you to take care of what needs to be done in Albert's life to insure the proper healing for his future sight." He walked back behind the desk. "Albert's complete recovery time at home in a bestcase scenario should be about six weeks. After that we can gauge his new lifestyle to include both high quality life and health."

"When can we do the surgery?" Al wanted a date to focus on.

Now Dr. Elbac looked seriously at the white board he

just walked away from. "I am hoping for next summer. A year will give everyone involved time to prepare, physically and emotionally, but that is not what I'm really concerned about. I want to monitor your eye and entire health for a ten-month period. The last two months will include procedures necessary before the surgery can take place. How does that time table work in your frame of reference, Albert?"

Al was quiet for several seconds. "To be honest I was hoping for something sooner, but I have to work with you not against you. You're the man with the knife."

Dr. Elbac always enjoyed being disarmed by Al and told his own wife on several occasions that he looked forward to the appointments with the young couple.

"That's right. Let me get both of you into the examination room upstairs so we can complete Albert's physical and get you two back home to the boys." Dr. Elbac smiled at Elaine as all three were rising from their chairs and preparing to leave the office. "Mrs. Plevier, where are you working?"

"At County Memorial in the ER. It was the only position I could find that would allow me to do the day shift. I'll be leaving just before Albert and Larry get on the bus, and I'll be home when they get off the bus. I didn't realize how much I missed the work force."

"Congratulations. It is very satisfying for an educated woman like yourself to be back in her field." Dr. Elbac led them to the elevator. "You should be finished here in two hours."

Dr. Elbac was consistently accurate in his time estimated for office visits. Al and Elaine could plan their window of opportunity the car ride home offered to talk about the experience they just went through. Today's visit had taken an unpleasant turn for Al. He had thought of nothing more than the possibility of having sight for Christmas and Dr. Elbac confirmed that was not going to happen.

"I'm excited but very deflated. A year seems like an eternity. I had a fantasy about seeing all the boys together under the Christmas tree this year. I pictured the outside lights I was able to see on Lake Road and realized I don't have markers for our lights yet at this house. The boys deserve Christmas lights." The memory of the vision allowed by the corneal transplant made his heart ache.

Still not thrilled about doing all the driving for her family, Elaine had kept her eyes on the road when they spoke. "I'm sad for you too Al, but now that I understand more of what the surgery involves, I think we both need time to prepare. You will be regaining your sight, but you will be limited in mobility to a degree. The surgery to remove part of the shin bone is going to be a painful recovery."

Al looked at her surprised. "Compared to what I've been through, I should skate through it without difficulty."

"Don't be so sure. Dr. Elbac didn't go into a lot of detail about that part of the recovery for you. You can't be tumbling around with the boys while that heals even after your sight returns." The success of the surgery was no longer a question in Elaine's mind. "If you get an infection in your leg it will affect your entire recovery process. It will slow you down and could potentially harm the implant if an infection should travel throughout your body."

"I know you're right." He paused for effect. "We'll take this year to continue settling into the new house and do the prep work for the recovery period after the implant surgery next summer." Al started to say something, stopped and restarted. "Elaine, if I have to wait until at least the summer, I might as well wait for next September. Albert will be in third grade, Larry in Kindergarten and Chris will be in all day preschool. It would be less stressful than the summer."

Elaine considered this new option. "That would work better. We could take day and weekend trips with the boys."

Dread began to fill Al's mind. "Sure. I don't want the surgery to slow down the summer for the boys. I agree."

"I was thinking about maybe a trip that's a week long. I've never been to Niagara and Mom said that Dad wanted to go through the locks." Elaine felt her spirits lift as they discussed the trip, countering the serious and scary scenario she had been presented with all afternoon.

All Al could think about was how he would get through an entire week without letting his family see how miserable he would be. He would have ten months to think it over. "Aren't there bus trips available? I'm sure one of our parents would know about that. It would make it much easier and more pleasant for you."

Elaine became more excited at the thought of watching the scenery while she kept the boys entertained. "That's a great idea. It will be something to plan and talk about this year." She was lost for a moment as she stared ahead out the window. "This may be the last holiday you don't have sight. Each visit to the doctor brings us one step closer for you."

"There's a goal now. Again. Another light at the end of the tunnel." He realized what he said. "Forget that metaphor. It's a new feeling, a nice feeling to know I'm not just coping. I want to see my kids."

"I think you're going to be surprised at how much Chris looks like your baby pictures. He's your little clone." Elaine took the exit for their neighborhood and now had the night ahead on her agenda. "I'm kind of excited from this afternoon. Do you want to get pizza for the kids and go down town for the fireworks?"

"Fireworks? It's August. What's going on downtown?" Al's stomach turned a little. Watching fireworks was something he missed a great deal. He never had a chance to see them much as a child and as an adult he and Elaine made a point of going to see them together in the summer months.

"A late Founder's Day celebration. I think the actual day was supposed to be in June. It's such a nice evening I think it would be relaxing and I'm sure mom would like to get out of the house after watching the boys." Elaine pulled up to the stop sign and looked over at Al. "What do you think?"

"Sure. Do you want to call your parents too?" He tried to sound enthusiastic.

"That's what I was thinking. A family outing with pizza and a warm clear evening to enjoy the fireworks." Elaine was looking forward to a relaxing end to the busy day.

Al wanted to play pool and forget the frustration of waiting another year to see. There was nothing for him to see tonight when the colors filled the night sky.

"This will be a nice evening for the boys." Al felt his stomach turn as he began to build the emotional fortitude he would need to get through the night.

He struggled the rest of the evening as he gathered with his family to hide his moodiness and to find a way to dissipate his depression. Self pity was not something he dealt with in his youth and fighting its affects as an adult was a battle. Later, when he heard the crowds react to colors and sights before them he contemplated the year ahead knowing life would continue, his children would grow and the world would carry on regardless of whether or not he could see it. He was in life, but there were times when he felt his own experience of it was put on hold.

Each month that passed as the end of the year came to a close added fuel to his longing to see again and left Al feeling as though he were in limbo. Elaine noticed the change in Al. She watched her husband no longer living in the moment and instead replaced his normal disposition with a nervous air of anticipation that wafted along with his prescence.

This new element to his personaility was more apparent Christmas morning after the chaos of the boys subsided. Nick had caught on quickly to the purpose of the pretty boxes as Elaine and Al sipped coffee and stayed out of the way. Al had spent weeks putting together the toys so they would be ready to play with Christmas morning. The real trick proved to be hiding them. Over the years they had been successful at creating a surprise and retaining the belief that Santa existed.

"We did it again, Al. These boys are going to collapse into exhaustion from the sheer joy of this morning." She watched Al's smile and couldn't help but feel it was forced. "Are you ready for our presents?"

"Sure, sweetheart." He reached under the cushion behind him and handed her a box. "Your mom helped me pick this one out. I'm not confessing, I'm just speaking the obvious which you will figure out as soon as you open it."

She pulled the larger box from behind the pillow on her side. "Whatever you gave me I will love it. I always do. I hope you feel the same about this. Hold out both hands."

Al felt the weight of the two boxes put together in one present. "Oh, boy. I bet this is a new skill saw."

"Nope. Sorry. I'm going to make you work for it too. You can't tell what it is from the boxes. You'll have to get into them." She saw that the new lines on his forehead were not easing into submission.

Elaine opened her present first, a bottle of her favorite perfume, extra large. She kissed him and gave him a strong hug. "I love this. Mom hit the nail on the head."

"Hey, whoah. I knew which kind I just needed her to pick it up for me." He felt himself get a little defensive.

"Ooops. Sorry. I realize that. Now hurry up and open your boxes." Just at that moment Chris came up to his parents holding one of his new toys and trying to see what they had gotten.

"Daddy has a new phone." Chris pointed at the box.

Al was struggling to hurry getting into the box and was relieved. "Thanks, Pal. Now Daddy can work on putting it together." He finally got the top opened and pulled at the contents. "This is no ordinary phone."

Elaine smiled and laughed at his obvious excitement. "It's two cordless phones. One for the kitchen and one for our room. I figured we are going to need two when one inevitably goes missing. It says on the box that they have a beeper system you can press on the base to help you find the phone."

"Excellent. We are definitely going to need that." Chris reached up to touch the phone and try for a grab. "Sorry little guy. For the time being this is Daddy's toy."

Not bothered in the least, Chris walked back to the pile of toys encircling his brothers.

"Elaine, I'm glad now that you went back to work. At first I was just happy for you to be doing something that gives fulfillment outside of us, but the extra money really made this an extraordinary Christmas." He leaned over and kissed her cheek.

"I think we all adjusted well. I missed you guys and I still do but I like my job. When I come home I'm thrilled to be with you." She sniffed at her new perfume. "The chance to be doing Christmas dinner for our families is great too."

Al felt the phone and all its paraphernalia. "The family is going to do the clean up and a lot of the prep, Elaine. I don't want you doing it all."

"Al, it's okay. The only person overwhelmed this year is Ronnie with a new baby and husband. The first couple months as a new parent is always a strain. Remember how we used to feel when Albert was first born?" Elaine reached over to grab a cookie off the tray she had brought in for the family.

Al was momentarily lost in thought at Albert's first and second Christmas. He had to shake himself out of the nostalgic sadness he felt and focus on next Christmas when he believed he would have sight again. The excitement of this moment and his new phone dissipated, only serving as reminders of what he had lost.

"Are you cold? I felt you shiver." Elaine took a sip of her coffee and watched Albert carefully examining the box that held his new airplane model.

Al tried to move past her question. "No, I'm good." He returned to their discussion of Ronnie and new baby Peter Jr.. "She'll be back to normal in a couple more months as he grows. I had to laugh when she was nervous about me holding him. It wouldn't matter if I had sight or not. She thought I didn't know how or wouldn't hold his head up properly. Your mom came over, she heard her sneeze and asked her if she had the flu." Both of them laughed at the same personality traits they exhibited when their first baby was born. "Look at us now. Four little monsters tearing the house apart and bringing us more joy than we could ever have imagined." He was, in his mind, enjoying next Christmas, taking mental pictures of all three boys under the tree. Unknown to his entire family, that is where his emotions stayed.

The winter of 1981 passed with the anticipated doctor visits coming on schedule in their mundane quality and at the end of each one confirmed that the surgery was no longer a possibility but imminent. When Elaine had begun her new job, Ronnie was on maternity leave from hers. She had helped Al get adjusted and into a routine. The four boys were excited to have a new cousin. Secretly, Al thought they were lining him up as the last rung on their peer ladder.

Al spent the winter building the wood working business and watching the boys while Elaine worked in her nursing career. The family had not had the celebration last year they should have upon her graduation from nursing school because Elaine didn't want a party or any acknowledgement. She felt this was more of a career move and was not the monumental feeling of elation she felt when she graduated with her Bachelors degree as a twenty-two-year-old woman on the cusp of an adventure.

She enjoyed getting out of the house and the shift work enabled her to still be present for her family. She and Al fell into a routine with the forward momentum of a working middle class family. They were pulling together as a team with the unspoken goal of life after his sight returned. The marathon of acceptance was almost at an end.

Elaine knew the vacation she planned for the summer was really for her, but she and the boys needed it. The family took day and local trips more inexpensively than people could imagine and when they fell short of the cash needed, their families helped out as they came along for the ride. There was nothing Mr. Hinds enjoyed more than time with all his grandchildren.

Ronnie and Little Peter decided to join them also on the trip to Niagara in July of the summer of 1981. The parents and grandparents sat back and watched the boys interact and find their way among each other as they explored the boundaries outside their home world. Little Peter had not yet started to started to walk so Ronnie knew she would be able to enjoy the trip and help keep an eye on her nephews.

"It's all becoming clear to me now." Ronnie hoisted Peter a little higher on her hip. "You guys brought me along so you could relax." She smiled brightly at her family all seated on the Maid of the Mist boat ride.

"Mommy, when are the fireworks starting?" Albert looked adorable in his plastic, blue 'rain coat' as he hung onto the railing with his chin just reaching over the top rail.

"Boys, they will start later, after our boat ride." Elaine leaned back against the wall of the boat and looked over at the beautiful colors from the sun radiating down on the falling water.

"Aunt Ron, how come we have to wear these stupid coats?" Albert tugged at his hood.

"You'll find out in a minute. Keep that hood off and you'll be sorry." Ronnie pulled the cover she had over Peter and stepped back to sit next to her parents along the side of the boat.

Mr. Hinds caught Larry trying to sneak away. "Hey! You stay right here in front of our bench. You can see the falls from the railing."

Larry hung his head and smirked and he sidled up to Albert who was quick to set his brother straight. "Told ya not to try. They're watching everything we do."

Al listened to his children's chatter and grew introspective and uncharacteriscally quiet. Elaine noticed immediately.

"Al we're getting close to the water. You're about to get doused." Elaine pulled down her hood. "Boys, hang on, here it comes!"

The water showered the three boys at the rail as Nick climbed into his grandfather's lap giggling as the boat moved through the mist close to the tons of water falling over the falls. Al felt the mist shower him as the boat lived up to its name. The only thought in his head was that he felt like he was in a rain storm.

Jayne Kelly

The boys screamed with delight. Even Peter laughed and giggled as the cool mist rained down on him. "Everyone is getting into the act." Ronnie smiled and kissed her baby's head. The sun was setting and the lights of the falls came on as their boat made its way back to the Canadian dock.

"Al, the lights are magnificent. The tour book said they shut them off immediately before the fireworks so each of us will have to hold a kid. The last thing we want is for them to be disappearing in the mist." Elaine and Al laughed together and she noticed how forced his laughter was.

"Let me know when the boat tour is getting close to the end. I will grab my designated kid before the boat docks." Al was glad for something physical to hold his attention. "Maybe give me Albert. He knows better than to try anything when I have hold of his hand."

Albert heard his name mentioned and turned from the railing. "Daddy, what are you talking about me for?"

"I was just telling Mom what a great time you and I are going to have watching the fireworks. You're going to tell me about the colors and shapes." Al knew he could zone out during the fireworks show if Albert was with him. The little boy would be so entranced he wouldn't notice.

"Am I going to have to hold your hand?" Suspicion emanated from Albert.

"Of, course. You don't want to lose me, do you? Who's going to coach you next season if you leave me at Niagara Falls?" Fresh mist covered his face.

Albert turned back to the water and lost interest in the challenge of how he was going to out maneuver his parents during the fireworks. He stayed at the rail with his brothers until he felt his father's hand on his shoulder ten minutes later.

"Albert, you're going to stay with me now and help me navigate the dock. Hold my hand tight." Al reached down and felt around until he grabbed hold of the little boy's hand.

Albert gave up quickly as he watched four adults he traveled with each grab one of his brothers. He wanted to be with his dad. "Okay, Daddy. I'm staying with you."

236

Al squeezed Alberts hand. "Play follow the leader. Stay behind Mommy. She always gets the best spot for the fireworks."

The family navigated their way off the Maid of the Mist and walked up the dock and toward the park where the crowd was gathering. Albert did not fuss, staying with his dad as dusk passed and the sky darkened.

He pulled Al along to keep up with Elaine and the rest of the family. "Come on, Daddy. They're going to start!"

"Okay, Albert." He felt the little boy pulling him downward. "Where's the blanket, pal?"

"Here. Sit right down." Albert plopped down and gazed skyward.

Al felt around to make sure he landed on the blanket. The last thing he wanted tonight was a damp butt. Suddenly he heard a collective 'OOhhh' come up from the crowd.

Albert squealed with delight. "Daddy, they shut off the lights!"

"Looks like we made it to grandma's blanket just in time." Al always marveled at how women were always prepared. He knew Mrs. Hinds had carried the blanket on the boat ride and thought it must be the Mom instinct in them.

Suddenly booms and crackles filled the air. The crowd reacted after each explosion so Al knew when the fireworks happened. Albert had already forgotten to describe the fireworks to his dad as he enjoyed them with his brothers, but he never let go of his dad's hand.

Al tried with all the resolve he could muster not to act moody as he did in Cooperstown. He had always wanted to see Niagara Falls as a poor child in Patterson. The irony of his life now was that even though he had a beautiful wife and children to travel with and the assistance of family financially for the moment when they needed it, he couldn't see the places he always dreamed of.

"Look at that. Wow. Albert, look, look!" Larry pointed at the star bursts of fireworks.

"Boy!" Chris smiled, laughed and covered up his ears with both hands.

Al sat quietly trying to maintain the smile on his face. He felt like they were never going to end. As he sat there he thought back to the bicentennial fireworks he heard from the operating room of the hospital as he waited for the corneal transplant in 1976. He thought he was missing a great party the entire country had, now he was glad he missed it.

Thirty minutes passed like an eternity. Al heard a boom and then applause from the gathered crowd and he knew the show had ended. "What do you think, guys?"

The boys cheered together. "What's next Mommy?" Larry jumped up and down even though it was now close to ten o'clock.

"Bed, for everyone. Adults, grab a child." Elaine let out a large yawn and reached for Chris.

Al felt Albert's hand in his. "Come on, Daddy. Night's over."

Al breathed out slowly. "Yes, it is. We have another boat tour tomorrow."

The second part of their trip was a tour through the lock and canal system of New York. This was something Al always wanted to see as an engineer. He wondered if once he had sight, the family would have the time to visit these places again.

He sat passively in his seat during the boat ride and drifted off until Larry shook him. "Daddy? Mommy wants to know what you want to have for lunch."

"Whatever is fine." He leaned back against the seat and felt a sandwich touch his hand. "Thanks."

"Your welcome, Daddy." Larry squeezed next to his dad in a seat meant for one person. Before long Al was laughing, but still looking forward to tomorrow when they would ride the bus home to New Jersey.

He climbed into his seat on the bus the next day, not feeling any difference from all the seats he sat passively in during the trip. Once the kids had calmed down, Al and Elaine had the chance to talk like they always do at night.

Elaine looked around at the sleeping family before turning to Al. "Are you awake Al?"

"Yes." His voice was a whisper. "I'm enjoying the quiet captivity of the boys."

She leaned back against the bus seat. "This was a great trip."

Al still couldn't give away how he truly felt. "Yeah. It was just what we needed."

"I'm glad we had this time before the surgery. This time next year you'll be able to see all the boys." She looked over at the expression on his face.

"It's been impossible for me to live in the moment. All I've been thinking about for the last couple of weeks is the day I can see again." He turned toward her. "When we get home, I'm going to start marking the days off on the calendar."

"I understand." She was thoughtful. "It's only two months away." She paused. "Al, I put in for a leave of absence. I'm part time so there may not be a job for me when the leave is over."

"As long as you're sure that's what you want, we'll be okay." Al's mind traveled to the years immediately following the accident. "The days when the neighbors, our family and friends brought over meals for us were the most humbling. I couldn't even do telephone sales yet. It was scary, but we were together."

Elaine's mind also traveled to the early days where one moment they were building their financial future and in the next moment it was all gone. "They were scary days. I always knew that, should we hit the complete bottom and lose the house, we could always live with my family. That safety net kept me sane at the worst moments." She smiled broadly. Looking from one head to another of the sleeping figures, Elaine took inventory. "I want to enjoy every moment."

The children were growing quickly. Nick was running as fast as his little legs would carry him to keep up with his brothers. The boys would try not to include him in their games and he would fight his way in, never being left behind. All the boys were thoughtful, but Al had to admit that when he would drop something and was crawling around on the carpet or grass looking for it, Larry seemed to appear out of nowhere to hand it to him. In the next second he would disappear again with his brothers creating havoc as they discovered what the world had to offer.

The family returned from the Niagara adventure in one piece, refreshed and ready to enjoy the remainder of the summer. For Al, it had been one more event he had to endure and survive that strengthened his resolve to see again.

The hospital where she worked had reduced Elaine's hours to part time since she could only work day shifts. Since it was summer she didn't care. For two days, the temperature had dropped down into the lower seventies and she and Al were taking full advantage of it.

"I'm going outside to get the mowing done so we can picnic outside." Al strode outside in his work clothes.

Ten minutes later Elaine was busy with putting together the food for a picnic when Albert came into the kitchen from the living room. "Mommy, Dad is outside yelling at the lawn mower."

She rolled her eyes in response. "Good. Let him get it out of his system. We'll have a fun afternoon."

Albert shook his head. "Mom, he sounds pretty mad."

She had heard the mower putter to a stop and waited for the evitable march back into the house. He came in carrying a ragged piece of material. "What do I have in my hand?"

Elaine, knowing his sense of humor, tried not to laugh too soon. "Looks like it used to be your sweatshirt."

"Whaaat?" Al ran the shirt through both hands.

Albert had heard the door open and came back into the kitchen. "Dad can we go outside to play now?"

Al tried to sound angry. "Albert, what do I have in my hand?"

"A torn shirt." Albert looked passed the shirt and through a window at the tree house.

"What did I tell you guys about leaving stuff in the yard

when you know I'm going to mow?" He shook the shirt a little for effect.

"Daddy, it's your shirt. Mommy borrowed it last night 'cause it got cold when we caught fireflies." Albert inched his way toward the back door.

Al paused for a moment. "Thanks for the help, Buddy. You guys can go play. I'm done mowing for the day."

Al ran from the room yelling for his brothers. A door could be heard opening and slamming as Al and Elaine continued to square off.

"Seriously? If you're going to leave stuff in the yard, make it your stuff. I don't pick up before I mow." He tossed the shirt in the garbage next to him.

"You were carrying it for me when I took it off. It was warmer than we thought, remember?" Elaine piled the sandwiches inside the bag. Picnics for them did not include grilling unless Mr. Hinds was around. Al was not a proponent of open flame of any kind.

"Wait a minute. This is my fault now?" Sweat formed on his forehead.

"Yes. You must have dropped it and forgot. That'll teach ya." Elaine raised her chin in victory.

Al stood there for a moment. "I got nothing. You win. I'm going to take a shower. The grass is half mowed. Is that good enough?"

"Perfect. The boys don't care. This may be the day Albert, Larry and Chris let Nick in the tree house. We have to be there to keep an eye on them." She headed for the door.

"Those boys are really mad that I put the picnic table under the tree. They think they own every tree in the back yard. It will be interesting when they start exploring the trees at the edge of the property line." Progecting into the future, Al saw the day his kids left the property confines completely as young adults in their own cars. He wanted to see that.

The boys came back into the house with Nick trailing behind. "Daddy, when are you coming out?" Larry was first in line with a frustrated look.

"I need a shower, then I'll come out." Al needed the momentum of the boy's energy and activities.

Lately his focus on the camera implant surgery led to a distraction. He tried to hide the distraction the best he could from Elaine and the children. When Dr. Elbac offered the hope of a return of his sight he promised himself he would work on finding joy in each day and for the most part he did. Depression would begin to settle in when he needed someone to transport him or when he was on trips. Traveling to places or vacations were useless for him, but necessary for the family. He brought himself out of depression by moving around physically.

The activity that helped him compensate for the lost sense of belonging during vacations was to create a park like environment for his children in their yard. It was unique and was his contribution to his role in their family. Parents of boys' friends could not believe what they saw when visiting the Plevier home. It was not unusual to have half a dozen children on any day of the week playing at their house. Al created the yard for that purpose and it amazed him that other parents did not desire the same level of chaos while their children were young. They were always grateful to drop their children off and Elaine welcomed them with open arms.

Today Elaine saw grumpiness in Al's disposition and knew without discussion what was really behind it. Every morning as he marked the days on the calendar until the camera implant could take place, he felt cheated of immediate sight. The boys sensed it too and did their best to 'make things better' as children do when they sense discord within their households.

One afternoon Elaine watched the boys exchange looks and circle Al quietly. Each boy put a finger to their lips trying to signal Elaine not to give them away.

Al sensed he was surrounded by the soft padded footfalls around him. "A smile spread across his face as he turned in the direction of Elaine. I feel like I'm in a trap." Al smirked and the room became deathly quiet as he reached out quickly grabbing at anything or anyone.

A happy shriek greeted him as he grabbed Chris and was then tackled by the remaining three. The cluster of arms and legs practically rolled in one great mass moving into the living room where the carpet made for a softer landing.

Calmly Elaine watched the progression as a shoe went flying and the giggles got louder. The rolling bodies stopped once, the boys looked at her and then took the moment to catch Al off guard. He landed flat on his back laughing before he had a chance to regain his ground. A second later he had Chris and Nick under one arm while being headlock by Albert.

"Big boys look out for Nick." Al thought he shot the warning too late but knew Elaine was probably watching.

Nick yelled out in alarm. "No! Nick play too." He slipped out of his dad's arm and dove for Al's middle helping to pin him to the floor.

Al was laughing so hard he lost hold of Chris. "You boys are going to have saw dust and garage dirt all over you like me."

Albert kicked the coffee table hard and froze waiting for the reprimand from Elaine that never came. She had already tuned out the all too familiar scene.

Al felt his shirt ripping. "Aw man, I am losing this battle."

"Yup Daddy. You're toast." Larry dove for Al's back as he watched his father gain ground again and raise himself up. "Nicky, grab his leg. You can do that."

Nick, always obedient to his older brothers, grabbed the leg with a toddler death grip. "I win!"

"Not yet." Al tried to stop laughing, breathed in deep and then raised himself up on his knees bellowing like a lion.

All four boys fell off him, giggled and looked for the next angle of attack. "I got his middle." Albert went for the dive and Al met him half way.

"Thanks for the warning kid." They rolled past the couch with the other three negotiating vulnerable places.

The tussle went on for another half hour. Happy screams came from the living room as Al roared up again on his knees. Al held his position as the four boys hung on him trying desperately to bring him back down. All that was left of his shirt now was the collar and one sleeve both hanging loosely over the Jobe shirt.

Elaine smiled at the memory and wondered to herself if that would bring Al out of his moodiness on this day as she watched Ronnie's car pull in.

She carried the picnic food on a tray as Ronnie met her at the back door with Peter on her hip. "Hey, guys. What's going on?"

There was a sad look on Ronnie's face and tears welled up in her eyes. "Elaine, can Little Peter and I stay with you for a while?"

Elaine stood in front of her sister holding her baby and looked at the confused look on the baby's face. She immediately put the tray on the back steps and opened her arms to take the baby with an over the top smile and high, pitched greeting meant only for babies.

"Of course! Come to Aunt Elaine. Give me that baby." Peter squealed with delight. "You want to go see what the big boys are doing? Or maybe I should say it more accurately, what havoc they're creating?" She looked around for the boys and spoke loudly toward the backyard. "I have a picnic lunch for everyone. Are you boys sure you want to wait?"

A stampede came directly from the tree house. "Well, that didn't take long." Elaine kissed baby Peter on the head as he pointed at the group and smiled.

The five stopped again and turned sheepishly to Elaine. "Hi Aunt Ronnie." Larry gave a wave to her.

This scene was exactly what Ronnie needed to forget last evening's decision by her and her new husband to separate. She had not called her family last night or this morning. In her

heart she knew she could count on her big sister to support her through the difficult time. Her four nephews would serve as a busy distraction.

"Looks like I arrived just in time." She saw Al approach

the group with a sad expression and wondered if they needed her as much as she needed them. "What's happening with you, old man?"

Al smirked and gave her an 'I know everything attitude'. "Where's the tribe?"

"Grabbing food off Elaine's tray." She crossed her arms defensively and caught Elaine giving a warning look at the four boys.

Al felt the palpable change in the mood. "I'm just fine." The boys smiled at their mother in relief. "But, I need a shower. Everybody stay outside with Mom and Aunt Ronnie. I'll see you in a little while."

"Daddy we're all dirty like you now." Boys and adults included, held their noses.

"Then you might as well stay outside and get dirtier or it's bath time." Al laughed lightly.

"Al, you're a mess." Elaine shook her head.

"Yeah." He laughed and ran a hand over the Jobe shirt. "I'll be out in a little while." He paused as he started to walk backwards until he felt the house wall behind him. "Ronnie, I wasn't ease dropping but did I hear that you'll be with us for a while?"

Ronnie began to feel anxious and hope Al wouldn't hear it in her voice. "If it's alright with you."

He smiled and shrugged his shoulder. "Of course, it is. The more, the merrier."

Chapter XVI: Continuation

"*Mr* Plevier did you see 'Star Wars after you had your corneal transplant?" The nurse smiled at the comparison she was about to make.

Al took a breath before responding. "No. My sight faded in January right before the movies release that spring. To be honest, we really didn't pay attention to the hype because we thought it would be a nothing movie."

The nurse laughed good naturedly. "Neither did my husband. Now we have all the paraphernalia he can get his hands on including the posters. He saw the movie five times." She laid another light blanket over Al anticipating his response to the operating room temperature. "I was looking at the C-3PO poster this morning. The camera implant you're about to receive is a miracle and you will resemble C-3PO."

"You're not planning on painting me gold, are you?" Al was always conscious of not wanting another person to be uncomfortable around him and she sounded young and socially inexperienced, not harmful or mean like Mary. "You and the surgeon are big fans."

The woman began to laugh heartily behind her surgical

mask. "Albert, you're a very handsome man. We don't need the women falling over you more than they already do. Your wife will sue us."

Al heard the door swing open and more than one set of padded feet entering. "Good morning, Albert." Dr. Elbac spoke with a focused tone, energized.

Someone moved close to his right side, wheels rolled and the anesthesiologist had taken his post. "Hello, Mr. Plevier. Are you ready?"

Al lifted his left hand slightly in acknowledgement. "Good morning, everyone. Let's do this."

Dr. Elbac reached out with his gloved hand to gently lower Al's left. "Albert, unless we encounter something unexpected, you will have 20/30 vision in your right eye immediately after the skin is cut away and the bandages are removed permanently in several weeks."

Al breathed deeply as he felt a needle inserted in his arm. "I'm okay, Doctor. I listened to all this information very closely on our visits. You don't have to prepare me again. I'm ready." The narcotic began to take effect immediately. "I want you to know how grateful I am for giving me this chance. It's true that in the larger picture of my life I would have to admit that because of my loss of sight I no longer see the trash in the gutters."

The doctor and the nurse assisting Al exchanged looks. "Relax, Albert. You'll be asleep in a few moments."

Al continued where he left off. "I experience the world through hearing and feeling. I feel with my hands and now my heart feels more." He knew he was on a soap box and he didn't care. His heart was so full of gratitude and sincerity he couldn't stop letting the man in front of him understand how appreciative he was. "If I had to choose between losing my sight or my hearing I would have to choose my sight. I've found beauty in music and in people's voices. Without hearing I would just have been looking ahead. I would see expressions and that would clutter my discernment." Al was slipping further away as his speech started to slur. "I'm just excited to know that the return of my sight will not be gradual. It will be immediate from the moment the bandages are off." Al felt himself drifting and knew that the man to his right was doing his job. Drapes were placed on his face. With continued slurred speech, he tried to hang on.

"Albert, count down from 100."

"Three, two, one. Hey, I'm still awake." A second later he was unconscious.

Dr. Elbac became stepped closer to his patient's head. "Immobize the head."

The beeps of the heart monitor were the only sound in the sterile room besides the requests of the doctor and responses from the support staff. Al was released into their hands and through them into the hands of God.

The surgery lasted hours. There were two stages, one to remove the small portion of shin bone and the second to complete the camera implant. Al did not dream. Suspended in a void, he heard nothing and felt nothing until a voice beckoned him.

"Albert, Albert. It's time to wake up. You're at Mt. Sinai Hospital. You've just had the camera implant surgery." The female voice came from a distance. "Albert. We want to wheel you to recovery to see your wife. You have to wake up first."

At the thought of Elaine his mind began to clear. He felt he had only momentarily been unconscious and tried to form words. "How?"

The nurse watched him stir and checked his IV line. "You're doing great. The surgery went well."

Al groaned again and then felt the accompanying pain from the surgery in his leg and his head. He wanted to return to the oblivion of a few moments ago. "Elaine?"

"Your wife has been waiting in a private area the doctor found. Someone is bringing her to you now. You will spend the afternoon in recovery. I'm going to step out to let her know you're awake. Stay with us. I'll be right back."

Al tried to focus on the soft padding of her feet. It

seemed unfortunate to him that the outside world would forget that he needed stimuli to stay awake in moments like this. Even with the pain, his desire to drift back to sleep began to envelop him.

"Al? It's me." Elaine stood next to his gurney with a surgical mask on.

Through the pain and fog he focused on her voice. "Hi."

"Hi, Sweetheart. The doctor said the surgery went better than he expected. It was a success." Elaine chocked back the tears.

Al breathed out deeply. "Amen."

Twenty-four hours later Al awoke fully in his private room as the pain, still very present, began to subside slightly. The right eye was covered with a thin skin and then bandages. Elaine sat next to the bed as Dr. Elbac unwound the bandages and examined the camera implant.

"The eye looks great. I see signs healing is taking place." Doctor Elbac wore a surgical mask and Al could hear the paper like fabric respond to his breathing.

Dr. Elbac leaned over him creating a shadow allowing to differentiate light and dark. "Doctor, I can see shadows and figures through the skin covering the camera lens."

Al felt the chill of excitement creep up his arms at the same time a huge palpable weight of relief was lifted from his shoulders. The anticipation of the last year and a half dissipated the instant he knew the surgery was successful.

Elaine stared, mesmerized by the surgical results. The procedure the doctor had described to her months earlier was nothing short of miraculous from her perspective. Dr. Elbac stepped back to retrieve something and she got up from her chair. She saw the thin skin stitched over the eye and the camera lens underneath.

"Elaine? I see your outline. I know it's you, but it's weird. The shadows are in reverse." Al kept his gaze forward. "Is this normal, doctor?"

Dr. Elbac did not hesitate. "Yes. Your eye is adjusting. If I'm understanding what you said, your vision right now is equivalent to viewing an x-ray."

The inverted perspective was making Al a little nauseous and he could not nod his head in agreement. "Yes. That's exactly right. Will it always be like this?"

The doctor moved to the end of the bed. "No. The eye is adjusting. Eventually you will have 20/25 vision in the right eye." The doctor waved to Al from where he stood. "You will still be bandaged for several weeks after you go home. We want to prevent any infections as the eye heals."

Al waved back to the doctor and everyone laughed. Neither the doctor or Al, with his limited sight, saw the tears cascading down Elaine's cheeks.

"You will always wear the glasses you will be given before and after the bandages are removed. Remember that the eye has no pupil contraction or dilation. This is a camera lens, not a normal eye."

"It's normal enough for me." He felt the pain in the eye thrumming. "I am still in a lot of discomfort. Should I give the eye a rest for now?"

The doctor stepped back up to the head of the bed. "That's normal. Just let us know how the discomfort is progressing. If it is subsiding even slightly, we are right on track. If it increases, we need to know right away."

"If I have increasing discomfort does that mean the implant is failing?" Al leaned into the pillow as the doctor put the bandages back in place.

"It could mean many things. Let's worry about that if it happens. At the moment, the implant looks perfect. The surgery went perfectly." He finished replacing the bandages over the eye and started to examine the right leg. "You're beginning to heal nicely. I'm very pleased with everything."
"Me too." Al felt the doctor replacing the leg bandages. "There is something else weird going on. I heard you move before you moved. Does that make sense? It's a little scary."

The doctor focuses his gaze on Albert and tried to hide any expression from Elaine. "Yes. We'll monitor whether that progresses or fades. You have sensory readjustment taking place and that is as simplistic an explanation as I can give you."

Al's head hurt too much to question Dr. Elbac further. "Fine. That explanation works for now."

"Mrs. Plevier. I'd like to give him time to rest. You are more than welcome to stay, but he needs to rest to alleviate the discomfort." Dr. Elbac wrote on the chart as he spoke.

Elaine walked to the chair, which in this room as in all the other hospital rooms Al had been in before, sat next to his bed. "I brought lots of magazines with me. My sister and parents are watching our children so I thought I would stay the afternoon."

Upon hearing this Al rallied around the pain. "What time is it?"

Dr. Elbac answered as he continued to write. "It's 1:30."

"Elaine, have you been here all morning?" His thoughts continued to clear and the pain in his leg battled for hierarchy against the headache.

"I've been here since 10:00." She watched Al's face and recognized the tense lines as he adjusted into the discomfort from surgery recovery.

"That's two days of driving into the city. I want you out home before rush hour. Please." He acutely felt the pain in both his leg and head. "I need to know you are safe so I can rest."

Elaine was always touched by the way Al tried to protect her even if it was from the dreaded task of driving that she always relied on him to do when he had sight. "If that's what will give you peace of mind I will." She stood next to the side of the bed and leaned down to gently kiss his lips. "I would prefer to stay, but I'm not going to argue with you." She turned to retrieve her the bag she brought with her. "If you need something for the pain, please tell them."

"Don't worry about me. You know I'm not shy when I need something." Al felt himself getting agitated. "I love you and I don't want to think of you stuck in all that traffic. Call the desk when you get home."

Elaine stared down at him. "I'll be back in the morning."

Al grew more tense. "If you want to skip a visiting day and stay home, I'll be fine. Driving back and forth every day is too much."

Elaine stood next to the bed with a bag over each shoulder. "Al, I'll be here tomorrow and the next day and the day after that. The children are being watched by our family." She decided to lighten the mood she could see Al retreating into. "Albert thinks he is in charge of the house while you're in the hospital. He's become quite bossy with his brothers."

A small smile appeared at the corner of Al's mouth. "Remind him that his dad will be home soon. I'll literally have my eye on him."

Elaine was at Mt. Sinai hospital in Manhattan every day of Al's stay. Each morning she passed through the front doors and was greeted sometimes by the sound or sight of children in the waiting area. The memory of the children in the waiting room Manhattan Eye and Ear never left her. Whenever she or Al felt heartbroken over their own predicament, they would, together, think back to the first time they heard the cries of the children waiting to be healed. Together, their faith held clarity in such moments. Elaine was always the first to say, 'There but for the grace of God go I'.

Each day when Dr. Elbac would visit, the skin covering the camera lens began to pull back. "Doctor, the shadows are starting to correct themselves. I still have that weird sensation of hearing what you're saying before I see your lips move, but at least life is beginning to look less like an x-ray."

"The sensory is correcting itself. Try to work with it. Your brain is incorporating a device. I'm very happy to hear that the shadows are beginning to reverse." He walked to the end of the bed. "That was my biggest concern, and it signals that the operation is a complete success. The time table I have for your recovery is two more weeks. You should have 20/25 vision when the remaining skin over the lens is cut away and the bandages are permanently removed." He lifted Al's leg slowly. "How is your shin discomfort?"

His jeans rubbed against the bandages that wrapped around the healing shin bone. "It is starting to diminish. The shin still hurts like the devil and the headache thrums. That's the closest way I can describe it." Al felt the doctor take away his hands and he eased himself off the bed. His toe stubbed the wheelchair brought for his discharge.

Part of Elaine couldn't believe the miracle she was witnessing. "Al, I can't wait for the moment you see the boys."

"Me either. I picture them in my mind every day. I wonder how surprised I'll be at who each one looks like." Everyone laughed.

"That's a nice team you're building." Dr. Elbac smiled broadly.

"It's built, doctor." Al deadpanned.

The doctor raised his eyebrows. "Are you two finished?"

This time Elaine chimed in. "Yes."

Dr. Elbac rebandaged Al's eye. "Sorry to hear that, but I understand. Your family certainly has enough on its plate."

Al shook his head in agreement and defiance. "We made up our minds that we would not change the trajectory our lives despite the accident. We trust our faith that the accident was just that, an accident. It's God's will that we live our lives to the fullest. He didn't cause the accident. His will is not vicious."

Dr. Elbac looked steadily at his patient. "You are the strongest couple I know. This situation alone may have broken another couple. The two of you not only grew closer, you enhanced your life together."

Elaine now felt the need to jump in. "This is the man I married. For better or worse we love each other. If the situation was reversed, it would be no different."

The doctor swallowed hard past the lump in his throat. "Let's get you home. I've signed off on your chart." He looked at Al sitting on top of the covers fully dressed and the bags next to Elaine on the floor. "You look ready to go. I'll get a chair in here." He reached over and took Al's hand. "Congratulations Albert. I'll see you in my office next week for the follow up exam. If you have any problems or questions, please call my office anytime."

Al shook the doctor's hand firmly. "Thanks Dr. Elbac, for everything. This was very important to me." Al held onto the doctor's hand.

An hour later Elaine pulled slowly into the driveway, always wary of the four small humans in their household who might be playing outside. "Al don't wrestle with the boys yet. We don't want any accidents."

Al turned to Elaine and answered her sarcastically. "No, really?"

"Alright, Al. I just think Albert will understand but the little guys probably won't." Elaine felt like Al thought she was mothering him and truth be told, she knew she was being overprotective.

He started to get out of the car. "I miss our family. Let's get in there." Al looped his cane over his arm and walked confidently into the house.

Ronnie walked toward him carrying Peter. "Hi Al. How are you doing?"

"I'm doing fine. The bandages will be on for another couple of weeks and the pain has all but disintegrated into a dull ache." He continued further into the living room.

Albert and Larry heard their parents come into the house and greeted their dad with a nonchalance that surprised both Al and Elaine. "Hi Daddy." Larry looked up at his bandaged eyes and large dark glasses.

Al felt in front of him and tousled the little boy's hair. "Hey, Pal. Daddy missed you."

"How are your eyeballs, Daddy?" Larry pointed at Al's glasses.

"They are still sore. Daddy still has to keep them covered." Al stood straight.

Larry stared blankly up at him as Albert ran across the

254

living room where they stood. "Hi Dad. Can you play ball?" Albert made a move to run and tackle Al as Elaine cut him off while dropping her purse on a table.

"Guys, you need to give Daddy a break for a little while longer. His eyes need more time to heal." Elaine began to tickle Albert lightly.

"When can you pitch again Daddy?" Albert, appropriate for his age, was very self involved.

"The doctor will tell us. For now, I still have to keep the bandages on. I'm gonna count on you to help me remind your brothers that Daddy can't wrestle around. Nicky might not understand and his feelings could be hurt." Al placed his free hand on Albert's shoulder hoping his oldest son would feel like a big boy.

"Aww, Daddy. I don't want to take care of them. Can't that be Mommy's job?" Albert gave a disdainful look toward Larry, who scowled back at him.

"He doesn't have to watch me, Daddy." Larry stared back at Albert and then he saw the toy behind him that they both fought over earlier. He made a mad dash for it, followed by Albert.

"What just happened?" Al stood still and turned his head in Elaine's direction.

"The usual. We're on our own." Elaine turned to see her mother laughing.

Mrs. Hinds jumped into the conversation. "Not entirely. We're going to stay with you until the bandages come off. There is no point to taking any chances with your latest miracle." Mrs. Hinds looked proudly at Al and Elaine. "You're both so brave."

The two boys were yelling and tugging at the same toy. Chris came in from his room, took one look at the mayhem his two older brothers were involved in and started laughing.

"Chris, Daddy's home from the hospital." Elaine tried to stop what she knew was about to turn into a three-kid pileup.

Chris turned absently toward his parents. "Hi Daddy." He saw that Larry and Albert had not stopped their fighting and he smiled again right before he ran over, picked up a blow-up bat and hit Albert with it.

Al listened and felt the pounding in his head start. "I'm going to relax. Call if you need a referee."

"Nice move." Ronnie watched her healing brother-in-law walk confidently toward the master bedroom.

Al called over his shoulder. "I'm hiding before it really gets weird."

Ronnie looked strangely at Elaine. "What are you talking about."

Al stopped and turned around. "With my new camera implant, I hear things first before people move or I assume, their lips move." He stood still. "I get to keep my bandages on for another week or two and hopefully that sensory input conversion will have corrected itself. I can't imagine what kind of chaos my mind would have to sort through with those three yelling and fighting. I'm going to take full advantage of the bandages."

"Whoah. That is crazy. Crazier than this house is normally." Ronnie shook her head and laughed. "I didn't think that was possible."

Chapter XVII: Details

Elaine lined all four boys along the wall in the living room and waited for Al to come out of the bedroom. She looked behind her as he confidently walked out of the master bedroom unbandaged and wearing his glasses. He lifted the glasses and looked directly from one boy to the next as he stood before them.

Elaine broke the silence. "Boys, your Dad can see you with his right eye."

The four boys stared at Al. Albert was the first to step forward. He walked to the right and watched his dad follow him with his gaze. Albert waved to his dad and Al waved back.

Albert stood in the spot for a moment then turned to his three brothers who stared back to him. "Parties over."

All four boys hung their heads and walked back to their toys.

Al watched them walk away and then turned to Elaine. "Chris looks like me. Albert looks like Dad. Larry looks like the mailman and Nick looks just like you." He had a lump in his throat and paused before he could speak, breaking into a smile. "And yes, the parties over."

Elaine was still staring at their little backs. "How much do you think they got away with the last couple of years?"

Suddenly she felt that their household was not completely in their control.

Al watched the boys and fought breaking down completely in front of them. "Relax. There were enough bottoms spanked that I feel confident that we are still in control. For the most part." Al let out a laugh and hugged her fully. "You look just as beautiful as you did in the hospital." He stared at her and overwhelming emotions started to build making his chest tighten.

She read the expression on his face and tried to counter the moment with brevity. "When I looked like an x-ray?" Elaine gasped.

"You look great any way I can see you." He focused on her with his camera implant. "How do you feel being married to C-3PO?"

She laughed. "I can't believe how accurate that description is. When the doctor first mentioned it, I thought he was speaking metaphorically. I think we should paint your face gold and put you on display."

He raised his eyebrows. "This is one tough family. I'm glad I'm the leader." He started to slip away from her as he flipped his glasses on. "I'm going to get my regular glasses now that the surprise is over."

"Hey, wait a minute. Who elected you leader of the pack?" She followed behind him as the boys looked absentmindedly at their exchange. "Are you sure it's alright to wear the regular glasses yet? It's a bright sunny day."

Al was still snickering. "We're inside. The glasses will be fine." He stopped and watched the four boys who had established a temporary peace accord.

The strange phenomenon of hearing people and then feeling them move had thankfully passed completely. He stared at his four boys, watching their chatter and observing how Albert tried to be leader, but each of the other boys, even Nick, held their ground. They were a team.

His family was new to him. "Hey boys. Who wants to play ball?" To his surprise the boys did not jump at his initial offer after spending the first two weeks of Al's recovery at arm's length from him and banished from all the usual activities.

Albert spoke up for the group. "Daddy, can we finish our armies first?"

Al was momentarily mesmerized by Albert's little face looking up at him with his big brown eyes. He felt pure joy.

"Daddy?" Albert was growing frustrated.

Al shook himself. "Sorry. You guys play. I'm going to see what our new house looks like with my camera eye." He took a moment to look closely at their living room and the family pictures.

Albert was giggling and pointing at Al. "Daddy you look like a robot."

Al smiled with them. "Laugh while you can. I'll be able to wrestle with you soon."

A look of excitement spread over Larry. "Can we wrestle now Daddy?"

"Not yet. The doctor said my eye needs to heal a little bit longer. The doctor has to make sure the camera won't fall out." Al thought a simple explanation would work.

"Whoah." Albert was on his feet immediately and pointing at Al's right eye. "That can fall out? Will your eyeball come out too Daddy?"

"No. My eyeball is staying right where it is." The color of the couch in all its red brightness drew Al's attention.

"Daddy, I like your new eyeball." Albert held up his tiny C-3PO.

"Me too." Larry never missed a chance to keep up or better his older brother.

"Me! Me!" Chris jumped up still holding his tiny green army man.

"Yeah!" Nick, not completely understanding what was going on threw both arms in the air, but refused to move from his wall of wooden blocks.

Al dragged his gaze away from the couch. "Thanks, boys. Finish play time and we'll all practice ball later."

Jayne Kelly

All four boys gratefully plopped back down onto the carpet as Elaine came into the room. "Hey, what are you guys up to?"

"Honey, that couch is a great gauge for my sight. That color is ridiculous, but bright. As much as I hate it, I love it. It fits into the new house." Al looked around appreciatively.

"Then it stays. One of the neighbors was getting rid of her couch and asked if I wanted it. I'll tell her no." She walked over and sat heavily down on the well-worn cushions. "We can always get a slip cover if the color bothers you."

Al smiled and shook his head. "It matters not, my love." He looked around the room again. "I like the size of this living room. We can all hang out together and there is still room for the boys to play." He walked around and peered out the windows. "I'm going to walk around and check out the new place."

"Keep your glasses on, Al. It's your first day without the bandages." She hung over the back of the couch staring lovingly at him as he stared back at her.

"I'll be careful. I'm not taking any chances. Besides, I won't be able to see anything without them since the lens doesn't contract." He saw his cane hung on the doorknob of the coat closet. He looked at Elaine and then back at the cane. "Maybe I'll take a bike ride." He smiled broadly.

"Hey Daddy, Chris is riding without wheels." Albert talked without looking up.

"I know. Remember, Daddy taught him right before he went into the hospital." Al felt this gentle reminder would keep the boys grounded in the fact that Al was there for them with or without sight. "Daddy's going to go for a little ride by himself. I'll be back." Al started to leave and then stopped. He noticed the expression on Albert's face had gone from stating a fact to annoyed.

"Chris can't keep up if you take all of us." Albert stopped what he was doing and stared at his dad.

Al felt a chill come over him. *The world keeps going. While I was coping with the darkness, the boys continued to*

260

grow up. Thank you Lord for this second chance. I may have missed the first steps of two of them, but you have given me some time. However long it lasts, it's time.

"I will take all of you at the same time. You'll have to learn to have patience." Al met Albert's gaze. "Let me get used to my bike again with a quick spin around the block." Al turned without giving Albert a chance to argue.

He slipped on the sunglasses and walked the short distance to the detached garage. The minute he walked through the side door of the garage he spotted the bike he had last ridden five years ago leaning against the wall in the dim light. It appeared to be more banged up than he remembered and he smiled at the thought that Albert had added to its seasoned appearance. In front of it, piled and scattered on the floor, were children's bikes. He saw the largest one and walked over to examine it pulling the sunglasses back up onto his head.

Albert has outgrown this. His legs are way too long. Larry is still a little short for it, but he must be standing to peddle. Connecting the dots, he knew when he had gazed upon each of his children in the living room he had taken a visual inventory of his family. *New bikes this year. For everyone.*

Excitement filled him. He hit the garage door opener and sunlight spilled into the space previously lit only with light from the opened side door and the one window to his left. Flipping down the sunglasses he had propped on the top of his head he bounded toward the ten-speed.

As he peddled out of the garage the asphalt driveway appeared to gleam. The circular driveway was on an incline that afforded the start up speed he knew the boys loved when they rode. Even Nick peddled his tricycle down the incline without fear.

He reached the incline and kept peddling. The wind smacked him in the face and it felt like he was flying free with unlimited potential. Constraints that he accepted and molded himself into melted away as the bright sunshine pounded down on his arms throught the Jobe shirt sleeves. Without warning today's date hit him hard and he almost tumbled off the bike as he made a sharp turn at the end of the driveway.

There was a short squeal of brakes as Mike, the neighbor several houses away, stopped his car as he was driving past the house. "Al! Are you crazy?" Mike knew what the family has just endured, but had not heard if the surgery was successful.

The neighbors in the Audobon Parkway neighborhood cared about the Pleviers. Al and Elaine knew they had made the right decision moving the family here from the Ridgeview Terrace home.

Al grabbed the hand brakes hard, skidded to a stop and turned to look at the face of the man who spoke to him. "Mike?"

Mike hung one arm over the steering wheel as he bent down to talk through the passenger window. "I'm going to assume since you're riding that bike that you can see." Both men laughed.

"Aww, come on. I'm not crazy enough to try a ride a bike without sight." Al watched Mike's expression as he leaned toward the passenger window.

"Now that you see me, are you disappointed?" The man's broad smile matched his personality.

"I'll learn to adjust." Al was not surprised to see the jovial face greeting him.

"How's your vision? Those glasses wrap around your head pretty good. Do they block some sight?" Mike was curious but also wanted to be informed as the neighborhood emissary.

"No, they're necessary. The camera lens doesn't dilate or contract. My vision would be a white out on a day like today." Al felt a need to explain how he almost let himself be killed. "I was just so excited to fly down the driveway, I never gave a thought to cars."

Mike whistled low. "How ironic would that be. Killed the first week you got your sight back."

Al shook his head laughing. "Yeah, it would. This is

the first several hours without bandages. You're one of the first people outside the family I'm seeing."

Mike was speechless and Al knew how unusual that was for him. He switched to the mundane topic of the weather. "You couldn't have picked a better day. We've been fortunate to have an elongated Indian Summer over the weekend. Not bad for the first day of October."

Al knew Mike had no idea how significant the day was to Al. "I intend to enjoy this magnificent weather."

Mike smiled broadly. "You deserve it. It's a good choice. Your family will still be there when you get back."

Another chill washed over Al. "Absolutely."

"I'm on my way to get coffee and then we're headed off to a pumpkin farm." He watched Al nod in acknowledgement.

Al was lost momentarily as the ominous feeling that had swept over him dissapated. "I think Elaine has pumpkin picking on our agenda for Sunday."

"Looks like you're ready to to take on anything Elaine sets up for you." The men laughed together. "Enjoy this day, old man."

Mike pulled away, Al waved to the retreating car and then hopped back on the bike.

Seven years later and I'm still here. It didn't beat me. Damn near killed me, but it didn't. I can see!

He peddled faster until he was flying by the cars on his road that were adhering to the speed limit. He stayed bent low over the curled handle bars. Breathing hard he felt his body respond to the first serious exercise it had in years. A stop sign brought him to a skidding halt. He stared at the brilliant red road sign for several seconds before leaning his head back and peering at the tree canopy above. Through the slightly, swaying branches he saw puffy white clouds drift. The blue sky took him back seven years to a choice and a day that started perfectly and ended in tragedy and pain.

Shaking himself free of the memory, he realized that in the excitement of this first day without bandages eyes, he had forgotten that he hadn't studied the front of his house. Pulling out of the garage on his bike, he had not looked back. Suddenly he turned the bike around and peddled toward the house as fast as he had peddled away. The view of the neighborhood that greeted him was spectacular, in his opinion. It was quaint, with new and old construction. There were no street lights in this rural area but the houses were as close to each other as the ones on Lake Road. Each one sat on a minimum of one acre. There were young, newly planted trees and older one mixed together on each lot.

As Al pulled back into the entrance of the driveway incline, he stopped both from a winded sensation in his lungs and from drawing in the presence of the home he always dreamed of as a child with a big circular driveway for playing and trees that surrounded the two-acre, property perimeter. There was a four-car, heated garage to gather the boy's paraphernalia with a workroom for him. The bright green grass was still vibrant on this fall day. The house stretched farther than Al had imagined in his mind. It was a two-story colonial style with a partially finished basement used for storage. There were large windows that were built in appreciation of the view over the tree line across the street. The incline of their property allowed for a peek at the small valley below. It was not a million-dollar view, but impressive none the less.

Their yard was entirely fenced in behind the house encompassing the back and side of the garage. He and Elaine would never worry again about the dogs eating hot dogs off a neighbor's grill although here in the Riverview Community it would probably make the family popular for decades.

He stared for a moment at the view, proud that his wife had chosen this house for their family. She was everything to him and he was everything to her. Their life together was chosen like this house. They had no regrets.

Suddenly he felt like he was on display. He turned back to the house and saw five faces watching him from the picture window in the living room. Four little hands went up and waved. He waved back.

Chapter XVIII: Days of Glory

" *C*ome on, Daddy. Harder. Throw harder. Overhand."
Albert's pleas had been reduced to whining as the afternoon
wore on.

"Patience, son. Daddy is getting used to his robot eye."
Al was surprised he found himself tentative about being hit in
the face.

The family took over the northwest corner of their yard
turning it into a mini ballfield. It wasn't long before the
neighbors heard the fun and begged to join in.

"Hey Al. You need some outfielders? Those boys are
getting good." Joe boosted his young son, Joe Jr., affectionately
known as JoJo over the fence. "We're climbing the fence now."

Al turned and met Joe's eye. "I can see you coming,
remember?" Al tossed the ball nonchalantly in his hand and
smiled.

Joe stopped short with one of his on legs over the fence.
"I was afraid to ask how effective the camera was." The man
felt emotional and swallowed hard as he lifted himself up and
over the fence and walked toward the group. "Is this the first
day without the bandages?" The Riverview Community, where

the Audobon Parkway house was located, gratefully welcomed the Pleviers back from the Ridgeview Terrace neighborhood.

"This is the first day. When we're finished with the game, we'll go inside and I can show you what the camera looks like. The family has nicknamed me C3po." Al watched Joe walk up and saw that he was about six feet two inches tall and, Al had to admit, handsome.

"Hi Joe." Elaine called loudly from her spot in the Plevier outfield.

"Hi Elaine. Congratulations on the successful surgery. I like the nickname." Joe gave a wave as he talked and watched his son take off to find a place in the field.

JoJo ran over to Larry and the two immediately started to wrestle, throwing their gloves on the ground and laughing uncontrollably. "JoJo, Larry, cut it out. We're practicing." Al realized his admonishment would have taken longer without sight. Now he saw immediately what was going on instead of hearing something out of place.

Larry stopped. "Okay, Daddy." He looked over to Albert and yelled. "Yup. Parties over."

Elaine, Al and Joe all looked at each other before bursting out laughing. "Are you kidding me?" Joe, older than Al and Elaine, was always surprised at how much kids knew and how honest they were about it. "Kinda scary to think about how much mischief you two missed."

"Kind of comforting too. I only know about the bottoms I spanked over the last several years. I guess that's a good indicator." Al lined up another throw from his place on the pitcher's mound. "Albert, pay attention."

Albert had momentarily lost interest and found a spot to dig his shoe into. "I'm ready forever."

Al acknowledged the phraseology with a furrowed brow and then readied the pitch when he saw the serious look Albert returned. "Here it comes." This time Al relaxed into a stronger throw to Albert.

Albert connected with the ball and smacked it over Al's head. "How's that, Daddy?"

Al smiled brightly into Albert's gaze. "Nice."

Joe retrieved the ball and pretended to chase Albert down. "Not a bad throw for your first day without the bandages.

"Daddy, you aren't playin' for real." Albert yelled with frustration.

"Albert calm down." Al watched his oldest son and how fast his little legs carried him as he ran the bases. "Maybe you guys are done playing." He watched Nick rolling on the ground heading for the property slope.

Four collective yells of protest went up. "No, Daddy! Pleeease. We'll pay attention."

Al smirked. "Then let's keep this game going." He looked from one to another of the boys for confirmation that they were all in agreement.

The practice lasted for another hour. Al looked at where the sun hung in the sky and decided to jump to another activity. He felt like a little boy let loose in an amusement park with a pocket full of ride tickets and another full of quarters.

"Who wants to play Robinson Crusoe?" Al tossed the ball he held lightly.

Larry shook his head. "Daddy, that's a tree house game. This is baseball."

"Yes, but if you boys want to switch games now you can." Al watched all five boys drop what they were holding and run toward the tree house. "Elaine, Joe and I can pick up the baseball stuff." He pulled off his mit and watched Joe pick up the baseball paraphenalia bag.

She started toward a ball laying near her and stopped. "This is a great afternoon, but I feel like I should say thank you for letting me participate in the baseball game. Everyone in the family knows I'm the weakest link in the team."

"Only in your ball skills." He looked at her lovingly. "I'm better at baseball than you even with my robot eye." He kissed her head as she came close. "Come with us while I show Joe the garage. He wants to go through the inventory for Christmas." Al continued to pick up all the balls and smiled each time he spotted one on the grass.

"Joe, I think Mary would love the Adirondak chairs Al made. They're sharp." Elaine loved the newest addition to Al's woodworking inventory list. "I was painting them white during my leave of absence."

"Mommy! Are we going to the pumpkin farm tomorrow?" Albert's head hung out the window of the tree house.

"Yes Albert." For a second Elaine wondered if he was going to tumble out.

"Can JoJo come?" Larry's head came out next to Alberts.

"Of, course." She turned to their neighbor. "Joe, see if Mary wants to come. We'll make a day of it. It's early in the month, but it will be the first family outing since Al's been home."

Joe nodded in agreement as he grabbed a bat off the ground. "I'm sure she would love it. Mary was wondering the other day if you missed working?"

Elaine sighed. "I miss the patients, but it's been nice to be with Al and the boys full time." The trio walked toward the back of the garage.

Al held open the small garage door for Elaine and Joe. "I don't remember how I ever managed without a four-car heated garage. My business takes up two of the bays." They stepped into the dim light filtering through the small window on the north wall and Al lifted the sunglasses on top of his head.

"I don't think that's a good idea." Elaine watched his reaction to her caretaking.

"We'll have to put up the door. I can only see shadows in this light." Their two dogs came running into the garage. "Where have you two been hiding?"

Joe leaned down to pet the two beagle mixes as the garage door opened. "Are these two going to run out of the garage?" Joe inclined his head toward the opening bay door.

Al stepped into the space and pulled his glasses down as the door continued to open up, flooding the four bays with light. "It's okay, Joe. They'll run back into the yard since the boys are back there." Al waved Joe over to his work area. "Check out these dog houses. I can't believe how good they look. I knew my craftsmanship was good, but these are sharp. We got a call this morning for a new order."

Elaine stepped over to another piece of furniture. "Al did the inlays of these book cases prior to the surgery." She traced a finger over the custom design Al had carved into the face of the bookcase.

"How did you do that without sight?" Joe examined the curved edges forgetting about the dog houses.

Al stepped closer and lifted his glasses a little to look closer. His gaze went from the right side to the matching design to the left. "I don't think they are that great. Passable and definitely worth the price I'm charging but they sure aren't perfect. I don't think I could do better with sight to be perfectly honest." He traced his finger in the rough edges of the design. "I love working with wood. When I was stuck in an office I felt like a prisoner."

Joe looked over the inventory stacked in the two right bays of the garage. "You certainly have a lot. Are you taking orders?"

Al gave Joe a conspiratorial look. "You have got to hear about the order I received today." He reveled at the fact that he could gauge Joe's reaction by his expression and not have to rely on the tone of his voice.

"What, tell me." Joe stopped admiring the furniture and turned to face Al, anticipating a good story.

Elaine stepped closer. "How come I didn't hear this?"

Al held up his hand. "A lady called to order a dog house and I told her I had some in stock. She says no she wants a custom order. I told her I just got my sight back and I could start on it in another week. She tells me she just wants to make sure she has it for Christmas and congratulates me that the surgery was successful. Kerry and Stephen recommended me and told her how unique it was to have something built by a blind guy that was finished so well." Al was building up as he repeated the phone call from this morning that he had answered before he saw his boys lined up.

"We had been so busy with the boys and the excitement of this day that I forgot about it." Al looked from one face to the other, thrilled to read the expressions as he built the story up. "The woman said she was excited because what she ordered would be even better since I could see."

Elaine snorted. "That was rude."

Al shook his head and laughed. "No. Not really. She tells me that she has one more request."

"What?" Joe spread his hands out when Al paused for effect.

"She tells me to build it large enough for me to be able to climb inside." Al started to talk fast and high pitched. "I asked her if she had a St Bernard and she said no." He paused for effect once more when they both looked at him quizzically. "She said no. She said she needed it large enough for her slave to climb into when he was bad."

Both Elaine and Joe let their jaws drop and spoke in unison. "Nooooo. That's crazy."

Joe knew Al's flare for exaggerating a good story for a laugh and looked at him with disbelief. "You're kidding."

"Hey, not even I can make this up." Al was shaking his head and holding his hands out in supplication.

"Are you going to make it?" The salaciousness of the story held Joe's attention.

"Yeah." Al exclaimed sarcastically and definitively. "Money is money. Why should I walk away from a paid woodworking job?" He looked over at several dog houses already built. "I was thinking I could alter the inventory I have. It is only a matter of lifting the roof and raising the sides."

Joe smirked. "Oh, that's bad."

Al shook his head and held his arms across his body as he laughed and when he stopped he waved a hand toward his inventory. "What's your pleasure, Joe? Elaine is right about the Adirondack chairs."

Albert came into the garage. "Mommy, we're hungry. Can we have chips?"

Elaine was staring at the dog houses when Albert came in. "Pick the chairs, Joe. Trust me. She turned to Albert. "You can't have chips but I'll make you guys either apples and peanut butter or half Pb and J sandwiches. We're going to order pizza for dinner. JoJo can stay if he would like."

Albert looked over at Al. "Daddy, are you doing soccer practice Monday? You didn't go last week."

Guilt washed over Al remembering it was vanity over his still bandaged eyes that kept him from Albert's practice. "Sure Buddy, but I'll be watching not coaching Mr. Chiltendon will." Soccer was the only sport Al had no talent for or interest in coaching.

Albert nodded his head vigorously. "I know. We're doing baseball practice too. Mommy knows." Albert looked over at Elaine pleadingly.

Al saw the exchange and realized Albert was not picking up yet on the fact that he saw everything. "I know, Albert. I'll ask the baseball coach if I can help. That's going to be a short practice. Remember. Both are after school and you boys will need to be home for dinner."

Albert's eyes lit up. "Good!" He ran back outside.

Joe turned back to the furniture. "I'll take two Adirondack chairs, but you have to keep them here until Christmas."

"Do you want them painted?" Al would not have considered painting the chairs before his sight returned. In his mind, they looked nicer in natural tones but with sight he could see why they were sometimes painted in either stores or by creators like himself.

"Painting them white like my house would be great." Joe looked around. "Are you going to amp up production now that you have sight?"

Al shook his head. "Actually, I'm thinking about going back to working construction for my old company full time." He and Elaine looked at each other and shared an unspoken

Jayne Kelly

agreement and the ability to do so warmed his soul. "Elaine might be working as a nurse part time now that I'm fully healed."

Elaine ran a hand over several of Al's pieces as she spoke. "I do miss my patients but I'd rather not work full time while the boys are little if I don't have to." At that moment, all the boys came into the garage for their bikes. "Guys, stay in the driveway." Elaine's tone suggested this was an order not a request.

"We want to ride bikes to Pop Pop's house." Albert grabbed the ten-speed bike Al had ridden that morning.

"No. It's too late in the day. Pop Pop and Grandmom will be over for pizza in a little while." All the boys, including JoJo made angry faces. "I mean it. Stay in the driveway." Elaine's no-nonsense tone made it clear the boys should not test her.

The boys now looked at Al for confirmation. Without peripheral vision, he didn't realize they were looking toward him until he was prompted.

"Daddy?" Larry stood still waiting for support.

Al jerked his head to Elaine and then the boys. "Listen to your Mom. She said no. Maybe we can ride there tomorrow after pumpkin picking." This time, the five boys made faces in Al's direction and instead of their obstinance annoying him, he relished it. "You guys have a basketball court, rope swings from the trees, a jungle gym and two dogs to play with. The only thing you can't do now is swim in the pool. Mommy said stay here and you are going to listen to her. Pop Pop will be over tonight."

Ronnie appeared in front of the garage with a sleepy Peter. "Hi Joe. When did you get here?"

"Hey Ronnie. We heard 'the team' playing ball so JoJo and I climbed the fence." Joe was still looking over one of the Adirondack chairs admiringly.

"I see Al's business is booming." Ronnie saw Al watching his family. "Al, there was a phone call for you. The tenant's wife from Ridgeview. She needs a lightbulb in the driveway changed."

Elaine looked at him with disbelief. "Al, aren't they a little high maintainence? She knows you were in the hospital for a serious operation." She felt herself starting to whine. "It's your first full day with sight. How much more can you do?"

Al shook his head. "I'm not complaining." He jutted out his chin like a man in charge. "It's good rental money and now that I have sight, I'm going to run over there. No need to put anything off." Al could now see that his enthusiasm and energy bordered on becoming annoying and was reflected in the faces around him. "Ronnie, will you give me a ride?" He scratched absentmindedly at his chest area.

"Yeah, but do I have to stay?" She handed Peter off to Elaine, anxious to move Al along and headed for her car where she always left the keys in the ignition.

"No. I'll walk back. I want to enjoy the fresh air." He was thoughtful for a moment. "Elaine, did they say when they want the pool closed? It's October first. That should have been done Labor Day weekend."

Elaine shrugged her shoulders, obviously annoyed that he was thinking of leaving even for an hour. "The weather has been so mild that they're enjoying it. I talked to them last week and they said if you would let them they would leave it open until the first week of November." Elaine jostled the baby.

Al shook his head. "That's not up to them. The realtor said as soon as the inspection is complete for the new buyers next week, I can close it. That's all I've been waiting for. Come on, Ronnie." Al turned to the boys. "I'll be back in a little while. Mind your mother." He held out a hand to Joe. "See you Monday at soccer practice?"

Joe stood up. "Yes. Thanks for letting JoJo stay for dinner." He ran a hand over his choice of furniture. "The chairs are one gift checked off my Christmas list before I head home." He turned to Al. "Both practices will be short."

"Are you taking off from work?" Al stepped out of the way of a bike and then began to shift from one foot to another.

273

"I'm done by two on Monday." He walked over to say good bye to JoJo. "The players are going to be thrilled that you can see." He watched Al shifting his weight. "You got ants in your pants or are the burns bothering you?" Joe was not a nosy neighbor, but in the tight knit community the area residents felt protective of the Plevier family.

Al smiled and waved off Joe's concern. "Just a habit from the old neighborhood in Patterson." He ran a hand over his shirt. "The scars are still bothersome, but they always will be. The Jobe shirt has been a God send. I'm healing just fine." He thought back to this morning and his soap choice.

He was finding that certain soaps would bother him due to the lye content. Even with the progress he was making because of the Jobe shirt, he had a lifetime of inconvenience and uncomfortable days that would be intermittent. Today, even with the Jobe shirt, he was itchy. He knew the scratching would lead to bleeding and the discomfort from the soap of this morning's shower was not lessened by the talcum powder he applied afterward.

Joe looked around at the happy mayhem the family had brought to the neighborhood. "I'll let you get back to the troops." He gave a short wave and headed for the fence.

Al gave Elaine a quick wink that did nothing to dissuade her anger and then he left with Ronnie. She dropped him off at the Ridgeview house without checking to see if anyone was home.

Al walked up and rang the doorbell and a beautiful blond answered. "Hi Albert. Thank you for coming over so quickly." She stepped aside to let Al enter. "Christian is going to be glad to have the bulbs changed. We're having a party tonight."

Al was a little shocked. This was the first time he had seen his tenant and she was a knock out. Speechless he followed her through the house, glimpsing the house for the first time with sight.

"Are you okay?" The young woman was confused. She knew Al's surgery had been successful and didn't understand why he was walking so carefully.

"I'm sorry, but this is the first time I saw this house. It's quite beautiful. My wife has good taste." He shook his head admirably.

The blond raised her eyebrows appreciatively and Al noticed that this made her more appealing. "We've been very happy here. I'll miss it." She unlocked the inner garage door for him. "Do you need anything else?"

"No, I'm good." He stuttered. "Is it the bulbs in the posts at the end of the driveway and the two by the pool?" He found himself nervous around the young lady.

"Yes, both." She grabbed a towel hanging over the back of a chair. "If you don't mind, I'm going to go back to sunbathe by the pool and take a swim. The weather is amazing. I've been out there all day." She smiled a perfect smile.

"Sure. Sure." Al stumbled as he walked. "I'll get out of your way as quick as possible.

Al replaced the driveway bulbs and walked around the garage to the pool area. The trees created a wonderful canopy and were beautiful with the setting sun behind them. As he opened stockade gate for the pool he made sure it locked tight behind him before turning toward the lights. In front of him fast asleep was the naked, sunbathing tenant. He dropped his bag and the tools.

The clatter woke her up and she started. "Are you okay?"

There's a loaded question. "Yes, sorry. Still getting my footing. Believe it or not there's an adjustment to having sight." *Thank you Lord for this day.*

She rolled over. "I'm going inside in a few minutes. The sun is amazing."

Al turned to go to work. *Don't look. She's European. She'll think you're a pervert. Elaine's going to freak out.*

Al never changed a bulb so fast. The young woman was getting up to go inside as he finished and walked right past him without a any clothing.

She gave him a huge smile. "Just in time for our party. Thank you again."

Al blushed and responded with a broad smile. "You're welcome."

He walked home to Audobon with the setting sun as a backdrop. When he reached the end of their driveway the lights were on in all the windows and it made a beautiful sight. He stood at the end of the driveway staring at it for a little while before going inside. The family and the pizza Elaine had ordered were waiting for him at the kitchen table.

"You look happy. Did you finish the AC unit for them too?" Elaine pulled his slices out of the oven.

"No. I'll have to go back next week for that." He sat down and started to eat greedily.

"Was she happy you showed up so quickly?" Elaine pulled a toy from Larry that he had hidden under the table and stared into his face. "I'll keep this. No toys at the table during dinner." She looked at the boy's plates where only crusts remained. "You boys go play." The ensuing stampede now included a toddling Peter.

Once the boys were out of the room, Al jumped into his story. "I think we just got even with the snotty Ridgeview Terrace neighbors." He was nervous about Elaine's reaction and hoped diverting the target might help. "They thought we were uncouth? They must be flipping out."

Elaine looked at him quizzically. "What are you talking about? What happened?"

Al broke right into the story. "The tenant is still enjoying the pool and the warm weather." He started to laugh uncontrollably. "She sunbathes in the nude. Completely nude." He continued the story with nervous laughter. "That wasn't one of the first sites I expected to see today, but beggars can't be choosers."

Elaine did not laugh but Ronnie had to turn her head. She couldn't believe Al told her sister this truth. It was one she thought he should have kept to himself.

Without a snicker, Elaine responded. "Find someone else to fix the AC." She got up from the table abruptly, nearly knocking over her chair.

When she was out of hearing distance, Ronnie turned to Al. "You're an idiot."

Al shook his head in acknowledgement. "Not completely. That was damage control. I'm sure one of the neighbors is going to call her about the tenant sunbathing in the nude. Those delusional high brow idiots always had our phone number handy for complaints." Ronnie shook her head in agreement as Al pointed his thumb at his chest. "This idiot is going to have an enjoyable evening to close out this truly remarkable day."

For the first time in seven years Al slept throughout the night less due to relief and more from a sense of accomplishment. The corneal transplant had never returned his sleep patterns to normal and without sight, it was constant struggle to first stay awake during certain events and then to be tired in the evening. There were many nights that he would get up in the middle of the night, start a project and wake up one of the children or Elaine.

Al awakened the next morning refreshed and with energy. He had stepped backward in time, with the body and presence of mind he had before October 1, 1974.

Chapter XIX: Still Me

$\mathcal{A}$ looked at Ronnie. "Peter's peg board table birthday present came. Big Peter is coming over tomorrow to put it together."

Ronnie's expression hardened. "Thank you for the warning. I'll make myself scarce.

The tension between Ronnie and Peter had lessened but was still palpable since they had agreed to separate after being married a short time. Part of continuing to do what was best for her son was to allow Pete his time to be part of Peters life and today that meant putting together a childs peg board table they had ordered together for him, with Al.

Al watched Ronnie walk away and smiled to himself. He had opened the box this morning after the delivery truck had dropped it off to make sure all the parts were there. Within minutes of sorting throught the barrage of child sized parts, he had an epiphany.

He found some pieces of wood that resembled the parts to the table, added them and a few extra screws to the mix after tossing the directions in the garbage. He even painted one side of a board and drilled a few extra holes in the packaged wood to complete the match. He then repacked the box making sure to include the final picture of what the table should look like upon completion. A little bit of meanness, a little bit of protectiveness for his sister-in-law and a large amount of Al's comedic nature sealed itself inside the box of extra parts and mislabeled paraphernalia that morning.

The next day an apprehensive Peter arrived and Al led him inside the heated garage. "Relax Pete, I think Ronnie went out shopping with Elaine." Al saw the lines in Peter's forehead disappear.

"Do you think the little monsters are going to come in here?" Pete looked cautiously over his shoulder.

"They're not monsters, but you're safe. They went out with Elaine and Ronnie. I begged my way out of that." Al couldn't help letting out a small laugh.

Pete gave him a cross look. "This is going to be one cool little peg table for Little Pete." Pete opened up the box and dumped the contents on a work blanket Al had laid out.

"Everything is here." Al spread his hands wide and looked over each part.

Pete looked at the pile skeptically. "Paint. We need paint, brushes and screw driver."

Al shook his head to stop from laughing. "They're behind you."

"Why don't I run down to the hardware store and make a beer run too." Pete started to get up.

Al held up his hands. "Nah. You'll want to have this done before the girls get back."

"Yeah, yeah." Peter sat back down.

Al watched Peter look over each piece as he picked it up. "I have a few things to do inside. The picture of the table is under the pile of parts you dumped out. Yell if you need me." Al made a hasty departure.

Fifteen minutes later Al came in to find a perplexed Peter holding up a piece of wood. "I don't know where to start. I can't believe this didn't come with directions."

"Start from the bottom. It's only a peg board table. I counted the parts. Piece of cake." Al cocked his head sideways.

Peter gave him a frustrated look. "You think this is a piece of cake because you do construction."

Al didn't miss a beat. "No, I was asking if you wanted a piece of cake. I found it in the kitchen." Al really felt like he owed the young man sitting on his garage floor a frustrating afternoon.

Peter shook his head. "I don't want anything." He dropped a piece of wood on the floor. "I thought this would be a quick job and I'd have an afternoon free."

Al shook his head slowly. "Anything involving a kid is never quick, easy or free."

Peter did not grasp the sarcasm or life lesson passed to him. "If Ronnie comes home, tell her I'm busy."

Al agreed with a touch of sarcasm. "No problem. I have to get back inside."

Peter looked at him in a panic. "You're not going to help me?"

Al surveyed the pile. "It looks like you have a good enough start." Al left Pete staring at the pile of parts.

Several hours later the family came running into the house, except for Ronnie. After seeing Peter's car still in the driveway, she thought he might hung around to visit and went into the garage.

Albert was first into the kitchen. "Daddy!"

Al looked up from the food he was eating while the stereo played in the background. "Hey Pal. How was your day?"

Albert jumped into the kitchen table chair as his brothers and Little Peter dispersed around him in the house. "We went to see Star Wars number two!"

Al looked questioningly at Elaine. "Really? I thought that was long out of the theatres."

Elaine dropped a bag on the counter. "They had a Matinee at the mall so we thought we would keep the boys out longer. Peter is still here?"

Al nodded. "In the garage still putting the peg table together." Al started to laugh.

Elaine looked around for Ronnie. "All this time? Get out there and help him. The sooner he's done the better."

Just then Ronnie came storming in the kitchen door. "You're going to have to finish the table, Al. He left." She continued past them into the living room.

Al dropped him sandwich. "I think that's called Karma. I'll be back in a few minutes."

Peter left the smaller garage door wide open and the little boy's table in a partially finished state. Al laughed out loud when he found that Peter had actually worked one of the extra pieces into the table structure. Within ten minutes the table was completed and Al covered it and placed it into a corner hidden behind one of his projects. He scooped up the unnecessary pieces and tossed them into the garbage with a smile. His first month without sight was glorious on many levels.

A week later Al stood behind home plate coaching both the batter and the pitcher. Fall ball practice was coming to a close as the cooler weather began to close in on New Jersey. Joe was by first plate as they tried to be as authentic as possible while coaching.

Al lifted his glasses for a brief second to test his sight in the cloudy sky and then called to the pitcher. "Across the plate, Christian."

"Whoah." James, the batter, was mesmerized by the first glimpse of Al's robot eye. "That is cool. What do you call that, Mr. Plevier?"

"It's a camera, James. I usually don't let anyone see, so let's keep it our secret." Al was amused by the young boy's amazement. "It helps me to see."

The young boy nodded conspiratorily. "Like a robot." He nodded again. "Do you have a robot brain too?"

Momentarily stunned he tried not to laugh. "I have a great memory that I worked hard at in school. Robot brains are for computers. Do you know what a computer is?"

The young boy lost interest. "Nope." He looked at the pitcher. "Hey, throw it."

The pitch was high. "Ball one." Al called out.

The young boy turned to him. "Should I have gone for that Mr. Plevier?"

"No. Unless you think you could get a piece of it. You have to go with your instincts and roll with the game. Remember, if he is going to throw balls, you can let him walk you." Al watched the boy's face.

"If you can see the pitch now, Mr. Plevier can't you tell me for sure?" The frustration on the little boy's face was transparent. "You couldn't do that before."

Standing behind the plate and seeing the pitches for the first time in years was thrilling to Al, but he held strong to his ethics. "I can't tell you what to do. I can tell you that the best way to play the game is to build your ability to hit and throw the ball. If you want me to tell you what to do every pitch, you're never going to learn."

"I just wanna get a hit." The boy looked back to the pitcher.

"Everybody does." The next pitch came in and Al watched the boy swing and miss.

Banging the bat on the ground he turned angrily to Al. "You're not helping me."

Al took a breath and realized he needed to come down from his adult soapbox. "Okay, James. The pitch needs to come in between your chest and thighs, just like we taught you, right over the plate. It's not always going to do that. You need to step a little closer to the plate. Keep an eye on the ball and swing level if you like what you see." It was sheer joy for Al not to have to ask the boy or the other coach where the batter was standing.

Joe walked over to Al from his post at first base. "How you doing on your first day back?"

"I'm good, Coach Joe. Just getting used to seeing the pitch." The two men exchanged knowing looks as James began to kick at the bat now dangling from his grip.

"Get ready James. Listen to Mr. Plevier." Joe walked back to his post as the pitch was thrown and James swung and missed again.

The frustrated eight-year-old threw down his bat and began to stomp off. "Whoah, not so fast. Come back here. You're never going to get better at batting if you quit."

James looked at his shoes. "My turn is over."

"You're turn would be over if it was a game. This is practice. I say what goes. Pick up the bat and step up to the plate." James looked at Al first with astonishment and then with tears in his eyes and walked back to the plate. "You'll hit it. Remember not to swing at everything. Choose your pitches. It's going to take time. Don't quit. You have all winter to practice before spring little league. That's why we're here." The kid pitching looked frustrated and Al answered the sullen expression. "Hey, Christian. Over the plate."

Christian tossed the ball in his hand. "I know, but this is the first day I've been practicing since summer."

"That's why you're here." Al looked around at each boy holding their position.

Christian threw the ball and this time James did not swing at the pitch that went high. "Good eye, James."

"Thanks Mr. Plevier." The kid smiled for the first time. "You got a good eye too."

Al didn't know whether to laugh or cry. "Pick and choose what you hit." Al looked over at the other grumbling hitters waiting their turn. "Hey, everybody will get to hit. It's practice. Watch and learn." This latest bit of wisdom did not go over well with eight to ten-year olds, among them Albert. "James, you'll have to learn to adjust. You can't hit every one, you have to watch."

James had a puzzled look on his face. "What's a-jus mean?"

Al felt himself shrinking. "It means you're getting the hang of the game and I told you how to stand and when to hit, but anything can happen. Right? You could become the greatest hitter of all time and the pitcher will know this and throw balls you can't hit so he can walk you."

The little boy shook his head. "That's not fair."

"Nope, it's not. Just do the best you can. You doing better than the spring." Al hoped this encouragement worked.

"How do you know? You couldn't see me then." James looked over his shoulder at the boys waiting to bat.

"Coach filled in the parts I couldn't see." The young boy was getting him at a disadvantage. "Come on. No more talk. You can do this."

"I'm sorry Mr. Plevier. My Mom doesn't know how to practice baseball with me and I don't have a Dad." James hung his head a little.

Now Al wanted to cry. He bent down to the boy's level and spoke low so that the other boys would not hear. "Son, you listen to me. Don't pay attention to those other kids. You're doin' just fine. I didn't have a Dad either when I was your age. I had to learn baseball myself. My coach never let me quit." He knew he was glazing past a few pertinent facts but this little boy didn't need to know them.

James face lit up and when he talked, he stuttered a little. "I won't quit. I just wanna hit it."

Al privately thanked God he could see James' face at this moment. He knew just how much this practice, soon forgotten by the other kids, meant to him. "Watch what comes in." Al looked up at Christian. "Put one down, Christian."

Christian nodded and put a determined look on his face. He wound up, threw the ball, watched it go high and then watched James connect with it anyway. It didn't go far, but since Christian had to run to retrieve it, James made it to first base. No one cheered, it was practice after all, but Al had the pleasure of seeing James smile as he ran.

Joe patted James on the head when he hit the base. "You got a piece of that one."

"Yup." James waved to Al from first plate.

Al waved back.

The next boy started up to plate. It was Albert. "James finally hit something."

Al looked hard at Albert who stared at his dad. "Yup, he's developing a good eye no matter where the ball goes."

Chapter XX: Team in its Entirety

&ach Plevier boy was bundled up. Fighting with true spirit, they begged Elaine to let them out the door in their sweatshirts, but she was tougher than her five-foot-two-inch frame would suggest.

"It's thirty-eight degrees outside. Put on your hats!" Each boy, hearing her tone and volume, ran for the closet.

Al walked out the door ahead of them down the driveway and yelled to them over his shoulder. "Pop Pop will be waiting on his front porch. Grab your bikes and let's go." The promised bike ride to Elaine's parents house had been delayed for over a month until this morning when the boys would not take no for an answer.

The thunder of many little feet stormed through the house and out the kitchen door which led directly to the open garage. "Daddy! Wait for us."

"I'll be at the end of the driveway." Al strode with his head held high gazing at the tree branches from behind his sunglasses. He stood at the end of the driveway at the bottom of the incline looking both ways for lumbering cars in the narrow neighborhood street.

285

"Daddy!" Albert was flying toward him down the driveway standing as he peddled.

Al watched as one by one Albert, Larry and Chris flew out of the driveway at full speed followed by Nick peddling as much as his training wheels allowed. "Stay to the side of the road!" He ran next to Nick.

"Daddy, come on. We go faster." Nick peddled as if he was ready for two wheels.

A minute later a car creept slowly up behind him. "Hey, are the boys aware that they need to stay to the side?" Elaine looked down sweetly at Nick's effort. They're probably almost there. Your dad was going to walk part of the distance to meet them." Al felt himself getting winded. "Honestly Sweetheart, sometimes I wonder if our neighborhood is ready for the Plevier boys."

"We're welcomed with open arms." She continued to ride slowly next to Al and Nick.

"Yeah, I get that. We may just need more room or a larger play area." He turned to watch her expression.

"We have two and a half acres that's enough." Nick picked up speed as he watched his brothers pulling out of sight around the bend in the road.

"It may not always be. I'm just saying." Al was becoming breathless and began to seriously consider the need to begin an exercise regiment.

Elaine started to get ahead of them. "I'll meet you at Mom's. I want to keep an eye on the boys." She watched little Nick pedaling with all his might. "You're almost ready to take those training wheels off big guy."

Elaine pulled away. "Hey, maybe Mommy is right. Do you want to surprise everyone and give the bike a try without your wheels?"

Nick stopped. "Yeth." Nick fought to keep up with his brothers.

Al watched the priceless expression on the little boy's

"When we get to grandpop's house you can hop off and I will unscrew the wheels."

Nick was standing on each side of his pedals looking very apprehensive. "Daddy?"

"It's going to be fine, buddy. I won't let go of the back of your bike, I promise. We'll go slow." Al looked down into Nick's eyes and second guessed his suggestion. "If you don't want to do it today, that's fine. The boys won't know. You can tell me when we get close to the house."

Nick looked away from his Daddy's penetrating camera eye that was hidden behind the sunglasses and stepped up on the pedals. "Good." He took off again peddling as fast as the training wheels allowed.

Al ran out of breath. "You're doing great. You're fast with the wheels on."

Nick stopped and looked at Al reproachfully. "I want to ride without them, Daddy."

Al was afraid he had created a monster. "Good. I'll take them off when we get there. Keep going."

The other boys were racing up and down their grandparent's driveway when Al and Nick arrived. Nick jumped off immediately and stood aside as Al began the process of unscrewing the training wheels with the pocket tool he always had on him.

Nick looked up as his brothers squeeled their bikes to a stop in front of Al. "Daddy, are you taking off Nick's wheels?"

"Yes. He wants to give it a try." Al pulled off the first wheel and began to work on the second.

Albert looked at Nick sideways. "You're kinda little to have your wheels off."

Nick put a fist on each hip and stood looking tough at his brother. "Am not. Watch."

Al turned the bike over. "Here you go, Nick. Let's give it a try."

Nick stood on either side of the bike and then stood on the peddles. "Don't let go, Daddy. Don't let go." Nick kept his eyes focused on the driveway in front of him and finally sat down on the bikeseat. "Don't let go, Daddy!" He peddled and took a second look over his shoulder.

"I won't. I promise. Hold the handlebars tight." Al ran behind as the little boy started to pick up speed.

Al was unable to keep up with him. The bike went down hard to the right and Nick landed face first. Al ran up to the over turned bike as a sick feeling crept up from his stomach. Nick, momentarily stunned, lifted himself up and tearlessly wiped his scraped hands on his jeans.

Picking up his bike he threw his leg over the bike. "Ready? Don't let go, Daddy."

Al shook his head in agreement. "Sorry Nicky. Daddy is so out of shape. You ride faster than I can run. That's good. You'll be riding in no time."

Nick looked steadily at Al. "Yes, Daddy."

When the boys saw Nick riding without his wheels they all whooped with delight. "You're ready for the hill now Nicky." Albert gave Nicky a sly somewhat dangerous look.

Nicky smirked back at his big brother with a little bit of fear in his eyes. "Yup," was all he could manage.

Al saw both looks pass between the boys. "Albert, he's trying to ride early. He's still little." He warned his oldest son with a deadly look.

Albert gave a nonchalant shrug and Nicky reacted immediately. "Daddy, I a big boy!"

Oh jeez. "Nicky, I know that. I know you like to keep up with your brothers, but it's Albert's job as your biggest brother to look out for you."

Nicky gave Al a scowl and with strong determination marched away pushing his bike up the driveway hill. Albert followed behind him as Larry and Chris circled on their own bikes.

Mr. Hinds walked down from the top of the hill of their driveway to greet Al. "Hey, Boss. Your mother-in-law has cooked up a storm. I hope you like lots of cheese and garlic in your ziti today. The house smells wonderful." Mr. Hinds rubbed his belly appreciatively.

The two men looked up to see all the boys gathered around Nicky's bike after he crested the top of the driveway.

Al could tell the little boy had his chest pumped out as he pointed to where the training wheels used to be before climbing onto the bike seat. Albert held the back of the bike as Nicky started to pedal down the hill and then he let go. Al watched in horror as the little boy smiled broadly and flew down the hill. Behind him his three brothers cheered loudly and ran after the bike.

"Don't forget the brakes," yelled Larry hysterically.

Realization now came across Al's face. "Brake Nicky!"

Nicky was balancing perfectly. He gave his dad a strange look as he smiled. He steered ever so slightly to the right as he came closer to his dad. Mr. Hinds stood with his arms wide ready to catch the mini turbo headed for disaster.

"Brake Nicky!" Mr. Hinds gave one last attempt to halt the impending disaster.

The bike and Nicky never made it to the end of the driveway and his Pop Pop's open arms. He went straight into the thirty-year old spruce whose deep branches swallowed him up almost entirely.

The only thing Al saw when he ran over was a tire still spinning elevated about six inches. "Nicky?"

A little voice came out from under the branches as Nicky crawled backward out of the forest he found himself in and toward the surrounding feet surrounding. "This fun."

A stampede ended right behind Al. "Is he okay Daddy?"

Al snapped his head around. "Why didn't you show him how to use the brakes?"

Larry shrugged. "We thought he knew."

Nick stood up and dusted off his knees. "Do 'gain." He furiously pulled the bike out of the trees and began to push it up the hill again.

"Show him the brakes or you're all busted." Al stood firm with his hands on his hips staring down Albert and Larry.

The two boys looked down guiltily and walked after Nick. "Those boys have a healthy respect for you and Elaine." Mr. Hinds shook his head and tried to hide his laughter.

Al watched the two boys meet Chris and Nick at the top. Chris was already showing Nick how to stop the bike. Nick nodded his head vigorously and jumped back onto his bike. Albert grabbed hold of the back of the bike and started to guide Nick down. Nick steadied the bike and peddled until gravity took over. For a second time, he smiled broadly as he flew down the hill toward his Dad and Pop Pop. Just when the two men thought they were going to have to grab the bike, Nick worked the brakes, too hard, and flew into the handle bars almost becoming a projectile over them.

"I did it. I ride!" Nick jumped off and started to push the bike back up the driveway.

Mr. Hinds stood with Al who silently shook his head. "What a tough little guy."

"They're all pretty tough. Elaine says that's my fault." Al inclined his head toward Nick. "Elaine bundled him up with so many layers that maybe he didn't feel anything each time he fell." The two men nodded and laughed.

Al thought of the Pocono house they had just purchased with some of the settlement money and how wonderful sledding would be in the snow. This was going to be one of the best winters the family had experienced in a long time.

Mr. Hinds smiled. "You and Elaine are a helluva team." He followed Al's gaze to the boys and knew his son-in-law was drinking in the sight of his children. "Not one of those boys looks like the other, but each one looks like someone in the family." It was a sense of relief to speak to Al with the freedom of not measuring his words in regard to the visual world.

Al looked at the boys and reacted. "I can't get over the color of Albert's hair. It hasn't lightened one bit since he was born. He looks just like you." Nick was on his way down again, but this time he tested his braking power and coasted to an awkward turn at the end right next to Al. "This one looks just like me with a little of Elaine. Seeing him and Chris for the first time turned me into a weepy mess. Chris is all me. Larry is all Elaine."

Nick looke up at the hill as the boys ran into the house.

"Daddy. Dinner."

The three of them headed toward the food. "Dad, you should have seen the looks on their faces after I built the rope slide. I had the tire slide on Lake Road but this new slide has wheels that run on the cable between the tree house and the landing port that I created at the other end. The seat is a tee shape similar a ski lift on a bunny hill. The boys went nuts when they saw it. It curbed their enthusiasm to go outside the property boundaries for now."

"Wow. I wanna play on that thing. How long is the run?" Mr. Hinds kept up with his four grandsons in everything physical.

"It's about one hundred feet long. They were playing Batman the other day. Adam West would be impressed." It thrilled Al to watch his kids play with the abandon their yard provided.

He created these playgrounds at each home they had lived in to compensate for not being able to take his children to play areas on his own. The irony after this last surgery that he didn't need someone to go with him was that the children wanted to stay in their own neighborhood. For them nothing compared to the contraptions their dad built.

At that moment, Ronnie pulled slowly into her parent's driveway with her Oldsmobile convertible top down.

Peter sat in the front seat next to her with his hands in the air. "Hi. It looks like we made dinner. I'm starving."

Al looked at the heavily bundled toddler laughing and smiling. "Aren't you two cold? Are you nuts?"

"It was just from your house. I felt like cheering myself up. Peter loved it." She reached over, pulling little Peter to her. Dad, will you take him while I put the roof back up?"

"Sure, Honey." Mr. Hinds reached for the happy toddler. "Let's get you inside and see what Grandma has for your dinner."

Al walked next to Mr. Hinds and mussed Peter's blond hair. "This blond hair, blue eyed guy is a heart breaker already." He thought Little Peter looked like Ronnie.

"He'll be running with your tribe shortly." Mr. Hinds hoisted the baby in the air.

"He sure will. We were all surprised as we watched him take his first steps last week. It won't be long until he's running." Peter laughed and struggled to get down as they reached the front door.

Mr. Hinds let the little boy down and Al grabbed one of his hands to support his big step over the door threshold. "You are the role model this little guy needs. I hope you realize that. He's going to look up to you and I."

Al watched the toddler teeter through the living room toward the cacophony his own children were making in the dining room. "I'm great with that Dad. He'll be holding a bat and ball before he talks. Trust me." Al smiled thoughtfully. "We'll take him fishing too. The boys are already bugging me now that I have sight."

Al thought back to June 1974, several months before the accident that changed his life in October of that year. That summer he was working a second job in construction and the company had sent him to a site outside Patterson. He was familiar with the town, but didn't immediately find the job site. When he was finally on the right street, he found himself staring at bridge with déjà vu. He pulled the truck over to the side of the road and felt compelled to walk across it. Looking down from the top of the bridge he felt that something was not right. There was a path leading from the west side of the bridge and he was drawn to walk down to the river. Once at the bottom he looked up and in an instant a memory came flooding back to him.

He knew he was four and the memory was right before his Dad had died. Clearly, he saw himself standing next to his father who was carefully tying a worm onto Al's kid sized bamboo pole. Al was so focused on watching how his dad attached the bait that the caught fish they would bring home. A clear image of that fish presented to his mom on newspapers felt like the ultimate trophy.

That warm, loving memory, long forgotten, had come

back to him four short months before the accident. It was the knowledge that his own father had died a short time later that drove Al to fight to live immediately after the accident and be the father his dad was denied the chance to be.

Al and Mr. Hinds sat down at the dining room table with the rest of the family. He watched Elaine and her mother systematically walk around the table scooping food onto the children's plates.

"Daddy, come on. Let's eat fast." Albert was shoveling the ziti Elaine had scooped onto his plate into his mouth.

Elaine stopped next to Larry and put a reproachful, but gentle hand on Albert's arm. "Slow down. You and Daddy have lots of time to play."

Chapter XXI: Infractions

*T*he month after the camera implant surgery Dr. Elbac gave Al clearance to work full time outside the home if he chose. Elaine had returned to part-time nursing and living with Al and Elaine allowed Ronnie to help with the boys. The woodworking business inventory in the garage filled all the orders for the Christmas holiday which was closing quickly on them. The ability to contribute to the family income as the main bread winner in seven years gave a resurgence to Al's sense of fulfillment.

In early December, the opportunity to return to the field he enjoyed presented itself. "Kenny called this morning. He has a contract for a job at St Joseph's Hospital. He can use me to frame. It will be great to be around the old neighborhood." He finished helping Elaine fold the continuous mountain of clothes they were always conquering. "I can start Monday."

"That's good. We can take the rest of the week and the weekend to get our schedules together. Ronnie isn't going back to work until January. By then we'll have Nicky in nursery school." She lifted one of the tall piles and walked toward the master bedroom.

He followed her with three combined stacks of little boy's clothing. "I can't wait to get my hands dirty again."

"You do that around here all the time." Larry pushed past her as he ran up the stairs to his room.

"I know, but this reminds me of why I liked construction better than management. It's the confirmation that I enjoyed being outside, meeting new people, not being stuck in the same place each day and, at the end of the day, I get the satisfaction of creating something. When I'm done, I'm done. No more being on call." Chris was in the hall chasing after his brother.

"You might be glad to get away from the chaos. Work can be cathartic." Elaine was thinking about the break work gave to her.

"It will be good to be around the guys. If I had the time I'd join the ball league. Kenny's company still has a team." Both boys came out of their bedrooms and then ran back in when Albert started down the hall.

"Do you feel bad about missing out on softball now that you can see and play the game?" She heard a rumble and laughter coming from Larry's room.

"Not one bit. Every second of sight I have I need to make up for what I missed." Absentmindedly he made their bed after coming into the room.

Little things like making their bed meant a lot to Elaine. Without sight, he had not thought to do that simple chore unless she asked and she never did. In the larger scheme of their life it didn't seem important.

Now it was important to her that he noticed. "Thanks, Al."

"No problem." He pulled the covers up in a haphazard way. "Since I have the construction work coming up, I'm going to stop the telemarketing. As the winter progresses I can work on developing a business I can run from home. I've been thinking about that for a while. I needed sight to work through the paperwork. The last thing you needed was more to do. I can handle that." He had been working on a small service company in his head, and before the surgery had thought about proposing it to his brother-in-law. "Now that the surgery has been success I can start creating a business while I bring in a paycheck from the construction job."

The smell of something burning reached them. "Al, what is that?"

Al followed the smell and began to run down the staircase closely followed by Elaine. "Boys! Boys!"

They could see a light gray smoke coming from the open door of the half bathroom. Albert, Larry and Chris ran from the house leaving a confused Nick standing outside the door staring at his parents. Al dove into the half bathroom to find the toilet on fire with the seat down. Momentarily confused he looked wildly around the windowless cubicle.

The smoldering fire was fueled with mounds of toilet paper with little flames licking at the edges of the faux wooden seat. First Al pushed the handle to flush and caused some water to come down the edges, but the flames started to lick higher and over the edges further. It was obvious the water tank was empty probably from continuous flushing. Lifting the lid with his foot, he grabbed the plunger and stirred and pushed down on the mess until the fire was completely out.

Al looked around the bathroom and spied a box of matches on the sink. "I'm gonna kill those kids." Where did they get the matches?" He pointed at the abandoned miniature match box.

Elaine shook her head in astonishment. "They're kept in the cabinet over the refrigerator. I didn't even realize the kids knew they were in there." Her voice became louder and high pitched.

White hot anger began to spill out of Al. "I didn't realize they knew how to strike a match." Even with his sight returned Al still had a healthy fear of fire instilled in him since the accident. The new house had a fireplace that they had installed an insert into that did not allow the family to be exposed to live flames. "When I'm finished with these kids, they will never touch a match again."

Al and Elaine cleaned up the bathroom before they went on the hunt for the boys. Nicky had slunk back upstairs to the room he shared with Chris, playing quietly on the carpet waiting for his parents. Al knew the little boy had been too slow to keep up with his retreating brothers and he marched upstairs to look for him first.

Finding Nicky on the carpet, Al tried to tone down his anger so that it wasn't misplaced on the toddler who did not understand the gravity of what had happened. "Where are your brothers, Nick?"

Nicky shrugged his shoulders. "Out Daddy. I sorry."

Al glanced out the window to the backyard treehouse. "Nicky, playing with matches is very, very bad. You could get hurt."

Nicky rose slowly and sniffled. "Sorry Daddy."

"I know you are sorry, but you are still getting spanked." Al patted the little boys bottom very lightly. "You are not to leave your room unless you have to use the potty. Call Mommy or me for that. We have to go find your brothers. You stay here, understand?"

The little boy sniffled loudly. "Yeth."

"Aunt Ronnie should be home in a few minutes from Pop Pop's and we'll tell her to check on you while we find the boys. Don't come out of your room." Al watched the little boy climb onto his bed and he bent down to hand him some toys to keep him occupied. Al turned on his heal and ran quickly from the room. The second he hit the top step of the stairs he heard Elaine yelling. He followed the voice as quickly as he could to the kitchen door.

Elaine had found the boys hiding in the treehouse and pointed angrily across the yard. "Get down here now! Albert first!"

The boys had pulled down the canvas window covers Al had made for them and pulled up the rope ladder. Al stormed past Elaine and the two of them ran to the tree house.

Al reached it first. "Get down here! If I have to come up there to get you it's gonna be ten times worse for each of you."

The rope ladder fell down the side of the tree. Larry was the firstone to respond to his parents. He stood in front of them bravely with his head up and eyes downcast.

Al towered over him. "What were you thinking? You're old enough to know not to play with matches. Mommy and I have told you never to play with fire." Al smacked the little boys bottom hard. "There will be no more play today. You are going to spend the day in your room. Since you boys decided to hide in your tree house, you won't be playing in it for a week."

There was an audible groan from the Albert and Chris still inside the fort. "Albert! Get down here!" Elaine yelled at the top of her voice.

"Hey, what's going on?" Ronnie had pulled in the driveway and heard the yelling as soon as she and Peter were out of the car.

Peter pointed at Elaine looking for facetime and he received it as she momentarily became gratefully distracted. "Hi Sweetheart. Aunt Elaine is very angry right now, but not at you." She turned her gaze back to the treehouse. "Ronnie, the boys are in big trouble. They set the toilet on fire."

Ronnie tried as hard as she could not to laugh. "Oh, man. That is crazy. I'll stay out of your way." She began to back away.

Al looked over at her. "I need you to escort this one to his room and check to make sure Nicky stays in his. The boys are on lockdown for the day without any playing."

Ronnie shook her head in agreement. "Come on, Larry. Playing with fire is a dumb thing. You could have gotten hurt."

Larry rubbed his bottom, but no tears came. "I am hurt."

She didn't respond, because she had witnessed the spanking he just received and felt it was completely justified. The two walked away quickly with Peter munching on his fist and trying to squirm out of his mother's arms.

Al turned to see Albert slowly come down the rope. When he reached the ground, Al reached for him. "You are the oldest." He smacked the boy's bottom hard, four times. "Get inside and go to your room. I can't believe you would play with matches. How many times have I told you how badly I was burned? You see every day how much that hurts me. Do you want that to happen to you or your brothers?"

Albert hung his head. "No Daddy. I'm sorry."

"Why Albert? Why? You know better. You could have been hurt. Were you the one to get the matches down from the cabinet?" Al felt his fury rise again.

"Yes Daddy. I didn't think it would be bad 'cause we could flush the toilet paper. But the toilet water stopped." Albert rubbed his butt.

Al looked hard at the boy, amazed that he thought his experiment through. "Not exactly how you planned it. Let me ask you something, Albert. If this had worked, would you have tried it again?" Al didn't want to spank the boy anymore.

Albert hung his head down. "Yes." The single word came out low and soft.

"Go upstairs. Right to your room. Your Aunt Ronnie is watching." Al turned and saw Chris come down the ladder.

Chris looked up at Elaine with guilty, scared eyes that did not assuage his mother's anger. "Chris, I can't believe this. You and your brothers could have gotten hurt. You are not leaving your room today and you are not playing in your tree house for a week." Chris' eyes grew wide at the two punishments he had already heard. Elaine leaned over and spanked Chris hard. "Go upstairs." Chris ran to get away from his parents.

Al watched the little boy run, gave a quick, hard yank on the rope ladder and watched it fall at his feet. "I'll put the access to their tree fort back up after their prison terms have ended." Al shook his head and put his hands on his hips. "I never thought fire would be something our boys would be curious about. I just assumed after growing up with my hospital visits and scars, that was something they would fear."

The anger Elaine had a few moments ago had transformed. "I believe these boys are fearless and that scares me."

Al was thoughtful for a moment as he stared up at the tree fort. "It scares me too. We'll continue to set boundaries and reinforce the consequences." He gave her a smirk. "The good news is they're fearless. The bad news is they're fearless." Elaine did not laugh. "What do you want to do while we police these kids tonight?" He bent down, scooped the rope pile and rolled it into a ball.

She breathed out heavily. "I don't know. I think I'd like both of us to calm down first. My day just turned upside down."

"Looks like we're all on lockdown." They walked quietly to the garage until their mind's cleared.

She brightened slightly. "Let's take the afternoon to plan our next trip. I need something to look forward to. Mom's been talking about Disney."

Al dumped the rope inside the garage door and they both stomped toward the house. "That seems like a strange diversion to the boys nearly burning down our house."

Elaine turned and looked directly at him. "I need a vacation."

Al laughed. "Doesn't that defeat the purpose of punishment tonight if they hear us talking about taking them to Disney?"

"They won't hear us. I think a trip will work well for everyone-a short vacation like a week." She looked up before going through the kitchen door and saw Chris' little face peeking out between the curtains of his bedroom before he jumped away leaving the curtains moving. "Ronnie could use a quick trip away from Jersey. This has been a tough couple of months for her."

"You're right. It will be good to see her getting back to her old self." Al showed genuine concern.

"Mom and Dad have vacation time coming up from work. I'll call her and coordinate that before I put in for time at my job." It started to dawn on Elaine that she was going to need a vacation from planning her vacation. "We should try to get to the Pocono house more this winter. They're having a good snow season."

"Absolutely. I was thinking about Christmas week." Al

stopped as another little head stuck out from the curtains of the next bedroom and disappeared when it saw Al's gaze. "My sight is better than I expected. I can live without peripheral vision if I get to watch our boys grow."

Elaine walked closer to him. "We're blessed, now let's talk about vacation."

Al shook his head in agreement and held his hands up in surrender. "You don't need to convince me. The Ridgeview house will be sold before Christmas and this mortgage will be paid off so we might as well enjoy some of the money I earn in construction."

They walked up to the house as the milk truck pulled in. The milkman waved to Elaine and was shocked to see Al wave back to him. He parked the truck and walked up to the couple.

"Mr. Plevier, can you see me?" He waved a hand in front of Al's face.

"Yes, for a while. I usually miss you in the morning. You're running pretty late today." Al set eyes on the man who delivered milk to them at the Lake Road house since Albert was born. He noted that he hadn't changed much.

"I'm so happy for you. I watched this family go through many changes." Tears welled up in the man's eyes. "Let me get your order. You're right, I'm running late. They had a problem with one of the trucks and I had to combine deliveries." They watched the man climb quickly into the truck and gather their order. "Mr. Plevier are you still making furniture?"

Al walked over and received the milk cartons off the truck-something he hadn't done in seven years. "I sure am. What do you need?"

"I'm interested in a cherry wood cabinet for my wife. She has a lot of collectibles that are scattered all through the house." The delivery man was climbing back into the truck. "I can call you tomorrow with the dimensions, but I have to get going." The delivery man gave a wave and started to pull away.

"Sure, whenever you have time." Al watched the truck leave. "He hasn't changed. Doesn't even look older."

"Looks like you have another order. Will you have time to run the woodworking business and work construction?" They walked back to the house. "I don't want you to be overtaxed." Her thoughts went to the success of the camera implant and the potential risk an infection posed.

"I promise. Besides, we'll see if he calls." They entered the kitchen and heard scampering little feet upstairs. "For today we have little prisoners to keep under lock and key and a couple vacations to plan."

Elaine walked ahead of him stomping to give the boys plenty of warning that they were back in the house. "Al, the news last night said the snow is good in the Poconos."

"Has the Pocono getaway been marinating since last night? I know when I'm being hustled and I'm good with that." He stomped alongside Elaine. "Why don't we go up over Christmas vacation?" He followed behind her up the stairs.

"That sounds good, but I was thinking of January. Christmas is so crazy with these little guys. They usually just want to spend the week playing with their news toys at home and visiting friends. January and February is when they have cabin fever." They had both stomped all the way up the staircase.

He stopped at the top. "Wait, are we going to Disney first or the Poconos?"

The first room on the right was the room Chris shared with Nick and the two boys heard every word. "Disney? Yeah! Mickey Mouse! Mickey Mouse!"

Chris cheered loud enough for Larry and Albert to hear. "Yeah!"

Elaine gave him a very annoyed look. "I thought you were smart enough to talk in code. I didn't think I needed to tell you."

He held out his hands in defense. "Sorry. I didn't think they were listening."

"Are you kidding me?" Elaine spoke loudly as she stood in the middle of the hall. "Boys, there will be no Disney unless you all start to behave. You are being punished and if you don't listen and mind you will NOT go to Disney." Elaine walked down the hall and snuck up on a smiling Albert. "Young man, wipe that smile off your face. You're in the most trouble."

Albert immediately hung his head. "Yes, Mommy."

"You are not going to Michaels birthday party tomorrow." Al walked in behind Elaine.

Albert had a shocked and horrified look on his face. "But…" Albert knew he shouldn't try to argue. "Is Larry going?"

"No, of course not. You're both coming home from school and going straight to your rooms." Elaine caught the shadow of Larry in his doorway.

Al readjusted his temperament to the anger he felt a short while ago. "Mommy and I are going downstairs. You will each have dinner in your rooms. We'll bring it up later. And remember, you are not going to know when we are coming up to check on you." Al and Elaine walked downstairs without stomping and waited out the punishment they dispensed on the boys.

In the morning, Albert and Larry were grateful to go to school. Nick and Chris stood in the doorway, watched them load onto the bus and then mournfully turned to Elaine.

"Mommy, do we go to our room now?" Chris looked up at her with huge eyes but no tears.

"No." Nick was too young for another day in his room. All he understood was that they had done something wrong. "When your brothers come home they have to go to their rooms and so will you. For the day, you are not allowed outside. Play with Peter inside." At the mention of his name the toddler stopped eating his breakfast and looked to his Aunt. "Daddy has to work in his shop. Aunt Ronnie will keep an eye on you."

Ronnie was happy not to have to chase Nick outside. She had not started back to work yet, bargaining instead to help Al and Elaine with the boys as they adjusted to their life that included both of them working.

The phone rang and Ronnie grabbed it for them. "Yes?"

Oh, hi. Sure, I'll tell him. Bye." She replaced the receiver and turned to Al. "That was the milkman, Carl. He's coming by in an hour or so to drop off some plans he asked you about."

Al was genuinely surprised. "Really. I didn't think he was serious. We don't have a milk delivery today so he must want the new cabinet." He threw on his heavy coat and went out the back door calling over his shoulder. "I'll be in the work shop."

Ronnie looked at his back and then turned to Elaine. "People come and go so quickly around here." She watched her sister roll her eyes as she drank coffee.

Later that morning the milkman stopped by with a schematic. "Mr. Plevier this is the drawing. Are you able to build something like that and do you have an estimate of the cost?"

Al took the drawing from the man and quickly sized up the job. "I can build this for $300 in pine or $900 in the cherry wood that you requested. We can also do a combination of pine on the sides and cherry for the front for $300. The doors will be smoked glass to give the cabinet a richer look and I'll purchase them premade. The cherry is a much more expensive wood to obtain." Al thought it was a simple design. "Carl, I would suggest the pine if cost is a large factor."

Carl had a look of concentration on his face as he listened to the figures Al proposed. "Do you think the pine would look as nice as the cherry?"

"I'll stain it and create a natural look. Pine is a good sturdy wood but cherry is sturdier and has a prettier grain, that is why the cost is more." Al gave him a chance to jump in. "It really comes down to the cost."

"You're right. I can't afford the $900 so let's go with a combination of the pine on the sides and cherry for the front. Here's a catalogue picture of the cherry cabinet she had picked out. It cost $2500 retail." He handed the picture to Al. "Could you do the combination for $300?"

The job was undercutting the current market price for hand crafted furniture, but Al thought this piece was a nice example for other customers. "That is a beautiful cabinet. I can build something to the specs of you schematic and tweak your design to be more similar in appearance to the retail piece. The schematic is a bit different but not too much." Al tacked both pictures on the cork he kept above his work table.

"I'd like to place the order and firm up the details today so that it will be finished for Christmas. Is that possible so close to the holiday? The pine will be perfect if you can stain it to appear as cherry." Carl appeared anxious.

"I'm not going to raise the price if you go home and talk it over with your wife." Al had an uneasy feeling about the transaction.

"I've seen your work. You did a beautiful job without sight, I'm sure it will look wonderful now that you can actually see what I'm interested in." Carl spoke quickly.

At first, Al didn't know how to respond to the man's lack of tact. "I start on it tomorrow. That should give me time before Christmas. I'll work on it at night if time gets tight. There's no deposit necessary."

Carl smiled. "Great. I have to get back to my route. I'll see you tomorrow for your delivery."

"That's fine. I'll keep you up to speed on my progress on our milk delivery days." Al shook Carl's hand and hoped it would move him along.

After lunch, he started on the cabinet a day early. He had the rest of the week before he started back in construction on Monday and he wanted to finish up as many of his own projects as possible. The fact that the boys were on lockdown, helped free of his time further.

On Friday, he found out there was a delay on the part of the site supervisor that would hold Al back from starting at the construction job at the hospital. The company wanted to make sure he was cleared to work with the insurance for the construction company and the supervisor had neglected to file the paperwork. The simple cabinet design project kept him busy.

Three days into the work Carl stepped into the garage after dropping off the milk order. "Hey Mr. Plevier."

Al looked up from his work. "Hi Carl. Come over and take a look at the project."

Carl walked over tentatively. "Wow. It's sharp. I can't believe how much you've done. I'm surprised."

Al ignored the back-handed compliment. "My sons have been on lock down for the last couple of days. We've been shackled to the house while we police them."

Carl gave Al an odd look. He was aware at the ages of the boys. "Everything okay?"

Al laughed. "Yeah. They're doing five to ten for arson."

Carl shook his head with wide eyes and a confused look. "I'll check in with you at the end of the week."

"Good. See you then." Al watched him drive down the incline glad to see the man leave as he watched Elaine approach him from the house.

"Al, it's going to be a long weekend if we don't end the grounding for the boys." She crossed her arms and looked at the cabinet. "This is coming along nicely. That's a beautiful piece of furniture."

Al stepped back and took a long look at the cabinet. "I have to agree. It is pretty." He looked up as Fenna and Rose pull into the driveway.

Fenna came into the garage. "Hey you two. How's it going?"

Elaine answered for the family. "Albert and Larry are thrilled to get on the bus every morning." The women turned to Al.

"When does the lock down end?" Fenna walked over and ran her hand over the unfinished cabinet. "This is nice. A special order?"

"Yes. The milkman." Al touched the piece of furniture with pride. "Elaine and I were just talking about shorting the sentence for the boys.

Fenna, entranced by the cabinet, ignored his comment. "How much do you charge for these?" Fenna opened one of the newly installed doors.

"This is the first one I made. He brought over the schematic. $300."

Fenna whistled low. "That's cheap. When you finish I want to place an order for one. A beautiful cabinet like this would look great in my dining room."

"If I have time. I'm waiting to hear what my new starting date is for the construction job at St Joseph's in Newark. The cabinet project is for some extra cash and to keep me busy while we're policing the boys." Al tossed the rag he had in his hand on the workbench.

"Elaine, are you guys free this weekend? We were hoping to go out to the movies with all the kids." Fenna looked from one to the other.

Elaine answered first. "What do you think, Al? We beat them, took away a birthday party and let them know we don't trust them. Is that enough?"

Al shrugged his shoulders in defeat. "Yeah, I need to get out." He put extra effort into each stroke of the sandpaper.

Elaine and Fenna walked toward the house. "We'll let the boys know there is a light at the end of the tunnel." The two women laughed lightly.

Al watched them go and then stood back to look once more at the cabinet. *I'll finish this by the weekend. This could be the template for others. I can't wait to see the look on the milkman's face when he sees the finished product. I'll deliver it to him personally.*

That weekend as the boys ran excitedly around the house in anticipation of their release from their parents lock down, Al and Fenna's husband, Bob, loaded the finished cabinet carefully into his pickup. They gingerly laid it down in the bed of the truck where they had placed several old comforters and then surrounded it with cushions on either side.

"The milkman is going to be thrilled. I can't wait to see the look on his wife's face. I've never met her." Al felt like he had created something wonderful.

"Does this guy have a name?" His brother-in-law gave Al a weird look.

It took Al a second to recognize and acknowledge the fact that he was continuing to engage people with looks. "Carl."

Bob shook his head and looked over at Al suspiciously. "Did you get a deposit on this?"

Al waved a hand. "It's only $300. He's good for it. The job took less than a week. He should thank my kids for that. I was out here practically twenty-fours hours a day."

Bob raised his eyebrows. "It's your business, Boss."

When they arrived at Carl's house, they were backing the pick up into the driveway when the milkman came out with his wife. The two stared at the cabinet laying on its back with the grain, staining and smoke glass windows fully visible. The wife turned and went back into the house after whispering something to her husband. Bob saw the entire interaction, but Al had been watching the cabinet to see if it shifted at all. He jumped out of the truck before Bob could say anything to him.

"How are you folks today?" Al smiled broadly and offered his hand to the milkman.

The milkman hesitated and then shook Al's hand. "Hi. Looks good. Let's climb up there."

Al motioned to Bob. "Let us lift it out for you. Where do you want it?"

The milkman hesitated again. "Let me get a dolly from the garage."

"No need. We brought our own." Bob and Al unloaded the cabinet carefully. They had it fully onto the dolly when Al turned to the buyer. "What do you think? She's a beauty."

The milkman looked nervous. "We really wanted all cherry. It looks fine, but since you didn't build it completely in cherry we're only paying you $150."

Al stood stock still for several minutes staring at the milkman who had suddenly gone quiet and a little pale. He placed a hand on his hip silently and then slowly turned and lifted his head to Bob.

"Bob, let's get her loaded back up." Al didn't give the milkman a chance to negotiate.

Bob smirked as he carefully leaned the cabinet onto the padded tailgate. "We'll load her the same way we did at home. She'll slide nicely on the comforters."

The milkman looked down at the ground and mumbled. "It's not worth $300."

Al snapped his head as he held the weight of the bottom end of the cabinet. "It was worth $300 when I told you it would be made of pine on the sides and cherry on the front. You want all cherrywood, call me. The new price will be $2500."

Now the milkman snapped his head. "That's the retail price."

Al turned to finish loading the cabinet. "Yup."

The two men loaded the cabinet wordlessly, quickly, and carefully. They pulled away without acknowledging the milkman.

Al turned to Bob when they reached the end of the driveway. "I guess I can count on my milk being late or not delivered."

Bob burst out laughing. "Screw that guy. What an idiot. Put an ad in the paper for $800. I bet it goes within a week."

"You and Fenna can have it for $200. I don't care. At least I'll know you appreciate it. Tell her it's an early Christmas gift from you." Al reached for gum in his pocket.

Now it was Bob's turn to snap his head. "Really? Are you sure?"

Al shrugged his shoulders. "Yeah. I said $300 to him."

Bob smiled. "Fenna is going to love that. She was already planning on ordering one from you."

"Sold." Al leaned back and looked out the window. "Nobody screws me out of money. I learned my lesson with Elaine's Pontiac." He shook his head slowly. "People never cease to amaze me. I cut this guy a break and he tried to take advantage for $150 bucks." He smiled. "I'd give it to you for free, but Fenna and I have had an agreement since we were kids-

I ain't the bank." They both laughed. "Did she ever tell you how I used to charge her interest on loans?"

Bob laughed uncontrollably. "Yes. You're nuts, Buddy."

"Yup." Al turned to Bob. "Let's take this to your house. It will be a nice surprise when you two come home tonight after the movies."

The two men set up the cabinet at Fenna and Bob's and then hurried back to the house to pile the children in the cars for the movies and everyone's release from lockdown. As they watched the boys run chaotically around the waiting area for the theatre, Elaine and Al wondered if they shouldn't shorten the next prison sentence.

"I've never seen them with this much energy." Elaine shook her head and watched Al smiling. "What is so funny?"

"Nothing. I'm just glad to watch them." His head followed the circles they and their cousins made around them."

Fenna grabbed at her daughter and Albert. "Enough. There are other people in this movie theatre and if you don't calm down you're both grounded and not helping with the Christmas lights tonight." The two horrified children froze.

Al had forgotten about the chore. "Bob, you still want to hang out and help with the lights tonight?"

Fenna's husband smiled and shrugged his shoulders. "Free dinner?"

Al watched Albert trying to escape Fenna's hold. "Unless Elaine has started charging."

The line moved forward and for two hours the children stayed transfixed and quiet as the collective movie of choice played out for them. Driving home, the two cars of adults and children sang Christmas carols in anticipation of a night that included pizza and decorating.

To Al's dismay, the deocorating started the second he stepped out of the car. "Sweetheart, why don't you and Bob get the boxes out of the garage? I'll order the pizza's."

"Thanks, Dear." Al and Bob dragged out the clearly marked Christmas boxes and started hanging the lights on the porch.

"Al, the left line is drooping." Bob stepped back to look at the progress they had made after fifteen minutes.

"Pull the other ladder over and we'll try to get this done in one shot. Hammer the nails and clips in tight. I don't want to have to line these lights up again next year." Truthfully, in the back of his mind, Al was always preparing for the possibility that he would be returned to darkness. "The hooks I had permanently nailed on Lake Road made it easy to hang the lights without sight."

The ladder banged against the house. "Al, relax. The surgery was a complete success. You have your life back without a timeline of the implant's failure that you dealt with before."

A soft clip as the light string popped into place resounded in the still twilight. "I'm planning ahead, just in case." Shutting down the conversation, he slid down the ladder like an experienced construction worker.

Bob stood on the ladder and watched his brother-in-law haphazardly pull another string out. "Do you have the strings marked for color?"

Al stared at the string dangling in his hand. "Nope. Elaine never mentioned it. Looks like all of us are in for a surprise when the switch flips up."

The two men laughed as the pizza delivery truck pulled into the driveway. "Hurry up, Al."

"Let's do another one and finish the rest fo the strings after dinner." They hung the latest string he had fished out and ran in to join everyone.

The two men finished up after dinner as darkness descended. "I'll go gather the troops for the unveiling."

As Bob was folding his ladder an army of little pounding feet could be heard inside the house and toward the front door. "Daddy! Did you finish Aunt Elaine's house?" Bob's daughter stuck her head out the door as Fenna was forcing a coat on her.

Jayne Kelly

"Yes, Honey. We're all done. Who's throwing the switch?" Bob stood back and rubbed his lower back.

The stampede funneled out the door and Ronnie handed Peter to Al. "I got the switch. When you're all lined up give me the signal."

Elaine squeezed passed Ronnie among the little running bodies. "Thanks, Ron." She rushed out the door to the group of darting children and tired, smiling adults.

The line formed by the group had inadvertently placed Al at the center with his arm around Elaine. "Hit it Ronnie!"

The house burst into light accompanied by a collective cheer from the group. Every string hanging on the house had been hung on the two previous homes they lived in and each twinkle caught Al's breath.

Elaine felt his stillness among the controlled chaos. "Do they look clear to you, Sweetheart?"

"Crystal clear. Part of me wondered if I would ever see them again."

"This holiday is just starting." She kissed him lightly on the cheek.

The lights burned bright each night for the next two weeks before Christmas Eve and then for three more weeks after Santa's arrival. Much to their parent's surprise, the four boys were on their best behavior with the threat of a delivery of coal from Santa. A shocking and entertaining moment came when Albert wrote an apology letter at school to Santa for the burning toilet. His teacher called Elaine when she realized what the little boy was apologizing for.

"The letters were to be mailed to the NorthPole from school. If I send it home with him he'll know it was never sent. I thought you might want me to read it to you."

"Yes. Please." Elaine felt like she was the one going to the Principal's office. "To be clear, the boys were severely punished and we're confident playing with fire is never going to happen in our home again." Silence greeted Elaine.

"Here is the content of the letter, Mrs. Plevier." The teacher read from the letter, pausing to correct the language the immature writing reflected.

Dear Santa,

I was bad. I'm sorry. I tried to make the fire stop. I won't play with fire in the bathroom again.

Love, Albert.

Elaine had to cover the receiver. "My husband and I will discuss this tonight. Thank you for letting me know. Please send it with the rest of the letters."

"I will." There was a pause. "Albert is a nice boy who gets along with all the other children. He's doing well with all his subjects except Math. He may be acting out because he needs more attention at home."

Elaine clenched her jaw. "He gets plenty of attention from his Dad and I. We're both very involved in our boy's lives. Additionally, we have always kept the matches hidden, but our children are not only smart, they are resourceful. I appreciate your help. It's great to know there are teachers that will take the time to reach out to the parents."

The tone of the teacher's voice became condescending. "I understand."

Elaine felt her temper rise. "I'm not sure you do. My husband coaches Albert's baseball team in the spring months. He has regained his sight, but he coached last spring without it. He plays with our children. He works to support his family. This is a man who spends more time with his boys than men I know with vision." She caught her breath. "I have four young boys who like to test the limits of their world. Much like their father. We're working to harness the creativity and energy together as parents."

"Mrs. Plevier I certainly didn't mean anything offensive. I was just concerned."

Elaine saw an opportunity and ran with it, greeting the teacher with the same condescension she had given Elaine. "I understand. Thank you and have a good week."

"You also." The teacher hung up.

Ronnie heard Elaine laughing from the other room. "Hey."

"Hey."

"What's so funny?"

"Your nephew sent a letter to Santa apologizing for setting the toilet on fire. His teacher thinks he needs more attention at home."

Ronnie joined her sister in laughter. "Did you tell her you have half your family living with you at any given time? How much more attention could these kids get?'

"Maybe she doesn't have children of her own. I thought for a brief second telling her about catching Albert on riding his bike on Route 23. She would have called Child Protective Services on us."

"That is a day that will live in infamy. That boy turned eight and thought he was king of the world."

"Wow, I didn't even mention that we believe in corporal punishment in this house. That would have definitely put her over the edge." Elaine laughed through the guilt she had about how hard she had spanked Albert when she caught him with his best friend on the busy four lane highway. "Following him home with the car after screaming at him gave me all the time I needed to build up my reservoir of anger. I heard Michaels mother blamed Albert but still gave Michael a good spanking."

"Al thought you were losing your mind. He has his sight back for one month and witnesses his wife giving Albert the thrashing of a lifetime."

"That was right after the toilet incident." She was thoughtful for a moment. "Albert didn't apologize for that in the letter, according to his teacher. Maybe he doesn't think that was as bad." She and Ronnie exchanged looks. "That little boy is not to ride his bike without an adult with him until he's a teenager."

A week later as the family sat watching wrapping paper fly in all directions, Albert reached into his stuffed stocking and felt a letter at the top. He saw his name on the front and Santa's return address. He snuck a peak under his eyelids at his two

parents who were trying not to stare at him. Slowly he opened the letter before reaching further into his stocking.

Dear Albert,

If you ever play with matches again or ride your bike on Rt 23 I will come in the night and take all your toys.

Love Santa

Albert's eyes grew wide with fright before he peaked further into the stocking. Seeing no coal, he continued to dig. Elaine watched him try to hide the letter. That Christmas afternoon, as the boys were occupied with their new toys, Elaine retrieved the letter. It hung on the outside of his bedroom door at eye level for the next twelve months.

Chapter XXII: Of Skin and Bone

*Onc*e again Elaine and Al found themselves at a table with neatly stacked files and papers in front of them. "You would think we were rich with all the goings on in our lives." Al turned his head, slowly taking in the entire table with his right eye.

Elaine shrugged her shoulders in response. "We're rich in other ways, but this family is fine financially too." She lifted the stack of papers in front of her and tapped them lightly to align the collection.

"Time flies." Al thought back to the frustration and disillusionment he experienced since the accident.

"The social security will always be granted and the house is paid in full now that we sold Ridgeview Terrace." The mention of their last home brought a stiffness to Elaine's back that Al saw.

"Still not over the naked lady incident?" It took all the restraint he had not to burst out laughing.

She ignored the comment and continued to discuss the finances. "We have money saved up. Let's do Disney with my family this summer."

He immediately thought of the hot sun on his Jobe shirt. It kept him covered but would be hotter than Hades in Florida's summer heat. "Whatever you want. We can hold the trip over the boys all winter to keep them in line."

She sent him an annoyed look. "It will also be a great family adventure and fun to spend time with my side."

Al began to stutter. "Who, who from your side is going?"

Elaine confidently waved her hand. "Mom and I have been working on this. So far there are fourteen people."

The thought of fourteen people from one family traveling to Disney seemed ludicrous to him. "That's going to be a fun plane ride."

"Don't be ridiculous. You'll be taking the train with Albert and Uncle Charlie."

"Whaaat?" Al was stunned as the conversation went from ludicrous to impossible and then a car horn sounded. "I have to go to work." He jumped up from the bar stool. "When is your shift starting?"

Elaine kissed him lightly good-bye. "Noon. One of the older women needed my morning shift."

"I'll have the kids bathed and a private dinner for the two of us by the time you get home tonight. How does that sound?"

"Like a fantasy." She returned to going over her paperwork as he bounded out the door. "Have a good day at work."

The energy and enthusiasm with which Al greeted his work day was equal to the annoying boundless energy of his first day with sight. "Every day is good. It's nice to go to a hospital for work and not to be worked on."

The construction job at St. Joseph's Hospital in Patterson had opened for bid last year. His old company that he had worked for before and intermittently while at A&K Chemicals had won the bid. The job had been going on since the fall of 1981. Al's old boss, Ken, had initially been reluctant to rehire Al. Ken was aware of Al's woodworking business, having hired him to cut headers, and to cut and bundle bridging for sub floors as he needed, but the insurance liability gave him pause. It took two months after the camera implant surgery to secure a face-to-face meeting with Ken. The two men discussed the issues of what Al would and would not be allowed to work on and a strategy for hire was enacted. Desperate to work outside his home again, Al was willing to fold to the concessions offered by the company. In order to prove to Ken that he would make money for the company and not just be a symbol of a goodwill gesture made to an old employee and friend, Al worked harder, longer and more effectively in the areas he was allowed, than half of his co-workers. This cold January day he would be working on the hospital's seventh floor, a new wing that did not yet have the heating system operable.

"Looks like they have everything done on this floor but the environmentals. I'm starting to get used to freezing my butt off." Al looked over the room they were sent to and then to his co-worker Steve. "Let's get started."

"Al, what do you think of my cabinets I lined up yesterday? You've installed cabinets a million times." Steve ran a hand over the top. "The doctor is supposed to come in for inspection today."

Al gave Steve a quizzical look. "What doctor?"

"The Chief of Staff." Steve leaned against a wall and crossed his arms.

"He's coming in here? Why?" Al reached for a level in his tool belt.

"No idea, but he's not coming. He's going to look the job over from behind the partition." Steve pointed to the one undraped section between the older section and the new floor they were working on.

"Good. That piece of plexi glass will keep him out of our way. It's not in my job description to deal with the brass." Al and Steve went back to work and were so busy that they did not notice when the Chief of Staff and another man watched them from behind the partition.

The Chief of Staff pointed out several areas to the man with him. Al and Steve were looking over a printed directive from their boss for the day. Due to the low light level Al had to take off his glasses to see the print. The Surgeon General had a full view of his camera implant.

Al looked up from the paper he was reading. Two stunned faces on the other side of the glass partition greeted him when he lifted his hand to wave. The Surgeon General's face was white. Before Al or Steve could walk over the doctor came through the door without the other individual. He was momentarily stunned when the cold air from the construction side hit him, but he never took his eyes off Al.

"What the hell is in your eye?" The man brought his face close to Al's.

Steve jumped in to protect the friend he had known for many years. "Excuse me, Doctor, is it necessary to stand so close to my friend?"

The doctor was not deterred. He moved even closer to Al's face looking dumbfounded by what he saw. "What is that?"

Al didn't want to embarrass the man, but could not contain himself. "You have no idea what this is? Aren't you the Chief of Staff?"

The doctor answered him without sarcasm or annoyance. "No, I don't and yes I am." He continued to visually inspect the camera implant. "I can see that your left eye has no sight. You obviously have a field of vision in the right that allows you to work in your chosen field."

Now Al laughed. "It was my chosen field originally and it should have stayed that way. I was a chemical engineer in another life that led to the mess you're looking at." He paused thoughtfully. "You never know what you got 'til its gone."

The doctor stood straight. "What happened?"

Al held up a gloved hand. "Not important." Al paused, grateful that his Jobe shirt was covered under heavy coat. "You've really never seen this procedure on a patient before? Recognition of the quality of care given to him in Manhattan flooded his consciousness.

"No." The doctor continued to stare. "It's a camera, right?"

He held out his hands. "Isn't it a shame that you're the top guy here and you don't know about this?" Al dropped his hands and began to shift from one foot to another. "I don't mean any disrespect, I am just talking about the seeming lack of communication once you cross the Hudson."

The doctor stood back slightly. "Oh, that explains it. Is this what they're doing over at Manhattan Eye and Ear?"

"No, this procedure was performed at Mt. Sinai by Dr. Elbac." Al jumped up onto his soap box. "Shouldn't the larger medical community know when this type of experimental option is available?" He stopped shifting. "I'm sure Dr. Elbac and Mt. Sinai is not hoarding the technology for themselves."

The doctor continued to look over Al's right eye as he laughed softly. "I'm sure our staff has read the material concerning this."

Al didn't want to appear condescending or arrogant in front of the Chief of Staff and instead continued to speak about his progress. "The only sight I've had since my accident before this was a temporary corneal transplant that latest six months. My age and the condition of my right eye made me a strong candidate for a successful outcome." He looked the doctor up and down. "My vision is pretty good. About 20/30. I do everything except drive a car." The afternoon behind the wheel of the corvette popped into his mind.

The doctor smirked and crossed his arms over his chest. "This is wonderful. My hope is that you have vision indefinitely."

Al did not know how to respond to that comment from the top doctor at the hospital or the expanse of opportunity left open to ask Al questions. "Stop back anytime. This section should be wrapped up in another couple of weeks."

The doctor nodded and both he and the colleague left after a brief acknowledgment. "You're doing a great job, gentlemen. Thank you."

After they were gone Steve turned to Al. "Too bad he didn't ask you to talk to his other doctors. You love being a lab rat." Steve walked away laughing.

"You're a funny guy, Steve." The two men lifted a cabinet. "It is too bad he didn't check me out and talk to some of his staff." The cabinet landed with a thud on its lower level location. "Maybe it's easier to learn from a book than to look and observe the real thing for some people."

Steve leaned on the top of the cabinet. "Don't take it personally. You have lost your charm and appeal with that robot eye."

"Enough." Al's heard his stomach growl. "Where are we going for lunch? I was trying to get away from Elaine this morning and I left my brown bag behind."

"If I had a wife that pretty I wouldn't be running away no matter what she said." Steve looked Al over severely. "Let's hit the grease trucks by the College. That should bring back some memories."

Al nodded in agreement. "That sounds good, but I have to tell ya that I never ate off the grease trucks when I was at the Newark College of Enginnering. I always hit the coffee shops." A memory from another lifetime flashed in his mind. He watched the terrified, angry, blind man stumble across High Street in Newark on his way to class. Al shook himself free of the scene and the promise he made to himself never to embarrass his family in any way. "Let's get this day over with, Steve. I have a family trip to Disney to help plan."

Steve gave him a horrified look. "That sounds awful."

"Fourteen people awful." He smiled at Steve. "I can't wait."

Steve was a man with a kind heart and loyalty to friends beyond measure, but he was unable to be tactful when necessary. "The one thing you can look forward to during that interminable trip is that being disabled means you get special treatment on the plane and I bet you are put at the front of the line on Space Mountain. You got it made buddy."

Al felt that he and Steve were good enough friends and companions that he could speak his truth. "Steve, if I was disabled I couldn't do my wood working when I didn't have sight. I'm handicapped even with the camera implant. There's a big difference from my point of view." He paused, smiling at his friend. "Excuse the pun."

Steve smiled back. "Thanks for the clarity."

They walked out of the almost completed hospital wing toward the trucks and the banter turned back to the Plevier's upcoming family vacation. "The trip should be great." Excitement began to build in him when, despite the aggravation he knew was waiting for him this summer while trapped with relatives, the ability to see his children's faces in front of the castle would make it all worthwhile. "This will be a vacation for all of us to remember." Al saw an envious look in his friend's eyes. "You have a point. I probably will get to the front of all the lines."

"I'm just looking for an angle for you. You have to have an angle to get by in this world and get ahead." Steve scanned the horizon for his favorite food truck. "You call yourself anything that makes you happy. I'll call you Al."

Al realized he had tried to draw the wrong audience for his soap box. "Next time just pop me on the head when I get irritating."

Steve gave him a side look. "I'd be popping you all day long."

Chapter XXIII: Blameless

The construction job at St. Joseph's hospital ended in April. Similar to all the other men he worked side by side with, Al became unemployed, in the traditional sense. He did not apply for temporary unemployment while the company negotiating its next contract bid. Al and Elaine felt that would be unfair. She was working full time as a nurse and Al's woodworking business was doing well. Ronnie was starting back to work full time after the planned Disney trip in June. They were blessed in many ways.

Financially they were blessed with common sense and a strong work ethic. Al's long list of jobs he had been working since he was eight competed against Elaine's list which was just as extensive and ran up to this moment in time. Al had started at eight years old as a paper boy, Elaine babysat. They had utilized the lawsuit settlement to buy a home for their family and were now in a position, while they both worked, to shoulder the financial responsibility of family vacations. It gave both of them joy to treat extended family members as a show of appreciation for all that they did for them.

The upcoming June trip to Disney was less than a month away. The total number of Elaine's side of the family that was participating had grown to seventeen.

Al breathed deep as he held the guest list from Disney in his hand. "Me, you, the boys, Ronnie, Peter, Mom, Dad, Cousin Steve, Carol, their two kids, Grandmom, Granddad and Uncle Charlie." He whistled low. "This ought to be interesting."

Elaine looked up from an episode of 'The Waltons'. "It's going to be fun. A trip to remember."

"If we all survive." He rubbed a hand along his beard stubble. "Let me get this straight. Albert and I are going to Florida on the train with Uncle Charlie. You, Larry, Chris and Nick will be flying on one plane with your parents. Ronnie, Pete, Grandmom, Granddad, Steve, Carol and the kids are going on a separate plane." He held two pages of itinerary in front of his right eye. "Are you sure we're all going to the same place?"

Elaine walked over and shut off the television. "Al, Uncle Charlie does not fly anymore. He became afraid of planes early. It's impossible for him to consider now that he's in his sixties."

"Albert and I are in charge of a mentally challengd man who doesn't travel well. So really, eight-year-old Albert is in charge of a mentally challenged man and a handicapped man." He looked at her over the top of the paper. "Who made up the travel list?"

Elaine waved off his concerns and sarcasm. "You can see fine. I thought it would be some quality time for you and Albert."

He dropped the hand holding the paper. "Quality time? As long as we don't lose Uncle Charlie I guess we can squeeze in a few laughs."

She gave him a long hard stare from her position on the couch. "Al, Uncle Charlie really wants to go. His life is very quiet and he counts on Dad and Grandpop to bring a little joy into his life. Spending time with you and Albert will make him happy."

Al felt guilt wash over him. "I'm sorry." Uncle Charlie was Elaine's grandfather's youngest brother and family was everything to their tribe. "That's good to know. It will be good for me to practice gratitude for my own life." He pulled the itinerary in front of his face and added some levity to the moment. "If one of us gets lost, I guess Albert will get us home."

Elaine gave him a deadly look. "Not funny."

Al looked over the top of his glasses at her. "It wasn't meant to be funny just truthful. I hope Albert doesn't mind hanging out with a couple old guys."

"Albert is going to be thrilled to have his dad all to himself." She waited for him to respond. "If you're insisting that Albert is going to be in charge of you two old guys then you might want to let him know. That will make him feel like a big boy."

"Whatever you say dear. I'm going to go along with the family flow on this trip. The only thing I ask is that I be standing in front of all four boys when they see the castle for the first time. I can't wait to see the expressions on their faces." He put the papers back in Elaine's Disney file and pushed it to the side. "Is the hospital going to hire you back after the summer leave of absence?"

"Yes. At first they weren't happy but I want to enjoy the summer with our children." She flipped the TV back.

"How can you watch that?" Al scrunched up his face.

"It's good wholesome Americana. No more talking. Let me enjoy my show." Elaine stared catatonically at the 'Waltons' and then switched to a sitcom. "I do believe this is the last season of my favorite show. It's not the same now that the children grew up."

Al smiled and looked at the calendar hung permanently next to the phone and then over to the black radio on top of the refrigerator. Staring at the simple black box radio that had been his connection to the world and kept track of the time and date for him, he realized he hadn't listened to it since his sight had returned in September. He had no need. Now he could look at

Jayne Kelly

the calendar for the date and the clock on the wall for the time. He still had not returned to wearing a wrist watch since the day of the accident. That October 1st afternoon he had looked at the clock on the wall and ignored the wristwatch he wore. He had never gotten that watch back.

"Elaine?"

"What?" She hoped the annoyed tone conveyed the fact that he was interrupting her program again.

"Whatever happened to the watch I was wearing when the accident happened?"

She turned and looked at him. "What made you think of that?"

"No idea. I had forgotten I wore one that day until I looked at the calendar."

She gave him a strange look about his stream of thought. "It wasn't in the bag from the hospital. The bag was very sparse. Your clothes had been cut from your body." Their eyes met the way eyes of victims brought together after a trajedy meet when they first see each other again. "Your watch might be in the box from the plant."

Al became angry at the thought of someone cleaning out his desk while he was fighting to live. "Maybe it ended up in the sink or fell off on the floor while I crawled. It had to be broken up or at least destroyed by the chemical." He was rubbing his wrist absentmindedly. "What was in the box from the plant? I know that makes sense that they would clean out my desk, but I never thought about it."

"It's in the attic. I never had the heart to look through it while you were recovering and then when I saw it again during the move from Lake Road, I decided to ignore it. They had Dad pick it up a couple weeks after the accident took place. I guess he may have looked through it." Elaine now stared blankly at the television screen.

"Is it in the attic?" Al sounded hopeful and he wasn't sure why.

"Yes. It's a cardboard box, sealed with packing tape from the last move. It's marked." She lost the storyline among feelings long buried that were rising to the surface along with Al's.

He looked up at the ceiling. "Maybe I'll go through it tomorrow, if I remember." He knew it would be the first thing on his mind when he woke up.

The next morning Albert and Larry's faces reflected the end of the school year as they boarded the school bus. "Have a good day, boys." Al waved as the door closed and the lumbering bus continued its journey.

Elaine had left early that day joining in the excitement of the ending school year and the approaching time off. Al stared at the house as he walked up the driveway incline listening to his sister-in-law preparing to leave for her work day. The box containing the last vestiges of his previous life sat under the eaves of the house, somewhere on the border of hope and reality.

"Al, I'm late." Ronnie stood at the kitchen door with Peter dressed for daycare, his diaper bag over her shoulder.

"I wish you would leave him with the boys and I. Give yourself a financial break from the daycare costs." Al winked at Peter who buried his nose in his Mom's shoulder.

She smiled warmly at him. "Peter needs to be around other children outside the family. He's growing fast. The boys will have plenty of time together at Disney."

"How did your boss feel about you taking the time off?" Al heard something hit a wall softly inside the house.

"Oh, please. I should take four weeks off. I jumped in there and got them back on track with their receivables. See you guys at dinner. I'll tell you about the new apartment I found for Peter and I."

"Elaine mentioned that. We sure are gonna..." A loud crash came from the living room. "I was going to say we'll miss you guys but I bet you will appreciate the peace and quiet."

She laughed as she walked to her car and Al tentatively went into the kitchen. He looked around and it didn't take long to find the bookcase with three shelves on its side. Nothing was broken but the contents were everywhere. He lifted it quickly looking for protruding limbs and when he didn't see any, he went looking for little bodies.

"Boys? Where are you? Don't hide. Disney is coming up quickly." He heard little feet running overhead and then down the stairs. Chris and Nick stood before him obediently waiting to be yelled at, but they watched their father continue to stare toward the top of the stairs.

"Daddy, you can yell now. We're right here." Chris pulled at Al's pant leg. "Daddy, we're right here."

Al dragged his gaze away from the stairs and looked from Chris to Nick. "Yes, you are, Pal." He felt himself readjusting somehow inside. "Who wants to tell me what happened?" Both boys started talking at once until it became white noise to Al. "Sounds like it was an accident. Am I right?"

Both boys looked at him dumbfounded. "Yes, Daddy." They spoke in unison and with a mask of innocence.

"That's a good thing because I want both of you to go to Disney World with Mommy and your brothers. Bad kids don't get to go, right?"

"Yes, Daddy." The two voices together sounded like two characters in a sitcom.

"While I pick up the shelf, I want both of you to behave." He tried to look at them sternly.

"Yes, Daddy."

Al tried not to smile as he turned around and lifted the lightweight shelf from the floor. He pushed it against the wall and turned to start picking up the books. Standing behind him Nick and Chris each held out one of the books that had ended up on the floor. Their big wide eyes burned into him and nearly burst his heart.

"Thank you, boys. You're both being a big help. I need you to help me put all the toys away in the house later. We want to leave the house neat the day we go to Disney."

Without a clear concept of time both boys took a quick intake of breath and smiled. "Yes, Daddy."

That morning the two little boys worked hard pushing

toys under their beds and into closets. They both fell asleep in front of their peanut butter and jelly sandwiches leaving Al to carry them to their beds for naptime. As he slowly closed Nicks' door, Al stopped and looked at the attic pull down stairs in the center of the hallway. Without pause he pulled on the short rope handle activating the easy release. The springs that held the stairs creaked slightly and Al winced at the thought of waking either boy. He had a small window of opportunity while they slept and no one else was home.

More squeaking accompanied his steps as he climbed the ladder and reached the attic. He hung his head down to determine if he heard any movements of the boys before he delved into the subject of his search. The dim light of the attic required him to take off his glasses but still he fumbled for the switch he knew was hung on the rafter in front of the ladder.

The dim daylight streaming up from the eaves gave way to visibility with the overhead light. Unable to fully stand in the low space, Al crawled over the plywood floor he had laid when they first moved in. He maneuvered past Christmas decorations and boxes labeled 'Elaine' until he found the one with his name and A&K written in sharpie across the side. He pulled the box to him and ripped it open.

Staring back at him were scattered pens, his nameplate, family pictures and the book he read on his lunch hour. It was rare that he would be able to take a full lunch, but when he did he made sure he had reading material unrelated to work. In that fall of 1974 he was reading "The Godfather".

Al picked up the book and tossed it aside. He remembered he had never finished the book, be he had seen the movie before the accident. His nameplate stared back at him. The white engraved letters against the black background was ironic to him. If his name represented him, he had been positioned in front of a very dark future every time he walked into his office.

He reached down and pulled out the pictures of Elaine and Albert that had sat on his desk. Forever frozen in time was one of his favorite picture of Albert and himself. Elaine had taken it when Albert was six months old during his first snow. As far as Al knew it was the only copy and he had not seen it for almost eight years.

Next, he pulled out the framed picture of Elaine from their honeymoon. She was smiling on the beach. He looked down at the picture and knew from this moment forward it was going to sit on his nightstand.

Al moved papers at the bottom of the box around and spotted an address of a travel agency he had written down on a piece of scrap paper. One of his softball buddies had recommended the agency because they had worked very hard to get the best prices with the best accommodations when traveling abroad. He was going to surprise Elaine that Christmas in 1974 with a trip to Italy for January before their second baby was due. The trip, the book and unfortunately the two pictures had been forgotten by Al in the months of survival and then years of recovery he and his family had endured.

He pulled his knees up to his chest, hurting for just a moment with what was lost. The moment didn't last long. Holding the pictures against his chest he flipped over, leaving the box open and crawled back out of the attic space. Daylight blazed up from the ladder opening. Flipping off the light switch he climbed down, released the stairs back up to close and replaced the glasses back over his eyes.

"Hi Daddy." Nick stood rubbing his eyes.

Al jumped, not expecting Nick to be awake. "Buddy, that was a quick nap."

"Hi Daddy." He shoved his thumb in his mouth and clutched his favorite blanket.

Al put down the pictures he carried on the small hall table behind him and reached down and picked up Nicky. "How about you and I go down and watch some cartoons until your brother wakes up." He kissed his forehead and clutched his son as passionately as Nick held his blanket.

"Daddy, too tight."

He leaned his head back and looked at his youngest. child. "Sorry kiddo."

Chapter XXIV: Adjustments

The noise level of the train station was beginning to wear on Uncle Charlie. He looked down and smiled at Albert, a young boy he thought was well behaved.

"Your daddy is fun to hang out with." He offered Albert the obligatory LifeSaver.

Albert took one candy from the multifruit roll. "Yup. We're going to have a great train ride, Uncle Charlie."

Al checked the boarding schedule above them. "Looks like we're boarding in fifteen minutes. Albert, I have a new match box car for you in my pocket when we board, if you're good."

Uncle Charlie looked at Al. "He's a good little boy, Al. He never complains. You're lucky."

Albert smiled sweetly at the old man. Visions of a burning toilet and bike riding on busy roads filled Al's head for a second or two. "Yes. Albert is a very good example for his little brothers."

Albert looked slyly at his dad. "I'll listen Daddy."

Uncle Charlie began to shift. "Al, I need to pee."

"No problem." Al looked around and spotted the men's room sign across the Amtrak waiting room. "Albert, would you like to go with Uncle Charlie while Daddy stays in front of the schedule board with the luggage? It's right there." Al pointed at the sign behind a row of plastic blue seats. "Uncle Charlie, there's a handicap room if you would feel more comfortable."

Uncle Charlie looked over at the large handicap bathroom door and then down at Albert. "Albert, wait outside for me, okay?"

Albert looked at his dad for confirmation and then back at Charlie. "Sure, Uncle Charlie."

Al watched both of them walk to the other side of the room and then turned in his seat to get a better view of the train schedule board with his right eye. The next time he turned back the handicap door was shut but Albert was nowhere to be seen. Panic set in. Al got up and walked away from their luggage not caring if anything happened to it.

He ran to the handicap bathroom door at the speed of light and began to knock. "Uncle Charlie, you in there?"

A shaky voice answered. "Yes. I'm not done."

Al's body went cold. "Is Albert in there?"

A confused voice responded quietly. "No. He's by the door."

At that moment Al turned to see Albert coming out of the men's room. "Albert, don't wander off like that, ever."

Albert made a face at his dad. "I didn't wander off, I had to pee too. Uncle Charlie was safe in the bathroom and I couldn't wait."

Al thought about the luggage, looked over to see it was where he had left it and yelled at the handicap door. "Uncle Charlie, I found Albert. He'll wait for you."

Uncle Charlie took a second to answer. "Okay."

"I thought you were watching me before, Daddy." Albert gave Al a questioning look and wondered secretly if more of these moments were going to become available to him.

Al turned his head to look straight at Albert. "I had to turn to see the board. Remember how I can only see in the right eye? I turned back and you were gone."

Albert looked at the closed bathroom door. "We can't lose Uncle Charlie, Daddy. He might never find us."

Al smiled down at Albert. "I can't lose you either, Pal."

The announcement for boarding their train to Orlando came in the usual fifteen minutes before departure. "How ya doing Uncle Charlie. The train is boarding."

A soft click came from the door handle and it opened and Uncle Charlie smiled brightly. "Let's go boys. Mickey Mouse is waiting."

Instead of smiling Albert took his dad's hand and the trio walked out of the bathroom area to retrieve their luggage. "Daddy, you got the tickets?"

"Of course, son." Once Albert's head was turned Al felt his pocket to make sure the tickets were there.

Uncle Charlie saw Al's gesture and smiled. "Good thing we got the smart one with us."

Al looked up at Uncle Charlie's innocent face with shock. He would make statement's like and it would bring Al nearly to tears. The family never spoke about Uncle Charlie's mental challenges. He was accepted for who he was and everyone looked out for him.

It was a long twenty-four-hour train ride for the three men. The had coach seats for the ride down and getting to the dining car was a challenge. The rhythm of the train kept Al up most of the night. When they arrived at the Orlando station, Al found a cab to take the three of them to the hotel to wait for Elaine and 'the troops'.

When they all gathered in the lobby later that afternoon the relief on Elaine's face was obvious. "Hi boys!" Albert ran into her open arms. "I missed you, Albert. How did you do with Daddy and Uncle Charlie?"

"Good. When do we got to the castle?" Albert looked around his mother at his brothers each making faces at each other.

Grabbing Albert's hand, Elaine walked toward Al and Uncle Charlie. "Hi Honey." She kissed Al lightly.

They took a few seconds to look at each other. "This is the first time I was away from you since the last hospital stay. I woke up, reached for you and sat up to see Uncle Charlie. I'm scared straight."

Jayne Kelly

Uncle Charlie, oblivious to the travel everyone had endured, walked toward his sister and brother in law, Elaine's grandparents. "Let's go to see Mickey Mouse."

A collective cheer went up from the children.

"That's good enough for me." Mr. Hinds was a man with a formidable physical precense. "Pop, grab Uncle Charlie's bag."

Mr. Hinds' father looked sideways at his son. "Hey, son, you're a lot younger than me or Charlie. You get it."

Mr. Hinds settled in for a light argument. "Pop, I'm keeping track of the kids."

His father gave him a hard look. "Son, you can do both."

Mr. Hinds' mother cut in to disperse the petty argument. "Who is going to make sure we stay together as a group?"

"Al and Elaine." Ronnie answered immediately.

"Will everybody please give it a rest." Al felt like he was listening to his four boys bicker. "Drop your luggage in the rooms and we will take the black van to the park."

"Al?"

"Elaine, please. I'm gonna kill them."

"Al."

The group began to move as one unit toward the open doors of the black van quietly ignoring the luggage piled in the hotel lobby. "Elaine, please. I got this under control. The whole group is quiet. Let's get them in the van and then they can argue all they want on the ride to the park."

"Al."

Albert and Larry jumped into the van as the attendant looked on with surprise. "Elaine, let's get the kids in first."

She laughed and held up her hands. "Enough. That's not our van."

The three eldest of the group began to laugh loudly. "Serves you right for being rude to the older folks. You're supposed to respect us."

Al hung his head a little and tried to tune them out. "This is going to be interesting."

The luggage was dumped in the rooms and the correct rental van was loaded with all seventeen family members together for the first time since they left New Jersey. Al was the last person in the family line for loading. The once daily Florida rain storm had arrived late in the day and was typically short finishing up as Al stood waiting for his turn to enter the van. He looked up as the rain lightened and the sun peaked out from passing clouds. An intense rainbow hung over the hotel and loading area. While everyone else went about their business, used to the common event almost daily accompanying Florida showers, Al stared. He walked away from the van to get a better look. It was the first rainbow he had seen in many years before he lost his sight. Rainbows were something he had taken for granted and never put much thought into. Today, the distinction between the colors was clear and sharp. Mesmorized, he never heard Albert walk up behind him.

"Daddy, come on. We're hungry and I wanna get to the castle." Albert grabbed Al's hand and started to pull.

Al didn't look down at him. "I'll be right there, Son."

Albert stopped tugging and looked up. "It's pretty." Then he turned to look at Al's right eye. "You can see it again tomorrow."

Al laughed. "You sound pretty sure."

Albert looked down at his feet. "Dad, can you be done?"

Al tore his gaze away from the rainbow and stared down at Albert. "Sure. Let's load up."

Al kept his face smooshed against the window on the ride to the restaurant until he saw the rainbow fade. It was late in the day and everyone was hungry so they decided to eat dinner first and then visit the castle that night and see the fireworks.

Larry jumped up and down, glad to be free from the constraints of his travel that day. "Daddy, can we eat fast?"

Al looked up to the sky. "I hope so Larry."

The van pulled up to a simple restaurant for hamburgers or chicken. "Al, this looks like it will do the trick." Uncle

Charlie was reaching for the door handle.

Al held up his hand in front of Uncle Charlie. "You guys stay here. I need to warn the waitress."

Uncle Charlie opened the sliding side door revealing the crowd inside to the occupants of the car next to them. "Uncle Charlie, I said for you to wait."

The driver next to them turned to his wife. "Looks like the circus is in town." The man behind the wheel laughed not caring if Al heard him.

Al stopped and smiled, disarming the man. "You got that right and I'm the ring leader."

Al went into the restaurant first to make sure it wasn't too crowded and to warn the staff. Three hours, four waitresses and eight frustrated kids later, they were entering through the gates of Disney World with full stomachs walking up Main Street U.S.A. Al's gaze went from each of his sons over and over looking at the expressions on their faces. When the full view of the castle was in front of them, the entire group stopped whining from their long travel day and stared.

Camera's were snapping pictures and the boys suffered through poses until they received clearance to go to Space Mountian. Everyone's wishes came true as the family darted from one fantasy ride and entertainment to another until they with the crowd in front of the castle waiting for the nightly fireworks

"Al, this is your first firework show since the accident." Elaine stared at a purple and blue starburst as the crowd reacted.

"No, I've been to many shows, this is just the first one I can see." He held a tired Nick who kept reaching over and poking his cousin Peter dozing on his mother Ronnie's shoulder.

"These moments of firsts for you catch me off guard." A green and blue starburst radiated over their heads.

"It's not like we can make a list. They happen as we're going along in life." The illuminated castle captivated Al.

A boom without an accompanied firework silenced their group. Even little Peter became fully awake. With their heads tilted backward, they stared waiting for the next set of bright colors against the starless black sky. Al blinked hard as he slipped off the glasses he wore. He had forgotten how quick and bright the colors were. His throat constricted and he wondered how he was going get through the event without crying. After a burst of brilliant purple, he smiled. The colors cascading behind and on top of the castle creating the fairy tale destination it was. Elaine snuck a peak at her husband. His gaze did not leave the sky the entire show and he even winced when the booms sounded for duds.

The show ended and the crowd erupted into applause. "That was amazing." Al continued to stare at the castle which had now turned on its night lights.

"Daddy I wanna go on the elephants." Larry pulled on his dad's pant leg.

"Where did you come from. You were supposed to be with grandpop on the bench."

Nick heard his brother and started to squirm. "Yeah, Daddy. Elfans."

He looked over at Elaine and they both shrugged wearily. "We have about an hour before they close the park. We might as well."

They were able to catch the last ride on Captain Nemo's submarine. Uncle Charlie giggled and looked with amazement as the water level rose outside the window.

Bounding down the exit ramp Uncle Charlie laughed with Albert. "I can't believe I went on a real submarine."

Al turned to Elaine. "This might be a very long trip."

The family wanted to make sure they enjoyed every second of their vacation. They were one of the first groups to enter the Magic Kingdom in the mornings and Epcot in the afternoon. When they left Orlando four days later to go to Cape Canaveral the children were ready for a new highlight.

"Where are the rockets?" Albert asked as he and the rest of the boys were in the first van with Elaine, Al, Ronnie, Peter and Uncle Charlie.

Larry reached over and hit his brother. "Dummy."

"Hey!" Al pulled down the visor to yell at the boys. "Knock it off you two. We have another hour of driving before we get to the Space Center."

Elaine rolled down the window for fresh air and recoiled when a wave of suffocating humidity smacked her in the face. "I can't believe we planned all this driving."

"What's this we stuff? You and Mom pulled this together." He flipped the visor back up. "I'm an innocent bystander. I knew it involved too much driving."

Ronnie grumbled from the back seat. "You had your chance to complain before we left Jersey, Al." Ronnie pushed Uncle Charlie off her shoulder for the third time. "Honestly, he was asleep before we got out of the parking lot at Disney."

Uncle Charlie awoke with a start. "I'm tired."

"Sorry, Uncle Charlie. I was just kidding." Ronnie checked Peter next to her on the other side. "Looks like I have two men asleep on either side of me. I hope they stay this way until we get to Kennedy Space Center."

Chris turned around to hang over his seat and stare at her. "Hi Aunt Ronnie."

She winked at him. "Turn around or I'll pinch you."

With that invitation, all four boys turned around and sang in unison. "Hi Aunt Ronnie." Peter woke up with the same start Uncle Charlie did.

"Great. Thanks, you little monsters. This trip will never end." Peter answered her with a whine as he cuddled closer.

The remainder of the car ride to Kennedy Space Center did nothing to quiet the boys. As the car pulled into the parking area, they passed the long drain ditches where alligators sunned themselves on either side of the road.

"Did you see that, Daddy? Did you see it?" Albert was bouncing up and down. "It was huge. I bet it was longer than the slide at the park."

"Everybody stay close when we unload. Do not run off or you will spend the day in the van." Elaine was the first one out. She opened each door and let the occupants out as the second rental van pulled up next to them.

"Does anyone want to warn Kennedy before we walk through the door?" Al reached down and grabbed Nick.

Uncle Charlie stretched his legs. "I think we are going to like the rockets. I can't wait to fly by Mars like at Disney World."

Al exchanged a look with Elaine as he tried not to laugh. "Sorry we didn't get to leave the rocket ship on our Mission to Mars, Uncle Charlie. I know you wanted that."

They moved as one unit as the boys kept their heads tilted back, looking at the iconic building in the distance. "Is that where the rockets are Daddy?"

Al looked at the direction the kids pointed. "Yes."

Chris became very excited. "Can we ride in one?"

Al turned his attention back to keeping the group in one unit. "No."

"Why, Dad?" Chris suddenly looked very bored.

"Because if you went to the moon, Mommy and I would miss you." There were three Plevier boys now calling him Dad instead of Daddy.

The scene entering the Space Center was reminiscent of the Cooperstown trip and Mr. Hinds was quick to point out that fact. "Kids, mind you Mom's, Dad's and us. If you behave there will be souvenirs but nothing if you don't."

The cousins tried to run circles with each other around their respective parents before being grabbed.

"I've heard that line before, Dad. Is this what they looked like in New York State?" Al took the entire scene in at once.

"Yup. Minus one or two of them. Now you can see what you missed." Mr. Hinds had Larry in one hand and Chris in the other.

Al whistled. "What a circus. The guy at the restaurant was right."

"What guy?" Mr. Hinds looked at him with curiosity.

Al realized he never shared that story. "Never mind."

Getting into Kennedy Space Center turned out to be a lot easier than getting out. The children did not want to leave and dragged out the departure by fighting over what sourvneirs they chose.

"Guys, we have to get Al, Uncle Charlie and Albert to the train station by seven. Let's start heading toward the parking lot." Elaine had one eye on her family and one eye on her watch the entire day.

Ronnie yawned and leaned her head back to the descending sun. "Tomorrow is going to be easy. Peter and I will hang at the hotel pool."

Elaine brushed hair out of her face. "I don't have that luxury. I have to get seven of us to the airport by noon. These people have to stay focused."

Al looked at his wife. "Next time you want to go on vacation, better make it two to three weeks on a beach."

She smiled at him conspiratorily. "I've been planning our shore vacation for next summer."

Ronnie lifted Peter from the bench where he sat and let him finish his ice cream on her lap. "Of course, you have."

Elaine was on her last nerve. "What's that supposed to mean? I did all the planning for this. You didn't give me much input." Elaine's tone shushed the whole crew.

"Nothing. We better hurry. We don't want Al, Uncle Charlie and Albert to miss the train." Ronnie shrank a little as she stood unanimously with their group to begin the exit.

Al thought a change of subject was in order. "Kids, what was your favorite part?"

The children answered almost in unison. "The shuttle."

"You didn't mind seeing it from the bus?" For Al staring at the shuttle from the tour bus window was a once in a lifetime experience for him. The threat in the back of his mind that he might not see it again nagged at him.

They moved together as they spoke around each other. "It was great."

Al watched the boys each holding their chosen souvenirs. All teasing aside, he marveled at Elaine's ability to organize the family trips and weekend outings. He knew that although she accepted input from anyone willing to give it, it was she that pulled it all together. After each family event, he tried to take care of her, when time and circumstances permitted.

The group approached both vans. "Alright, I've got Al, the boys, Uncle Charlie, Ronnie and Peter. We'll take the men to the train station and meet you guys at the hotel. The rooms are under my name."

Quick good-byes followed. Elaine sat behind the wheel of her van. "Al, I never told them to hold the double queen room for me and Ronnie. It's going to be musical rooms when I get back."

"Why should tonight be any different than the last four days?" Al looked around at the almost empty parking lot. "That train floor is looking pretty good right now."

Uncle Charlie chimed in from the back. "I don't want to go back to New Jersey yet."

Uncle Charlie's childlike demeanor touched Al. "Sorry, Uncle Charlie. These kids want to get back home."

Elaine began to move out of her parking spot. "Is the parking lot clear behind me, Ronnie? I can't see with this thing." Elaine tried to look out of the side mirrors.

"Wait another minute until our second van is gone. You want to give Dad lots of room with that thing." Ronnie craned her neck to watch the other van go and then returned her attention to a fussing Peter.

"Okay now?" Elaine was getting anxious about the time.

Ronnie pulled Peter onto her lap. "Yeah, go."

Elaine slowly began to back out of her space. She was out about ten feet and turning the wheel when she heard a crunch.

Al knew that sound. "Uh, oh."

A man screaming and yelling obscenities became louder as he approached the driver's side. "What the hell is wrong with you? Can't you ******* see?"

Al calmly snorted. "Now there's an irony."

Al's smart-ass comment didn't help, and the angry

driver stuck his head into the car window. "Is that supposed to be funny? That's a brand, new Mercedes you just backed into. I hope you have enough insurance on this rental you're driving."

Ronnie jumped over the back seat to get to the door. "Uncle Charlie, keep an eye on Peter." She slid open the van door and came around the back.

"What is wrong with…" The irate metro sexual stopped mid-sentence as the blond haired, blue eyed, Ronnie greeted him in a halter top, left over from her wardrobe of the 1970's."

"Excuse us. We have just spent four days in Disney World and we are anxious to get home. Why don't we call the local police or does Kennedy have its own security?" Ronnie knew the answer to this question, but hoped it would put out the fire of this man in front of her.

It did not. "I don't care if you call Mother Teresa. You're paying for this."

The four boys shrank in their seats. "Daddy?"

Al felt himself go tense. "Relax boys. It's just an accident. The police handle these things."

The man put up his hand as Ronnie tried to speak again. "Hey, Buddy. Why aren't you driving this cattle car? Come out here and look at what your wife did."

Al started to lose it. He hadn't been in a fight for over ten years and the last one was a friendly tussle at a construction job. He got out the passenger side and the man nearly knocked Ronnie over to get past her. As the driver came around Al took off his glasses.

The six-foot tall man stopped dead in his tracks. "What the hell is that?" He pointed at Al's right eye.

Al thought fast on his feet. "New robotics by NASA." It was at that moment that security pulled up."

The man continued to stare at Al as the security officer walked around and between them. "What's going on." The security man also stopped and stared at Al. "Are you okay sir?"

Al saw a golden opportunity. "I think so. My kids are A little shook up." He suddenly wished at times like these that he could walk around without his Jobe shirt.

The officer continued to take in the situation and caught a glimpse of Ronnie. "Anybody hurt?"

"No. This is just a little fender bender." Al snorted derisively. "Been through worse."

The two men were silent as Ronnie walked around carefully waiting for her opportunity. "Al, are you okay?"

The security officer turned around and gave her the once over. "Miss, maybe you should go back in the van."

Ronnie knew when she had the upper hand. "I'm concerned about my brother-in-law. We have to get him and our elderly Uncle on a train back to New Jersey. It takes a while to get him situated before we can leave." Ronnie got through making her statement with a straight face and the sweetest voice she could muster.

Al watched his sister-in-law closely and decided in the future he would double check any important information she had. "Officer, we apologize for the inconvenience." Elaine handed Al the rental paperwork through the passenger window.

Al passed the papers to the security officer. "Here, this should be everything you need." The officer barely looked at the paperwork before handing it back.

He turned to the irate man. "First, back that Mercedes up and get it off the van bumper." He looked around at the people watching the interchange. "There's an empty spot to back it into over there." He pointed several slots down.

The man looked dejectedly down the parking lot. "That's where I came from."

The security officer pumped his chest out. "Good, then you're familiar with it."

The man walked away with his head down.

Al jumped in while the man was out of ear shot. "Officer, we accept responsibility."

The security officer cut him off. "Relax." He looked over at a smiling Ronnie. "This is just a fender bender. I'm sure he has insurance. I have your plate and the rental company." He peaked in at the four small faces now glued to the window. "Maybe you should get to the train station. I got this. No need to call in the local Police."

Al was surprised. "Thank you. If you could guide my wife the rest of the way out of the parking space, we would really appreciate it."

The man held up both hands and smiled. "No problem." Al jumped in the van and they waited for Ronnie.

When she came in through the sliding door she was smiling and had a piece of paper folded. "Let's go."

Elaine started the van again. "Am I clear?" All the occupants including the little boys ducked their heads down. "Well?"

Ronnie looked up and waved to the security officer. "Yeah, you're clear."

They were four miles down State Highway 3 before anyone dared to laugh. "Man, I feel bad for the security guy. He's going to spend the next hour listening to that guy yell." Al leaned back in the seat and released the tension he felt.

Ronnie spoke up from the back. "Somehow I don't think he'll put up with that."

Uncle Charlie looked over at her. "Was that man nice to you, Ronnie?"

"Yes." She unfolded the paper and looked at the phone number and name written on it.

Elaine caught a glimpse of her sister in the rear, view mirror. "I'm sure we'll be down here next year." All five boys cheered.

Al held up his hands. "Let me recover from this trip first." He stared out the window at the passing palm trees.

The green of the Florida landscape was stunning. It was the first thing he noticed when they arrived at the train station in Orlando five days ago. As he watched it flash by his window today he observed every aspect. The highway was two lanes with businesses and then houses sprinkled in. He watched children playing in the front yards and thought about their lives.

"You got very quiet." Elaine caught a glimpse of him as she prepared to turn toward AIA.

"Just taking in the scenery." A pelican flew in front of the car. "You don't see that every day." He was not only enjoying the scenery but trying to tune out the mounting cacophony developing in the back of the van.

Elaine watched the bird disappear into the tree line. "That bird is out of his element a little."

Al made a face. "Florida?"

She shook her head. "No, the highway."

"It was good to see a bird like that. I don't think I've ever seen a pelican that wasn't on television or at a zoo." He thought about the alligators at Kennedy Space Center and a greater appreciation for the trip welled up inside him. "I realize I've been teasing you quite a bit about your trip planning but I need to tell you how much this trip meant to me." He turned, unbelted, in his seat. "Hey, keep it down to a dull roar back there."

"I know, Sweetheart." Elaine was aware of how boring Al had found the previous family road trips without sight.

"I could sit and watch the scenery go by for hours without saying a word." He turned again in his seat as the collective noise grew louder. "I said to pipe down a little. Anybody listening?"

"Me." Peter chimed in from the back.

The entire van burst out laughing. "At least someone respects me back there."

"He's still little." Ronnie smirked at Uncle Charlie.

"Al, I want to eat as soon as we get on the train." Uncle Charlie's world was singular in nature. "I like that dining car."

Al leaned back in his seat, watching the scenery. He Closed his eyes for a moment and then quickly reopened them.

He did not want to miss a thing.

Chapter XXV: Breaks

"And then we rode the Haunted House ride, and then we rode the elephants, and then we got locked in the stockade, and then we ate hot dogs, and then we walked right in the middle of the castle, and then we went to the island, and then we fed squirrels, and then we went swimming, and then we saw lots and lots of fireworks. Right Daddy?" Larry was wired from an afternoon of soda and boardwalk ice cream.

Rose Plevier sat next to Larry and listened with the attentiveness of a practiced Grandmom. "That sounds like a wonderful vacation. What is Mickey Mouse like in person?"

"Grandmom, he was real nice. He said hi to everybody. Even the big people." Larry sucked drips of ice cream off his fingers and hands.

"Did Daddy go on all the rides with you?" Rose looked over at her son. It never ceased to thrill her when he met her gaze.

"Yup." Larry laughed. "He screamed on Space Mountain. I didn't. It was short. Not too scary."

"Did Mommy like it too?" Rose took small scoops from her cup of soft ice cream.

"Yup." Larry was getting bored and at the mention of his mom, he looked toward the beach where Elaine sat with his brothers and began to eat in a hurry.

Al noticed lately that his mom was slowing down. "Mom, is your ice cream alright?"

She swallowed slowly. "Yes. It's delicious." Rose knew her son had noticed her digestive tentativeness. "I've been having some stomach issues since June. I have an appointment in October."

"You're the one who is always after me to take care of myself and not ignore anything. Don't you think it would be better if you went sooner?" Al wiped Larry's face.

Rose looked at her son with the eyes of a devoted mother. "I'm going to be fine. This is part of the aging process whether I like it or not." She took another taste of her ice cream before speaking. "You and Elaine will have each other to hold onto as you age into the sunset like I'm doing."

The full smile that Rose gave to Al took him by surprise. He couldn't remember the last time he saw her smile like that and was grateful he could see it. "We're here for you, Mom. Fenna and I will never let you be left alone."

Her full smile faded a bit. "I know that."

"I wanna go to the water with Mommy and the boys." Larry sucked the residue of his ice cream off his fingers.

"Let's go then." Rose stood up. "You have to walk with Daddy and me."

Larry stopped short from his attempt at running. "Are you going swimming Grandmom?"

"No, Honey. Grandmom likes to sit on the beach and watch." They reached the sand and Rose walked more carefully than she did last summer. "It was really nice of your other grandmom to rent the summer house for these last couple weeks of summer."

"Grandmoms are nice." Larry spotted Elaine and the boys among the sea of umbrellas. "Daddy, can I run?"

"No. You just finished your ice cream. Take it easy." Secretly Al had a nagging feeling this might be the last summer his mom would come to the beach and he wanted Larry to remember the walk with the sand between their toes.

"Let him go, son. She's right in front of us." Rose waved a hand at Elaine who waved back.

Larry took off at his grandmom's encouragement and Al acknowledged her generosity of spirit. "Mom, I'm really glad you came with us to Point Pleasant. This is a much more relaxing vacation than Disney. That was insane."

Al couldn't help but feel small pangs of guilt. He hadn't seen his mother since they had gotten back from Disney in June and the first thing he noticed when they picked her up were the deepening lines on her face. As they walked off the boardwalk he found himself following the handrail with his right hand. He couldn't break the habit of always guiding himself by touching his boundaries.

"The summer sun and the soft wind of the Jersey Shore are what vacation is to me." She looked at the cloudless sky. "I always wished your dad and I had come down to the beach on the train with you kids. Did I ever tell you that?" Rose became melancholy for a moment as she looked at the ocean.

"I don't think so. Did Grandmom Padula ever come down here?" The memory of the five-foot tall, Italian spit fire with a gold tooth and a hot temper stood in front of him.

Rose gave Al her wide smile one more time. "No. Back then if you didn't have much money, you stuck to your neighborhood. That's how I met Dad."

Al was thoughtful. "You met when you were out with the girls, right?"

Her smile remained. "You have your secrets, your dad and I had ours." She looked at her son. "I knew most of your secrets from childhood even though you thought I didn't." He gave her a wide eye look. "I heard from our neighbors in Patterson you used to push your bike to the arcade after we told you not to ride down there." They both smiled together. "You were independent, but I made sure you were looked after when I was at work besides the attention and guidance of Grandmom Padula. We had good neighbors. You weren't entirely a latchkey kid. And that is my secret."

"Mom, I never doubted that I was loved." He felt at this

moment it was very important for her to know he had no regrets about his life.

"I hope not. It was tough for us, but I'd like to think that was part of what gave you the strength you needed these last eight years."

"It was." He answered her immediately.

"The times you walked down to my house on Shore Road after the corneal transplant meant the world to me. Elaine and I would joke that she needed a break. I'm not sure who was helping who." She paused to catch her breath as they walked across the sand. "I planned out what kind of snacks I would have for you. Men always like food. In some way, I felt like I was waiting for you to come home from school, as strange as that sounds. It felt as if I was getting back what was taken away from me." Rose stopped to look at him fully. "Albert, I'm not bitter about your Dad's death at such a young age. Please don't misunderstand. I went to work and that is the way God carried us. I also feel he gave me time with you as an adult that I didn't have when you were a little boy. That is his grace. He always gives us a second chance. It gave me as much peace for you to have your sight back after the corneal transplant as it does now."

They reached the blanket and Elaine looked up. "What a day. Mom, I'm so glad you came down. We're playing pinochle tonight. I've got a nice bottle of wine."

"That sounds perfect. Helen and I will catch up. When will they be getting here?"

"They should be waiting for us at the house. Dad had a few things to check at their house and I think they were picking up subs for dinner." Elaine saw a calm look on Rose' face she hadn't noticed earlier. "Mom, is there anything you would like to do this weekend?"

"I'm doing it already. Just being here, smelling the salt air and feeling the sand between my toes is all I want." The boys began to throw sand at each other and accidentally connected with their grandmother.

Al felt a protectiveness for his mother that he could not explain when he saw that. "Knock it off. Get your buckets and

I'll help you build sand forts." Al started to pull off the long sleeve shirt covering his Jobe shirt out of habit and the overheating.

"Al, you should stay under the umbrella." Elaine looked nervously at him.

"Sweetheart, I'm fine." He started to rip open the Velcro fasteners of the Jobe shirt. "Dr. Grove said it would be okay occasionally to take the shirt off now. It's been seven years." He quickly grabbed one of the larger buckets and headed to the water. "Boys move the operation closer to the water. The tide is going out. This is going to be a fort to end all forts."

"Mommy, did you bring the camera?" Larry looked at her pleadingly.

"Yes, I'll get a shot of your fort for Chris's show and tell at school. Make it a big one." She relaxed on the sand as she watched Al working with the boys.

Chris did not have his show and tell time at class until a week before Halloween. Two days before that he had brought the notice home to Elaine completely forgetting about the sand fort he and his brothers had built several months earlier.

He sat at the kitchen table contemplating his choice. "I'll bring the dead butterfly from my room."

Elaine gave him a strange look. "Where is the dead butterfly in your room?"

"On my window sill," he said matter of factly. "Wanna see?"

Elaine shook her head. "Later. What about the pictures of the sand fort? Remember? You could bring the buckets and shovels you used also."

Chris's eyes lit up. "Oh, Mommy. Nobody ever brought that before. It was so big. I told Mikey about it at cub scouts and he didn't believe me. Wait till he sees the pictures."

Elaine was thoughtful and looked around the room. "You have to do something with the pictures. How about if I help you paste pictures from our vacation on a poster board? Your teacher will really like that."

Chris knew there was going to be work involved. "Why can't I just bring the pictures?"

"I think your teacher will give you extra credit if you do more. Wouldn't you like to get plus marks next to your grades?"

"No." Larry dropped his chin to his chest.

Elaine started to move about and not give him a chance to switch topics. "This will be fun. Go get the paste from the craft cabinet. I'll get the pictures."

Chris hung his head down as he walked away. "Mommy, my butterfly would be easier."

"Easier isn't better. Hurry up. I want all you guys to try on your Halloween costumes." She put aside the pile of what looked like loose fabric.

At the mention of Halloween Chris did as he was told and brought the paste Elaine asked for. "Here Mommy."

Elaine pulled a poster sheet from her ready supply and laid everything on the dining room table. "Look at these pictures, Chris. That is a huge sand fort you build with Daddy." The four, foot walls of the fort were impressive even to Elaine.

"Mommy look. Grandmom was the same size as the fort." Chris giggled at the size of his Grandmom Plevier.

Elaine looked at the image of Al's mother. From that angle, she looked about the same height as the wall. "The picture does make it look that way but Grandmom is bigger than your wall."

"Doesn't look like it." Larry grabbed the picture, smeared paste on the back and slapped in onto the poster board.

Elaine looked carefully at Rose' image. The picture was taken two months ago, and already she appeared to age considerably. She had stoically accepted the terminal diagnosis in September. Elaine wondered if Rose had felt there was something wrong before she made the appointment. It was the first time she had agreed to vacation with Elaine's family at the shore despite the invitations from Mr. and Mrs. Hinds over the years. Rose had always told Elaine and Al that this was time for that side of the family and she took the opportunity to spend time with Fenna. This was the first summer she had agreed without hesitation.

Chris' laughter brought Elaine out of her thoughts. "Mommy, look at Nicky. You can see his eyeballs behind the drawbridge."

"You could have held off all your enemies with that fort." Al looked like her fifth child in the pictures.

Chris slapped glue on another picture. "Daddy's a good builder."

"Yes." She stared at her husbands scarred chest in one of the shots after he had taken off the Jobe shirt against her protests, and tucked that picture back into its envelope.

"Can we show him the pictures?" Chris wanted an excuse to be finished with the work involved.

Elaine watched Chris' face closely. "He's at the hospital with Grandmom. We'll show him when he comes home."

Larry slapped another paste laden picture on the poster. "I bet he don't even remember this fort. It'll surprise him."

They had not told the children about the gravity of Rose' illness. The boys were too young to understand. She thought for a moment about how much the poster would mean to Rose and Al. "It will be a great surprise."

"When's Daddy coming home?" Chris inadvertently got glue on the front of a picture and gave Elaine a scowl.

"Tonight. He may be home after you go to bed. Grandmom is coming home to Aunt Fenna's tomorrow." She gently removed the picture from Chris' fingertips without destroying the image.

Chris slapped the last picture onto the board. "Can we see our costumes?"

For the moment, Elaine was grateful the children did not understand and were caught up in their own activities. "Yes, call your brothers."

Chris didn't move from his spot and screamed as loud as he could. "Albert, Nick, Larry! Come down. We got costumes!"

Rose had always been a big help to Elaine at Halloween. She had an old friend who worked in the prop department at a theatre. The two women had met while Rose was a seemstress after her husband died and before she had gone to school to be a bookkeeper. Last week before she came into the hospital for her procedure, Rose has asked her friend to bring Al something scary. Yesterday when she visited, she left a mask with Rose. Al sat with his mother that afternoon in her hospital room admiring the partial wolfman mask, wig and makeup.

"Mom, this is great. Thank Mrs. Shultz for me." He held the mask up to the light streaming through the window.

She smiled weakly at him. "I'm glad you like it."

Al stopped was he was doing and looked at her face. "They're excited to see you tomorrow at Fenna's." Concern flooded through him. "Are you sure you have the energy?"

She nodded. "I want to enjoy my time left. The children bring me so much joy."

A nurse came in. "Mr. Plevier, it might be a good idea to let your mother rest. She has a big day tomorrow."

Al dutifully started to rise. "Mom, I'll see you tomorrow."

The simple statement was very loaded with meaning. "Yes. Tomorrow."

Al left the hospital and caught a bus home without calling Elaine. He decided to walk to their house from the bus stop a mile away instead of having Elaine pick him up. The time alone allowed him to gather his thoughts. When he was approaching their driveway, he pulled the mask out of the bag and slipped it over his head. He crouched as he approached the back door and then threw it open in one movement.

Elaine had just pushed aside the poster aside she and Chris had been working on and began to lift the costumes as the kitchen door opened. "GRRRRRRR!"

Elaine screamed at the top of her lungs as Chris ducked under a bar stool giggling. "Al! I'm going to kill you." The dogs came running from the master bedroom on the attack. Elaine yelled to be heard. "You better get that thing off."

He pulled off the wolfman head and wiped the sweat off his forehead. "Isn't this great. Mrs. Schultz gave it to Mom. I have a wig and makeup too." The dogs stopped in their tracks still barking.

"Easy pups. It's your Dad. Whoa there." Al reached down to pet the basset hound. The dog backed away and peed all over the floor.

The boys came running into the room and stared at the mask in his hand. "Wow! Dad that is cool." Albert was very impressed. "I wanna be wolfman next year."

"Maybe. What are you this year?" Al realized he had been consumed with his mom's illness over the last several weeks he hadn't kept track of the things important to the boys.

Today at the hospital Rose asked him to not worry about her and be with his family. He looked at the mess the dog left behind as they ran and for the first time, did not mind cleaning it up.

Albert pointed to the costume Elaine was putting the finishing touches on. "I'm a pirate. Look."

Chris popped up from under the stool. "Daddy, I'm a cowboy."

Nick and Larry pulled their costumes of Batman and Robin from the bag at Elaine's feet. "Wow."

"I'm feeling like I need to wear this Wolfman costume over to the Ridgeview Terrace neighborhood." The boys laughed uncontrollably as they put on their costumes and watched their dad clean up the dog's mess.

"Al, they'll shoot you. Don't be stupid." She watched the two dogs cowering behind the children. "Your own dogs wanted to bite you before you took the mask off."

"Fine." He finished cleaning the mess and carried his head for the boys to play with. He noticed the poster on the table. "What's this?"

"Show and tell for Chris. Remember the sand fort from the shore vacation?"

Al looked over the pictures. He too had realized how frail his mother had become over the last several months.

354

"She's fading fast, Elaine. We're bringing her home to Fenna's tomorrow. Do you want to prepare the boys for her appearance when we go over to trick or treat?"

Elaine watched the four boys trying on their costumes and oblivious to the conversation their parents were having. "No. I think they will be too caught up in the candy to take notice. Let the visit unfold naturally. I want Rose to enjoy them."

Al swallowed past the lump in his throat to speak. "I'm going in my wolfman suit. What are you gonna be this year?"

"A nurse who wants to go back to teaching." She lifted the poster.

He nodded with encouragement. "Go for it. Keep sending out your resume. You're qualified for both positions. You'll make the transition smoothly." He watched the children's play erupt further into bedlam. "I can't believe you don't want to escape this every day."

She watched Albert and Larry attack each other and start to wrestle on the floor. "I live for this."

"Mom said the same thing when I asked her if she would prefer to stay in the hospital. She told me if she had a choice, the last sound she would hear as she left the world would be the laughter of the grandchildren." He had no intention of telling Elaine that conversation and couldn't believe it came automatically from him.

She could see the love for his mother he always tried to hide behind the tough façade. "Al, she will have that even if it's a memory she hears."

Chris came running breathless. "Our costumes are way better than anybodies."

Al was grateful for the change of conversation. "Your cousins won't agree with you. Mine is the best. I look real." He growled for affect.

The wolfman costume became a staple in the house before and after Halloween. Each boy wore it at one point or another. Halloween night there were various food crumbs, little tears and many scents of little boys imbedded into its fabric.

After canvassing their own neighborhood during Trick or Treating, the family landed at Fenna's house for an end of evening party in full regalia. He wanted to be the one to ring the bell.

"Grrrrr." He stood in front of her, claws out, fully posed,

"Hi Al." The boys and Elaine squeezed past him into the house. Fully deflated he turned to walk down the street.

Fenna looked at him strangely. "Where are you going?"

"I'll be back." He pulled the mask tight over his head and disappeared into the dark.

Carefully he went up to the neighbor next door that they knew very well. The young divorcee was sitting at her kitchen table when Al tapped on the window. She screamed and ran into the living room for her oldest son. Afraid he was about to get jumped, Al ran for the woods. When he came out the other side he saw his brother-in-law in the car. He flagged him down.

"Hey, Al." Bob looked worn out from the family events.

Al stood before him in an overstuffed shirt, pants and the wolfman costume. "How did you know it was me?"

Bob rolled his eyes. "C'mon."

The men went back to the house to let the kids unwind and when it was apparent that the night was too much for Rose, Al and Elaine took the boys home. "Elaine, I'll be in after a few more scares." He jumped out of their car before she could protest and before the boys would beg to join in.

"Please don't get shot." She watched Al run into the darkness before the boys ran into the house as a pack already trying to negotiate candy trades.

Al took off in the direction of the road. Audobon Parkway had a grass median between the opposing traffic lanes. The upperclass neighborhood was manicured but friendly and the home owners took pride in it's appearance. A car approached slowly, creeping along as it allowed the mini passengers inside to trick or treat. Al jumped on the hood the minute the kids were clear.

"Grrrrr!"

The driver threw the car in reverse. Al rolled off the hood and ran into the woods behind a neighbor's house to hide. When he was sure it was safe he found his way home and sat on the front porch, trying to look like a stuffed prop. A kid about twelve approached alone.

"Grrrr!" Al jumped up and watched horrified as the kid screamed, dropped his bag and never looked back. "Grrrr!" He gave another growl before walking over to pick up his spoils. Al lifted up his mask and stuffed his pockets with the large sized candy bars, the only ones he could see in the dim light. He left the bag and its remnants on the driveway knowing the kid would come back and went inside.

Elaine looked at him with a weird expression. "You went trick or treating alone?"

He stopped. "Sort of. Great costume, huh?"

She shook her head. "Where did you get that candy?"

"Not important." He pulled out the last bar and started to strip off the costume quickly. "We're done trick or treating with the boys, right?" Al turned to Elaine with a bit of fear.

"Yes. What did you do?" Shame clouded her face.

"Nothin'." He needed a distraction. "Hey kids I got you some more candy."

The five kids, including two-year-old Peter came running into the room. Peter was smaller than them, but he learned quickly that wherever the group went, fun things followed.

Nicky turned to give Peter a bar and Ronnie stopped him. "No Nicky. Thank you but he's still too little for that." Peter answered his mother's direction with a scream. "Fine, let him hold it."

Elaine watched Al strip to his street clothes. "Did you take that from kids?"

Al felt like he was twelve after he and his 'gang' had wrestled bags of candy from straggling trick or treaters in Patterson. "No."

She shook her head slowly. "I hope we don't have any angry parents coming to the door. This is suburbia not the mean streeets of Paterson.

Al looked over at the front door and then balled his costume up and shoved it into a paper grocery bag. "I'm nothing if not entertaining."

Elaine smiled at him. "Mom rallied today when she got home to Fenna's."

The doctor's diagnoses gave Rose only another month from the day she left the hospital. Al and Fenna felt she would try to hold on through Christmas and they were right. It was difficult for her as the cancer took control, but her strength and spirit carried her as she enjoyed her children, their spouses and her six grandchildren. She dressed for Christmas day, held at Elaine and Al's, and sat near the tree quiet. Her illness was the unspoken elephant in the room as the family determined that she would have a wonderful holiday.

"Mom, do you want wine?" Al leaned close to his mother and met her expression.

She was tired. "I better not. I'm sleepy. Do you have regular coffee to perk me up?"

"Absolutely. It'll take me a minute to brew. Elaine and I have become permanent tea drinkers." Al left hastily as Elaine came by with food.

"Mom, try these little mini quiches' that my mom picked up at Shop Rite. I was going to tell you she made them, but I knew you wouldn't believe that." Elaine held out the tray and caught her mother watching at a distance with a sad look in her eyes.

Rose took one mini quiche, the only thing she had eaten that afternoon. "Thank you."

Helen Hinds came over to sit with her friend. "What do you think Rose? They were only $5.99 for a box of twenty-four."

Rose took a bite. "Delicious. You couldn't have baked better yourself."

Elaine continued the rounds and left the two women alone. Rose was quiet for a moment as she sat with her friend watching the holiday activity. "Everyone will be alright when I'm gone. It's okay for me to leave." The children were playing noisily and just beginning to build to the level of toy overload that leads to fights.

Helen Hinds watched Elaine drop the tray on the table and pull two of the boys apart. "Elaine and Al have their lives under control, no matter what the future brings. They've proven that to you. The tragedy and their response to it as a couple stands as testimony to the strength of their marriage, love for each other and faith in God." Helen took her friend's small, frail hand into both of hers. "He is strong because you raised him. He is strong because of his family roots. He is good, kind, loving and wiser because of what he has endured and conquered."

Rose was humbled by the response of her friend. She knew Helen must have been scared at what her daughter faced in the waiting room of Overlook Hospital on October 1, 1974. Rose never heard Helen utter words of bitterness toward Al for the different life her daughter would now have to live.

"Helen, thank you for embracing my son as one of your own. I know he is and has always been loved and accepted. The first time I met Elaine when they started dating in Junior High, I thought she was the sweetest girl. A sense of peace came over me as I watched Al and your husband interact. Larry stepped right in to fill the shoes of a father that were empty for so long in Albert's life."

Helen took notice of Rose' latest transition of referring to Al as Albert, something she never heard her do over the years. "Al is the son my husband never had. When the girls were growing up he would sneak out on a Friday night to get away from all the females in the house." The two women laughed together. "He couldn't bond with Ronnie's husband no matter how hard he tried. With Al, it was instantaneous."

Fenna came up to the women. "Girls, can I get you anything?"

Rose smiled at her daughter. "Everyone keeps asking me if they can get me anything. The only thing I want today is to see the love and joy in my family. I have that." Her face was relaxed despite the pain she was in.

Nick came over and grabbed two handfuls of cookies off the tray on the coffee table in front of the women. "Hi Grandmoms." He smiled at them before he ran off.

The two women looked at each. "Blessings in pint sized packages," was the only thought that came to Rose.

Al came back with a cup of coffee. "Here you go, Mom." He stared at the Christmas tree. "I'll never take the sight of the twinkling lights for granted."

Rose smiled at her only son. "It means more to you than it does for some. I wish everyone could experience Christmas the way you do. Your face is so animated as you watch the children." They both looked at the children getting louder.

"They really keep us busy. I wouldn't trade a second of it." He never mentioned to his mother the various and numerous ongoing events with the boys that required behavior modification therapy for them by their parents. Based on his own childhood he assumed she probably knew.

"How long did it take them to open their presents this morning?" Rose asked.

"Four minutes. One minute per kid. Paper was flying, the boys were yelling, the dogs were barking. It was crazy. Elaine took a ton of pictures, but I wish I had it on video. We need to pick up one of the new cameras I saw at the electronic store." He shook his head at the crazy joy of their sunrise Christmas. They were still putting toys together at midnight Christmas Eve, but they didn't mind.

The blessing of the children eased Rose into her passing that January. Both Al and Fenna were at her side as she was released from the pain that had become her final days. The last wordless gaze Al exchanged with Rose convinced him of the peace his regained sight gave her. It was the second chance the Lord gives all of us that she spoke of. She could leave this world meeting the gaze of both her children.

Chapter XXVI: Fork in the Road

Saying goodbye to Rose required personal time granted by the hospital where Elaine worked and the construction company where Al was considered a permanent employee. The construction business had been steady since July, but Al had stayed on with the agreement that he have personal time last fall and into the beginning of the new year. He did not want to regret the opportunities to be with his Mom in her final days. Both he and Elaine returned to working full time in February. They felt once again like a two, career family balancing work around the activities of four boys.

This year would be Albert's admission to the PAL league. He was turning ten over the summer, but Al was able to sign him up for the spring season. Volunteering as an assistant coach brought a joy and sense of pride to Al as he accomplished the dream he thought he would have to relinquish with his sight.

April brought the first practice session. "Albert, come on son. We're going to be late." He carried over his shoulder a bag of bats and balls to be loaded into the car.

Albert came running out the front door nearly knocking over his dad. "Dad, I want the other coach to talk to me. The guys will think you're playing favorites if you tell me how to

361

hit."

Al was way ahead of him. "I spoke to Mr. Harritman. He and I both agree to give everybody the same instruction time. He has a boy on the team too."

Albert looked at him suspiciously. "Yeah, but he's older than me."

"Just relax. We'll do this one practice at a time." Al dumped the two bags he held into the open trunk of his father-in-laws car and yelled to Elaine who was out back with the three other boys. "Elaine, we're leaving."

She came around the front of the house. "You boys have fun."

They pulled away with a sullen Albert in the back. "Would you prefer I not coach next season?"

Albert shrugged his shoulders and Mr. Hinds jumped in. "You're lucky to have Dad and me. We can teach you based on how we played ball and learned from our mistakes."

Albert's head jumped up. "Dad, you told mommy that people don't learn from their mistakes or people would be perfect."

Al looked out the window trying to find leverage and then gave up. "Albert, enough. You're a lucky little boy to have a Dad and a Grandpop that want to be with you and teach you baseball. We like you. It's that simple."

He eyed his father suspiciously again. "Don't you love me anymore?"

Now Al turned around. "Of course, we love you. Enough. We are going to have a good time this season and your going to continue to get better and better at hitting." Al thought of one last reminder for Albert. "If you want the boys to treat you fairly make sure you call me Coach from the minute we step out of the car. That's a rule. I'm coach on the field and I'm not Dad again until we get back in the car to come home. Understood?"

"Okay." He thought this over as he stared at Al. "Are

we getting ice cream after practice?"

"Sure."

Mr. Hinds chimed in. "Hey, Coach. Did you bring enough cash to buy ice cream for the whole team? I think you forgot about that."

"You're right I did and no I didn't." Al shook his head. "See Albert, not perfect."

Albert gave a haughty knowing look and then stared out the window. "Good thing I remembered for you. You need my help Dad."

The fact that Albert called him Dad and not Daddy was not lost on Al. He felt a twinge in his stomach as he noted how full the two sentences Albert just spoke were. Al knew he was still a boy, who needed his help, but he was growing up. Day by day he got a little taller, a little wiser, a little faster and he would someday be a man with sons of his own. The always present nagging voice in the back of his subconscious hoped silently that he would be able to see these grandchildren.

"Albert, pay attention to Grandpop and me. Teach your brothers like we coach you." He hoped Albert would enjoy teaching younger boys.

Albert made an angry face. "I don't wanna teach those guys no more. They're a real pain. You do it Dad."

Al gave up for the moment. Talk was cheap and Albert would learn automatically from them without even knowing. He would pass this down to his kids. Sitting there on the way to coach, Al reminded himself that the platitude was right: 'Whatever will be will be'.

Al threw himself into coaching that spring. The last game of the season found the little league team at five wins and six losses. They hoped to win the last game, but so did the opponents. As a coach Al did not care about wins and loses. His main objective was to create an interest in each child and a skill set that would carry them to their age appropriate next baseball level. He stood before the preteen group prepared to make his final speech of the season.

"You boys did well this year and learned quite a bit. I'm looking forward to coaching next year. Some of you might be on my team again. Have fun today!"

"Thanks coach Plevier, thanks coach Harritman," the boys chanted together.

Al stood next to first plate during the third inning. "Paulie, you can steal second if you want to give it a try. Dennis is up to bat and he'll swing and miss on the first pitch. Ready, now. Go ahead." Al watched the ten-year-old go for his first steal and make it.

The young boy waved to Al from second base. He was surprised at how much that wave meant to him. Seeing the look of surprise and confidence on the face of a child that was not his own gave him a feeling of paying forward the second chance he was given at life. Albert talked continuously on the ride home that afternoon. Initially Al thought it was because of the fun he had that season, but if he was honest he began to think Albert was happy because he was free from both school and baseball for the summer.

Al decided to reduce his workload over the summer of 1983 and spend more time with the family. He was not sure why he made such a quick and decisive response to the reaction Albert had that day. The fact that Nicky would be starting PreK in the fall, weighed in on his reasons. He was becoming keenly aware that childhood is so brief for both parents and children and the time he lived without sight he could not replace.

Elaine had planned four weekend trips and a week at the shore. "Honey, I would really like to go back to Cooperstown this summer. I want to see what I missed."

"Let's work it in. I'm sure the boys would want to go back. Albert has a better appreciation for baseball and it will be new to Nick." She relaxed against the poolside chaise lounge in their backyard.

"It's seems almost ludicrous to go away when we have a great pool that half the neighborhood enjoys with our kids."

In front of them a group of ten children splashed happily. "I feel guilty," said Al.

"You won't feel guilty in August when the boys are complaining they're bored. It's just the way kids are." It was a perfect June day and not yet too hot. "I'm lucky the hospital lets me take time off in the summer. It's a good career that allows the flexibility if you have a family and a spouse with a second income."

"The boys are only going to be this age once. Unless you're planning on having more." Al looked at her sideways.

Elaine held her ice tea in mid air. "Not a chance. I love my kids but I'm done."

"Just testing you." The house phone could be heard ringing in the distance. "I feel like I'm running numbers. That phone never stops ringing." He got up quickly. "Is the answering machine on if I miss it?"

She nodded. "It's never off. That was the best Christmas present Mom and Dad ever gave us."

He returned shortly. "I'm going to shoot telemarketers."

She snickered at him. "Shoe is on the other foot now. How does it feel?"

"I have to get used to letting the machine pick up all calls. They never leave messages and after a while they take you off the list, like I did." He sat down in the same chair under the umbrella scratching at his chest. "I wonder some days if I'll ever be completely free of my Jobe shirt."

She looked over at him. "You've come so far. It's amazing."

"We've come so far. I'd have given up immediately if I didn't have you." He clinked his glass to hers.

Elaine dropped the magazine she was leafing through. "Do you really believe that?"

"Yes. I came back for us." He stared at the cloudless sky, always drawn the meanings nature offered. "You and our family was always the reason.

"Came back? You mean the vision? Do you believe

you had a choice or was the choice made for you?" She sat up and clutched her knees.

"Choice and free will is what we come back for and because of. We learn and grow. The Lord showed me a better place, but I had work to do here. It's like a parent that tells you to finish your greens before you get dessert."

She raised her eyebrows in surprise. "Nice analogy."

"Sorry. It was told so lovingly to me in the vision I had. 'Your job isn't finished.' I can still see and hear that voice. It felt like a melody being played over my body. I could see, hear and feel when I stood next to that man. I wasn't in pain, but my body was tired. Physically tired. It's hard to explain. Part of me wanted to push open the gates that were in front of me, but there was a 'knowing' in me that said I couldn't. It came from a feeling of sadness that 'strings would be cut forever'. I wanted to touch the doors, just to try. It was so beautiful, but when I looked at the man with me there was this incredible pull away from the gate. The pull was a loving pull. Happiness. Joy. Belonging. The same feeling on the first day of spring. I can only say that I ran toward the feeling, metaphorically." He stared off beyond the tree line of their property.

"Are you sorry you came back? You went through hell physically and emotionally." She knew he would tell her the truth. That was their binding tie. No matter what the answer, they would tell each other the truth.

"No. I understand that pull. Losing you for all eternity would have been Hell. We were just beginning. I had to correct the path I was on." He met her gaze, hard. "What I'm about to say to you I've never said before. I hope you can take it." Now he had her undivided attention. The boys were yelling to their parents to settle a dispute and Al and Elaine ignored them. "I'm glad some days that the accident happened. I wasn't while I was going through the pain of recovery, of course, because a mind and body can only handle so much at once. It's a long process."

Elaine was stunned. "How can you say that?"

"Retrospection. I was full of myself on a fast track to big money and ego to match. Don't get me wrong, I would give my right arm to have sight in both eyes, but I accept this miracle I have now." He stared at her blank look.

Elaine was sorting through how she wanted to respond. "I don't ask God why this happened. I did immediately after the accident when I was numb, but then I was grateful he allowed you to live." She swallowed and looked at the boys. "I can't honestly tell you I'm glad it happened. I don't believe I will ever do that, but I am glad to have you and I don't question why it happened. It's easy to do that now that you are whole and with us."

Albert came stomping up to their chairs, dripping and angry. "How come you didn't answer, Mom? Larry is being a brat."

"Albert, calm down. Your Dad and I were talking about something important." She looked how Albert had grown in the last several months.

"This is important." From behind Albert a war had erupted. "See. The neighborhood kids are getting mad too."

Al got up from his chair. Elaine thought he was going to start yelling at the kids. In an instant, he dove into the pool's deep end, fully clothed. The kids went crazy. All she could see was water, arms, legs, plastic water guns as she listened to the happy screams and chaos. Al was lost among the kids.

The magical summer Elaine and Al had proposed had come to fruition as one day piled on top of another. They never were able to squeeze in a visit to Cooperstown and instead put it on the calendar for the summer of 1984.

Nick jumped on the school bus that September. He had been watching his brothers leave him every morning for four years and was excited to find out why preschool was so great.

"Daddy, I'm sitting in the front seat. Mommy said so. The bus driver lets the new guys."

"You mean the little guys." Albert sneered over his cereal bowl.

"I'm not little! I go to school!" Nick held his ground

and looked around for something to throw across the table.

"Everyone calm down. It's the first day of school. You want to get off on the right foot." Al sipped his tea and looked forward to being at work and away from refereeing the kids.

Elaine came into the room in her nurse uniform. "It's a big day here. All the Plevier boys are now in school."

The three older boys grumbled and buried their heads in their cereal bowls. Nick was the only one to cheer.

Al tried not to laugh. "Did you guys have a good summer? The teacher is going to ask what your favorite part of the summer was. Any thoughts this morning?"

"No school." Larry spoke up without hesitation.

Elaine looked at Larry, seven years old and already with an attitude about school. "You loved school last year, Larry. What makes you think this year won't be just as much fun?"

"I want to stay home and play. The pool is still open and its hot out." He looked longingly out the picture window.

"You guys can swim after school. I'm going to be here to get you off the bus." Al was glad he made an agreement early with his boss. He took it as a sign that in reality, he was a disposable site worker.

"Promise Dad?" Albert eyed his father up from across the table.

Al could not get used to his oldest calling him Dad instead of Daddy. "Promise. If you behave we'll have pizza to celebrate the first day of school. Let's get a move on. You all have to brush your teeth, hair and get to the bus stop."

"The bus stops in front of the house, Dad. We have time." Albert dug further into his cereal.

"Enough of that. Let's go." Al stood and began to usher the boys into position.

Chairs slid and three sad faces dragged themselves to the bathroom. Nicky jumped up and ran past his brothers. "I'm gonna be first on da bus."

"Who cares." Larry sulked after him.

Al turned to Elaine. "I don't get it. They all do well. They should be glad to see their friends again."

She looked at him incredulously. "Are you kidding? All their friends come here in the summer. They don't need school to congregate. You've created their own personal amusement park. If we don't push them when they grow up, they'll never leave."

Al kept the fact that he would prefer that to himself. "It's a good thing I'm busy with work. An empty house after these busy years would be too much for me."

Elaine lowered her head. "Me too. I can't believe my boys are growing up. That wasn't supposed to happen so fast."

"I guess we should start planning our next move." He stared out the window.

"What? Are you serious?" Elaine was ready for a fight.

He shook himself out of his mood. "I didn't mean literally. I mean you and me. Our future. Us without the kids."

She rolled her eyes. "They're starting school, not moving to Mars."

They both looked at each other and smiled at their perceived melodrama as the boys stomped down the stairs. "I think we have time to plan the golden years."

After the boys climbed onto the school bus in one unit, Elaine and Al went back into the house to say goodbye to each other. "I have a couple minutes before my ride gets here."

She dropped a kiss on his head. "Good for you. I'm late." She looked around the quiet house. "I could get used to this as long as it isn't permanent."

"Bye Sweetheart." Al looked at the clock and thought he would catch up on the bills while he waited.

Paying the bills was a chore Elaine abhorred. She took it over when Al lost his sight and then happily relinquished it when the camera implant was a success. Al opened the cabinet over the desk area he had built in the kitchen and pulled down the ledgers. He started to close the door when he looked up at the monsters he had placed on the top shelf. Staring down at him was his stylist, the tool he utilized to write in braille and his folded cane. He felt a chill as he absurdly thought the cane was mocking him. Next to the stylist sat a stack of Braille cards he

Jayne Kelly

had been meaning to pass on to a member of the Blind group in Wayne.

Guilt washed over him as he acknowledged to himself the fact that he had all but forgotten his friends at the blind group. He and Elaine had been so busy with the children, returning to work and accomplishing what he considered rejoining the world, that he had left that life behind. Staring at the instruments of his survival while blind, he decided he would reconnect with the group in January when work slowed down again and the upcoming holiday craziness was behind the family. The people at the blind groups were friends and a part of him knew everyone would be glad to be in touch again.

He closed the cabinet as a horn beeped in the driveway. Grabbing his coat and lunch pail he bolted out the door turning the lock as he went.

The construction company kept the hired men busy throughout the fall of 1983. Al didn't have time to mull over lost ties and plan for the future. He was living in the moment of a nuclear family trying to stay one step ahead of school projects, packed lunches, wholesome dinners, cleaned bathrooms and a full tank of gas when you're late for an event.

September disappeared into October as Halloween rushed by. On good advice from the neighborhood, Al decided to forego the wolfman costume for some future occasion.

As he and Elaine unpacked and then repacked the costumes after the sugary event, he lifted the wolfman mask out of the box and put it on for her. "Grrrrrr!"

"What is wrong with you?" She laughed while admonishing him.

"Ah, come on. Don't hairy guys do anything for you?" Al shoved the mask into the box with the other costumes.

She was laughing loudly enough to draw the boys out from in front of the television. "Dad had the mask on. That would have been cool this year at Tommy's party," said Albert.

Al shook his head. "I was afraid one the kids there might remember me and demand their candy back." The boys did not get the joke and walked away unimpressed.

Elaine saw how deflated Al looked. "We'll have Thanksgiving dinner here this year. I think it will be easier on Fenna. This is the first Christmas without Mom."

The absence of Rose Plevier was not lost on Al. "It will be different." He let the statement hang in the air.

That afternoon the family began to make plans for the upcoming Thanksgiving holiday with phone calls and recipe exchanges meant to keep attention on the food. The strategy worked and carried into November while Fenna and Elaine shopped together for the children.

"I'm glad you took the day off." Fenna sat over lunch with Elaine noting the piles of bags between them.

"I would not have had time to hide the presents without it. I'm waiting for Albert to get wise about the attic and start investigating." Elaine looked over at the Orange Julius stand-Albert's favorite treat at the mall.

Fenna raised her eyebrows. "Would he go as far as pulling down the attic stairs alone?"

Elaine gave her a sarcastic look. "Are you kidding. I'm surprised he hasn't tried already. As soon as the kid on the bus ruined Santa for him, he had an edge on us. Al had to bribe him twice to not tell the other boys. Now, we've resorted to threats."

Fenna laughed. "That sounds familiar."

"If he spills the beans to his brothers, he loses half his presents." Elaine's tone was humorously adamant.

Fenna nodded in agreement. "That worked well for me in the past."

Later, in the early afternoon, Elaine climbed down from the attic stairs when she heard the kitchen door open. Thinking it was the boys she left the presents scattered without order on the attic floor and closed the stairs with a bang.

"Elaine?" Al came up to the second floor. "I thought we might have burglars."

Elaine turned around to find Al, with the right side of his face very red. "Al, what are you doing home so early? What happened to your face?"

He looked at her confused. "Huh?"

Fear crept into the pleasant day Elaine was having. "Have you looked in the mirror?"

"No. I just didn't feel right. I guess the guys on the job thought the red face was from the cold." He left her side to walk into the bathroom. "It's only on the right side. I don't remember hitting myself. Yesterday my face was itching a bit. I thought maybe it was from the insulation and kept scratching it."

Elaine looked at him hard. "I'm calling Dr. Elbac." She walked into the master bedroom without another word.

He kept staring at his face in the mirror and heard in the background Elaine hang up and make another call. She came rushing into the bathroom.

"Let's go. We have to get you to the hospital. Dr. Elbac will meet us there."

He ran after her retreating figure down the stairs. "The boys will be home in an hour." He took the coat Elaine held out for him.

"Julie down the street will get them off the bus and then call Dad." She headed for the back door. "We're going to Mt. Sinai."

Al's body went cold. "Why? What's going on?" He didn't slow down as he locked the door behind them.

They both ran and jumped into the car as he stared straight through the windshield while Elaine stuttered an explanation. "Dr. Elbac believes you have an infection. The doctor said they are worried about it traveling to the optic nerve and then to the brain. If it goes to the brain it will kill you. Do you have a headache?"

Al suddenly knew what was about to happen to him. He continued to stare straight ahead as the chill numbed his senses. "No. No headache."

"You have to let me know if you start to have a headache. We won't be able to go all the way into Manhattan then. We'll have to go to the closest hospital."

He heard her talking from a faraway place that his mind could not comprehend. His head turned as he watched the scenery fly by. The intensity of the green light of the intersection burned into his mind. When they fianally hit his favorite stretch on Rt 80, the silhouette of the city laid before him. He heard his childrens' voices in his head and wished he had stared at their faces a little longer this morning.

It was an overcast day without rain. Dreary in its entirety. Inside him something was dying. He turned his head to stare at his wife. It was the first time he had looked at her since they pulled out of the driveway. Her profile was beautiful. This is how he knew she would remain with him. There was nothing left to say.

She felt him watching her and turned for a second from her view of the highway. Tears formed in her eyes. There would be a time over the next hour that they would look into each other's eyes for the last time. It felt permanent.

Al stared at her and tried to remember that he had the left eye still available for transplants although the socket felt empty. An hour later their station wagon screeched to a halt at a parking garage. Elaine and Al practically ran together as they approached the emergency entrance. They walked in and people stared at the two able bodies walking as if they did not have a right to use those doors, until Al took off his glasses.

The nurse was waiting for them. "Mr. and Mrs. Plevier?"

"Yes." They answered in unison.

"Albert, you have to come with us." A wheel chair was brought as the nurse at the front desk paged a doctor.

"Wait." Al stood his ground.

"No. You have to come now."

"Not before I say good-bye to my wife." He lifted her chin as she no longer tried to fight the tears. "I love you. Let me see you smile before I go. Let that be the last thing I remember. Please."

She wiped away the tears as the nurse and orderly dropped their chins and turned away. She smiled the brightest smile as she remembered the day they met. "I love you too. We had quite a good run."

They both laughed, he kissed her hard and looked her in the eye. "Just remember, its your body that is burned into my memory not the hot blond from the rental house."

She shook her head and kissed him again. "Live, Al. Come back to me."

"We need to go now!" The orderly pushed him into the wheel chair and backed the chair through the double doors as a young woman with heavy makeup and a doctor jacket walked up.

Al stared at Elaine until the doors closed and they turned the chair around and ran him down the hallway. They made a right turn to a team that was waiting for Dr. Elbac. That was when Al cried. No one on the team said a word or tried to stop the man who had no tears to cry.

Chapter XXVII: Miles and Miles

"Do you have a headache?" The repetitive question asked by the young doctor in charge of Al's survival spoke an urgency in its consistency.

Al breathed deep as he tried to calm himself. "No." He knew that as long as he did not have a headache there was a small chance he would keep his right eye and the implant. He looked up and Elaine was standing next to his bed. "I thought they said you couldn't come into the triage area. Are you staying with me?"

The young woman spoke up, letting it be known to both Al and Elaine that she was in charge. "As long as she does not interfere with your care."

"The orderly came back while I was filling out paperwork and gave me permission to sit with you." She took his hand.

He stared at her. "Elaine?"

"Are you okay? Are you in pain? What is it?" Elaine was no longer calm.

Al was feeling the panic he saw on Elaine's face. "Who is this lady?" He inclined his chin toward the young woman wearing the heavy make-up.

The woman stepped closer to the gurney. "Mr. Plevier,

I'm your doctor until Dr. Elbac arrives."

Al's eyes went wide. "You're not much older than my son. Are you in training or something?"

"Al!" Elaine was mortified, but in secret she had the same reaction.

The young woman looked hard at Al. "Are you in pain?"

"No. Are you going to keep asking me that until the Dr. Elbac gets here?" The fact that she ignored is questioned worried him further.

The doctor continued to look at him hard. "Yes. We are trying to save your life." She came close and touched his face. "Dr. Elbac had the plane turned around in route. He should be landing in JFK within the next two hours." The doctor that was designated his watch dog and guardian stared at his face and the monitors attached to him under his hospital gown.

Al's mind was going in many directions. "Where was Dr. Elbac going?"

The doctor did not look up from the task she was performing. "Israel. Your surgeon is a very important man and has the ability to require the plane to turn around for a medical emergency. You're very fortunate to to have become a patient of his. Not all doctors have the ability to move mountains as that man does." She paused and looked into Al's eye. "Dr. Elbac has no intention of letting you die today. That is why he placed me in your care until he arrives."

With the thought that these may be the last hours he had sight, it pained him to be staring at the overhead florescent lights. "Elaine, I wish I could be looking at the boys before they put me under and take out the camera."

Trying to imagine how he got to this place from where he was last weekend raking leaves, wrestling with the boys and feeling invincible was incomprehensible. Twenty-four hours ago, he was happy, healthy and looking forward to a busy Thanksgiving, the first without his mother.

A wave of calming energy washed over him as the knowledge that his mother passed away thinking his returned sight was permanent or at least long standing let her rest peacefully.

"Can my wife continue to sit with me until the doctor gets here?" He wanted to see her face.

"We will allow it as long as possible." A note was handed to the doctor. "We just received word that the plane is landing sooner than expected." The doctor was all business. "Do you have any pain in your face, eye or head?"

"No, no pain." He couldn't believe the eyes of the doctor with too much makeup were the last he would see after Elaine was forced to wait in the emergency area.

"Dr Elbac was on his way to Israel for a family vacation. He will be escorted immediately off the plane and driven by the police to the hospital. Try to relax. We are doing everything for you that can be done. You must let me know the second any pain starts." She looked closely at him her face inches from his.

"Are you expecting the pain to start without question?" He glanced at the IV drip attached to his left forearm. "Is there a chance that the infection could halt? Could whatever you have in the IV stop it?" He thought he sounded like he was pleading and he didn't care.

The young doctor's demeanor did not change. "Dr. Elbac will answer all your questions when he arrives."

Elaine held his hand. "Just live Al. Just live."

Al stared at Elaine's face for another hour before Dr. Elbac was standing next to his bed and Elaine was escorted out quickly and unceremoniously. "Albert, how are you feeling?" The doctor began to touch Al's face.

Al looked hard at the doctor. "What is this infection?" He saw with dread that Dr. Elbac was in operating scrubs and watched Elaine step aside.

Dr. Elbac looked directly into the camera implant. "It's a staff infection."

Suddenly Al wished he was looking into the hard expression of the young doctor instead of the compassionate eyes of Dr. Elbac. He knew what that meant. "Will you need to operate?"

"Yes." He stopped touching Al's face. "I will be removing the eye. Albert, this is a race to save your life.

Elaine's words resonated in his head. *"Al, come back to us. Live. Just live."*

"I have no intention on dying here, Doc. Do what you have to. Work hard. I have four little boys at home that need me no matter what shape you send me home in." An immediate and paralyzing pain shot through his head and he could only see blinding light. "Oh, God. Knock me out. Please."

He felt the gurney moving quickly. There were voices, but the sounds blended nonsensically around the blinding pain. The only words he discerned clearly were optic nerve and spreading.

Chapter XXVIII: Rule of Law

*A*l did not fully regain consciousness for a week. He had been operated on four times in four days. He faded in and out of consciousness several times each day. The first surgery removed the camera and the eye. With the eye gone each subsequent surgery drained the socket of the infection and removed more tissue. Each time Al awakened he was hit with waves of nausea and pain similar to a hang over. Instead of getting better and alleviating the discomfort a little each day, it increased until it stopped its progression.

When he awakened fully, he was in darkness. "Elaine?"

Miraculously she was by his side. "I'm here, Al. You made it. You came back to us."

"I'm so sorry." He never had a chance to finish his thought.

"It happened. Maybe the camera would have failed eventually. Dr. Elbac told me after one of your surgeries this week, that some of the cameras implanted were 'blowing out' the optic nerves on patients."

"One of my surgeries? How many did I have? What day is it?" His head pounded.

379

"You had four. You've been here a week." She squeezed his hand. "You're coming home in another couple of weeks. That's all that matters. We're still a family."

He tried desperately to focus on the conversation around the pain. "How are the kids?"

"They miss you. Albert overheard a conversation I had with Mom one night. He realized how serious this was." She wondered why she mentioned this automatically without the thought that he should not hear anything negative yet.

Al focused on the last image he had of Albert. "Poor kid. He was probably scared."

She tried to buffer the last information she gave him. "The boys know you won't have your sight when you come home. Larry climbed up on the counter and brought your cane down. He unfolded it and placed it next to the back door. Chris put away all the toys, believe it or not. Nick is doing anything his brothers tell him to do."

Al could not bring himself to picture his cane. "Elaine, what about Albert?"

She closed her eyes. "He directed all the boys to help pick up. He's good at telling them what to do." Elaine looked across the room at nothing before continuing. "He must have hit a thousand balls into the net you set up behind the garage. He told me that when you get home from the hospital he will hit home runs every time." She paused again. "After he was put to bed one night I snuck up the stairs to give them all an extra tuck in and found him praying. Al, I've never seen him do that before without one of us being there. He wants you home. The next morning, he told me he would never do anything bad again, he promised."

Albert's face was a clear image in Al's mind despite the pain he was in physically and emotionally. "Poor kid. I'll talk to him." He squeezed her hand this time. "I'll explain that he should never tell lies." They both laughed lightly. "After I'm home for a couple of weeks I'll set the boys at ease. They can go back to being themselves. You know, a band of warriors out to conquer you and I." His head throbbed a little harder.

"Albert said he would help you learn how to be blind again." She couldn't hold back her tears. "Is that the sweetest thing you ever heard?"

Al's head suddenly cleared for a moment. "I'm the Dad, he's the little boy. I'll have to spend some time reassuring him he can count on me." Al felt something rise inside him. "This is their childhood. I am not going to let this slow them down. Maybe I'll remind them about how crafty they can be with a blind father."

"Al." Elaine could see his resolve to be a father to his children causing him distress and a machine attached to monitor him screeched in protest.

"No. I may be blind but I'm not useless. These kids have a father not someone they have to take care of. I'm going to let them get crafty and then I'm going to spank them when I catch them breaking the rules." The throbbing in his head eased as the machine noise continued. "I may not have control over what just happened to us, but I'm damn well not going to check out on my family." He took a breath feeling an exhausted energization. "The bad news for them is that I will be working out of the garage again. I'll be around all the time." The throbbing eased a little more. "This darkness is easier than the corneal failure." He breathed out. This was painful but happened quickly. The transplant failure was torture." The dimming surrounding the Christmas light was a memory in front of him. "I just wanted to live and come home to you."

A nurse came into the room, summoned by the steady machine noice. "Everything okay, folks?" She came next to the bed, looked Al over and shut off the machine. "Please try to relax, Mr. Plevier. You are still in critical care."

He responded quietly and slowly as the pain in his head resumed. "I promise."

On December 2, Elaine's Birthday, after several weeks in the hospital Al kept his word. Although he had not been given clearance to wrestle with the boys or play ball, he lined them all up against the wall just like the day he came home from the hospital with sight.

"Attention little soldiers. I'm back. Same old Dad, just different. Whatever you think you can get away with, I dare you to try. I need a challenge and I'm going to be home all day, every day with you. I'll be working from the garage like before." He stopped to give them a chance to say something. "Mom told me you've been very good boys, helping her and behaving. Are you guys sick?"

Albert was the only one who laughed. "Daddy, I'm going to hit home runs every time next season."

The fact that Albert called him Daddy, was not lost to Al. "Albert, you're doing great right now. You and I will practice when the doctor tells me my head is perfect."

Albert made a face. "Are you gonna make me practice for hours? I'm done in short times now."

Al wasn't sure what 'short times' meant, but the connection was re-established. He was the parent, Albert could go back to being a kid. "I'll let you know how long we'll practice."

"Fine." Albert stomped away and his brothers followed loudly, not really sure why Albert flagged them to follow his lead, but they were doing it anyway.

Al turned to where he thought Elaine still stood. "Sounds like we're back to normal."

She laughed with sarcasm and joy. "Whatever that is."

"Did you finish the Christmas shopping for the boys?"

"We're done. They're going to have a good year." She looked at the bare walls and wondered how the two of them were going to summon the enthusiasm to decorate the house this year.

Al answered for her. "I left the hooks for the outside lights." He started shifting from one foot to another. "Did you think I forgot what day it was?" He smirked at her through the headache he still suffered.

Tears gathered in Elaine's eyes. "You're my gift this year. Your home."

Al stood as tall as the headache allowed. "Nice try, but like I said to the boys, same old me, just different." He smirked again. "I'm not letting you hang a missed birthday over my head. I'm all about survival and winning."

Elaine cocked her head and tried to summon a response that countered his banter. "Whatever makes you sleep better."

"Oh no you don't. Trust me. I plan ahead." He paused. "I hid your gift in my underwear drawer with a card."

Elaine's eye's brightened. "Really? Let's get it." She turned toward the stairs with Al behind her.

When they reached the bedroom, Al went to his dresser and pulled out the small package with a card. "It's kind of a recycled gift."

Elaine opened the package slowly and under her fingers the image of Al holding baby Albert with snow all around them poked through a beautiful gold frame with pearls. "Al, it's beautiful. I forgot about this picture." The two smiling faces, one tiny, one adult looked remarkably alike before Albert became a toddler.

He sat heavily down next to her. "I found it in the box from the plant. It used to sit on my desk. I was going to put it among the family pictures but I wanted to show you how much it meant so I spent some extra money at the mall on the frame."

She had no words and hugged him tightly.

Al hugged her back and cleared his throat. "The doctor said physically I'll be almost back to normal in another week or two. That should give me the weekend before Christmas to decorate the outside of the house." He mentally calculated where each hook he had left in place the season before was located. "I feel like part of me knew that my sight was only temporary from the beginning."

Elaine was stoic as she stared at the picture of Al and Albert. "If I had to be totally honest, so did I. I don't know why I felt that way. Everything was going so well." She looked over his face. "After Dr. Elbac removed the camera and the eye, he discussed with me the failure of the camera lens implants on other patients. When I heard that, I became so angry. We were led to believe it was indefinite and there I was waiting while you fought for your life. This could have easily gone the other way and we would have lost you forever." She stared again at the image of baby Albert.

Al took her hand. "It's over. I pulled through." He was blunt in his finality. "It was worth all of it to see you again." Still recovering, he felt himself grow tired. "It's easier this time than when the transplant failed. This time I woke up in darkness all at once and it was a fight to live, like right after the accident." He held up his hands. "It's over. I've adjusted. Now, what should we do to celebrate tonight?"

"Al, you can't go out. You just got out of the hospital." She touched the card that she knew Al had picked out himself, knowing it was the last time he would be able to do that.

"Who said anything about going out? I'll call Mom and Dad and have them bring over a cake, subs and balloons. This family makes up a small army and a decent party."

Chapter XXIX: The Slide

"When you're feeling one hundred percent physically we can talk about a weekend getaway." Elaine took his arm.

Al pulled away from her in amusement. "A weekend getaway? I'm beginning to wonder if I turned into a prisoner of your will. Where exactly will I be taken to?

"Oh, calm down, it's the Poconos. You and I will need it." She watched him break free and wearily walk the stairs toward their bedroom to rest.

"I leave the details to you." He spoke to her over his shoulder. "Tell me where to show up and when." He left Elaine standing in the living room watching him ascend the stairs and listening to thunderous footfalls overhead. "Hey! What are you guys doing up here running football plays?"

Elaine looked down at her hands. The winter months were taking their toll with a stark redness against her gold wedding band. She rubbed them together vigorously feeling the coldness ease out of them. Al hadn't mentioned missing Thanksgiving and she hoped he wouldn't. Fenna had taken over the holiday and Elaine had marveled at her generosity of spirit knowing this was the first one without her mother. The holiday had played out much differently than anyone had anticipated. Christmas was different also.

The Christmas holiday passed in a more sedate nature than the previous year. Fenna's husband, Bob, assisted Al with the outside lights for the second year in a row and couldn't help but feel melancholy over from the memories of the previous year.

He watched Al closely and wondered if he should be climbing so close to the recent tulmultuous events. "Do you have a sixth sense Al?'

Al stopped with the string held in one hand and feeling for the next hook in the other. "Huh?"

Bob looked around quickly to see if Elaine, Fenna or the kids were in the vicinity. "Last Christmas you made a point of leaving these hooks in place even after I told you it was a waste of time. Remember?"

Al returned to stringing the lights. "I don't know, Bob. I think I just like to be prepared for all outcomes."

Bob nodded in agreement, forgetting for a second that his brother-in-law could no longer see the gesture. "You always have been resourceful." He saw the sad look on Al's face. "Hey, Buddy? I'm glad you're here. That last event was a close one. No more of those. This family, the entire family, needs you."

Al nodded in agreement and continued to finish hanging the lights. For him, there wasn't the sadness he experienced as the corneal transplant failed and he saw the shimmering Christmas lights vanish slowly. He had too much to do. Life was still waiting for him.

Concentrating on the vacation she was planning for the family in February during Presidents' weekend would be the bridge Elaine needed. Her parents would be there allowing Al to have one on one time with the boys and she could reflect and regroup.

The day they left for the Poconos a soft snow was falling outside. It was not predicted to amount to anything more than an inch, but that was enough to cause her stomach to tense. The only time Elaine enjoyed the snow was when she was tucked into the Pocono vacation house or someone else was driving if they needed to travel in a storm.

The view that afternoon from the vacation house was beautiful. It was on the slope side of a hill not connected with the local ski area, but overlooking Lake Hemlock. This allowed the boys a bit of freedom but still kept them close to home.

The New Year greeted them slowly and both Elaine and Al were glad they had planned in advance for the Presidents' weekend getaway in the Poconos. Al was fully healed and given clearance from Dr. Elbac to resume his life and activities by the end of January.

February 1984 offered a two-foot snow pack in the Poconos for the Plevier family. Al knew Elaine wanted some down time and he bundled up all five of the boys and with the help of Mr. Hinds trooped outside into the winter fun at the recreation area a decent walk from the house. Little Peter would not allow anyone to carry him. Within the little group, you kept up or fell behind and Peter kept up.

Each boy carried an aluminum sledding pan. "C'mon Dad!" Albert was in the lead as usual and impatient.

Al had a hand on Mr. Hinds shoulder. "Dad, you better jog a little."

Mr. Hinds was trying to catch his breath. "Al, these kids have climbed a hill. I'm not as young as I used to be."

"Are they far ahead of us?"

"Nah. We're on top of them."

"Dad, we're going first." Larry smiled mischievously at his brother never realizing his Al's apprehension at his words was from referring to him as 'Dad' instead of 'Daddy'.

The boys worked hard for a while sliding down and building a ramp at the end. By the time it was Al's turn they had created a hard, packed, channel that, in the sunshine, had the appearance of glass.

Mr. Hinds looked from one boy to the other. "Al, you're about to go on a little trip. You ready for that?"

"How bad can it be, Dad?" Al slipped out of his father -in-laws hand and felt his way to his son's voice. "Larry, lead me to the pan."

Larry grabbed Al's hand enthusiastically and dragged him the remaining several feet to a large tube. "Sit here." He reached up and tried to push Al into a sitting position.

"Relax. I'm going, I'm going." Al smirked, knowing he was being sacrificed and enjoying every second.

Albert yelled to the pack. "C'mon guys. Push!"

Al felt many sets of hands on his back the second his butt landed in the middle of the metal dish. "Whoa!" Al thought he was humoring his boys as the metal began to slide, taking off slowly.

A second later the dish picked up speed after Al felt a sudden drop off. He traveled faster and faster as the cheers behind him grew simultaneously. The smile on his face stopped the instant he was airborne. He hardly felt the ramp as he began to fly and let go of the pan with one hand. He leaned back when he hit the hill hard on the landing. Lying flat, he burst out laughing as he tried to work in his mind whether to kill the boys or congratulate them.

"If your dad is hurt all you boys are stuck inside for the day." Al heard Mr. Hinds yelling and soft foot falls around him.

"Daddy? You alive?" Chris poked Al's shoulder.

He laughed hard and felt his back reverberate with discomfort. "Yup."

The End.

For more information on The Albert Plevier Story please visit our facebook page: The Albert Plevier Trilogy by Jayne Kelly

Book I : "Beyond the Eight Foot World"
Book II: "See Saw"
Of the Albert Plevier Trilogy are available on Amazon and Kindle.

Made in the USA
Columbia, SC
08 September 2017